Arlene Fenlon, Ellen Oakes, and Lovell Dorchak are certified child birth educators in the Denver area who have taught classes in the Lamaze method of childbirth as well as classes on Cesarean birth and postpartum recovery. The authors have used the Lamaze method for the shared births of their own children.

In this book "he" and "she" have been used interchangeably when referring to the baby and doctor.

Arlene Fenlon
Ellen Oakes
Lovell Dorchak

Getting Ready for Childbirth

A Guide for Expectant Parents

Library of Congress Cataloging in Publication Data

FENLON, ARLENE.
  Getting ready for childbirth.

  Includes bibliographies and index.
      1. Pregnancy. 2. Childbirth. 3. Obstetrics—Pop-
  ular works. 4. Infants (Newborn)—Care and
  hygiene.
  I. Oakes, Ellen, joint author.   II. Dorchak, Lovell,
  joint author.   III. Title.
  RG525.F458   618.2′4   79-13442
  ISBN 0-13-354803-1
  ISBN 0-13-354795-7 pbk.

© 1979 by Arlene Fenlon, Ellen Oakes, and Lovell Dorchak

Printed in the United States of America

Foreword　　　　　　　　　　　　　　　　　　*xi*

Preface　　　　　　　　　　　　　　　　　　*xiii*

1

The First and Second Trimesters　　　1

Emotions　　　　　　　　　　　　　　　1

Sexual Relations　　　　　　　　　　　　2

Common Physical Changes of Pregnancy　　3

Fetal Growth and Development　　　　　　7

Nutrition　　　　　　　　　　　　　　　8

Nutrition Worksheet 1　　　　　　　　　*9*

Nutrition Worksheet 2　　　　　　　　　*19*

2

The Third Trimester　　　　　　　　　21

Changes　　　　　　　　　　　　　　21

Sexual Relations　　　　　　　　　　　22

Contents

Warning Signs during Pregnancy 23

Preparation for Childbirth 24

Breast Feeding 28

Buying for Your Baby 32

Things to Do before Your Baby's Birthday 36

Choosing a Doctor for Your Baby 37

3

Comfort and Exercise 38

Posture 38

Comfort Positions 40

Body Mechanics 45

Prenatal Physical Preparation 45

You Should Exercise during Pregnancy 46

The Prenatal Exercises 47

The Pelvic Floor 53

Practice Guide 57

4

Anatomy and Physiology of Childbirth 59

Anatomy of Mother and Baby 59

Uterine Function 62

Stages of Childbirth 66

The Maternal Pelvis 66

5

Labor 73

Going into Labor 73

The Length of Labor 74

Prelude Phase 75

Stage 1: The Labor Process 77

Early or Latent Labor 78

Active Labor 80

Transition 82

What You Should Take to the Hospital 85

Hospital Fees 87

6

Delivery 89

The Pushing Stage 89

The Pushing Technique 90

Stage 2: Delivery 94

The Delivery Room 95

Stage 3: Expulsion or Delivery of the Placenta 99

Stage 4: Immediate Postpartum 100

Emergency Home (or Car) Delivery 103

Things to Contemplate 104

Birth Day Procedures 105

7

The Newborn 108

At Birth 108

Characteristics of the Newborn 111

Special Babies 114

8

Relaxation and Massage 116

Active Relaxation 116

Learning Active Relaxation 118

Learning to Use Massage 123

9

Controlled Breathing Patterns for Labor 125

The Coach's Role 127

First-Level Breathing: Slow and Deep 127

Second-Level Breathing: Accelerated-Decelerated 128

Third-Level Breathing: Transition 130

Breathing for a Premature Urge to Push 131

Hyperventilation 132

10

Variations in Childbirth 135

Back Pain during Labor 135

Breech Presentation 136

Induction   138

Fetal Monitoring   140

Multiple Birth: Twins   143

11

Later Births   146

Pregnancy, Labor, and Delivery   147

Sibling Rivalry   149

12

Cesarean Birth   153

Reasons for Cesarean Birth   154

Tests of Fetal Maturity   155

Procedures before the Birth   156

Type of Anesthesia   158

Procedures during the Operation   159

After the Birth   160

The Fourth Trimester   164

13

Fourth Trimester   166

Common Feelings of New Parents   166

All Babies Are Different   170

Physical Changes in the Postpartum Period   170

Getting Back into Shape   171

Some Postpartum Advice   175

Sexuality   176

Contraception   177

Worksheet for Postpartum   *180*

Glossary   **183**

Suggested Readings   **189**

On Pregnancy   189

On Nutrition   190

On Infant-feeding Practices   190

On Childbirth   191

On Breast Feeding   192

On Exercise   192

On Newborns   192

On Siblings   193

For Children   193

On Cesarean Birth   194

On the Postpartum Period   195

On Parenting   195

Index   *197*

Childbirth was family-centered for centuries, and only in relatively recent times has there been a need to strengthen this concept. Advances in technology used in monitoring mothers and their unborn infants have widened the breach between the medical and the lay community. All too often, childbirth has been identified as a medical condition rather than a physiological happening. Expectant parents, once passive recipients of care, now ask to be participating members of their obstetrical experience. Health care personnel can be relieved that they are now able to share difficult medical decisions with an interested, informed couple.

If, indeed, patients are to be consumers of health care services, they must be given information as candidly and completely as possible, and by so doing, concerns and fears will surface and be discussed. The need for many couples to begin to assume parental responsibility surely begins before their infant's birth. Childbirth preparation can be one way of expressing their concern and excitement.

Getting Ready for Childbirth makes a valuable contribution to the education of the pregnant couple. The medical information has been thoroughly researched. Cesarean birth and nutrition, rarely discussed so completely, are carefully and accurately considered. Methods for evaluating the infant's intrauterine condition and maturity are concisely presented. The worksheets offer an excellent opportunity to experience pregnancy, labor, and delivery in a prepared fashion. This primer for childbirth coordinates the best efforts of the health care team with those of the family. I can think of no better way to assure a good outcome for all.

PAUL WEXLER, M.D.

Associate Clinical Professor
University of Colorado School of Medicine

Chairman, Department of Obstetrics and Gynecology
Lutheran Medical Center

Foreword

Childbirth is a time of new beginnings, renewal, and anticipation. It is the inception of a lifetime of joys, responsibilities, and warmth. It is an awesome event in the lives of the parents and important to the future of the baby.

We believe that childbirth should be experienced, not just tolerated; prepared for, not approached with ignorance; meaningful, not just undergone as it has been for years; but most of all, you should leave the experience with memories and feelings that are very special. We have written this book to help couples achieve these goals.

This book would not have been possible without the knowledge and sensitive teaching of our own Lamaze instructors or the learning that has taken place as we have taught childbirth preparation classes. The couples in our classes have taught us how to make practical what we knew in theory.

We would especially like to thank Dr. Paul Wexler for his encouragement, interest, and medical guidance throughout this project. He was generous with his time and knowledge. Not only is he sincerely interested in the well-being of expectant couples, but he is also empathetic and willing to help them realize their expectations for an emotionally satisfying childbirth.

We are also grateful to the following people whose assistance, suggestions, and encouragement helped us complete this book: Kathy Bernau, Cathy Callahan, Barbara Emshwiller, Heidi Lynch, and Mary Katharyn Oakes. Numerous instructors and other medical experts have read and evaluated our book, and we are indebted to them for their time and support.

This book would also not have been possible had we not experienced our own childbirths—so a special thank you to

Allyson, Erica, and Lindsay
Kristen and Sara
Greg and Katie

And our coaches—Jack, Len, and Jim

September 1978

Preface

Getting Ready for Childbirth

1

This chapter discusses emotional changes and sexuality during the first and second trimesters, common physical changes of pregnancy, fetal growth and development, and nutrition information.

EMOTIONS

Pregnancy is a time of self-reflection and growth for most people, both as individuals and as couples. Most authorities call it stressful and a time of change in identity and maturation. There appears to be a commonality to the process of adjusting to the reality of parenthood, although each person reacts in different degrees, depending on his or her background. You may find it reassuring to know that other couples have many of the same feelings and concerns that you have. Let's take a closer look at the process of becoming parents.

The Mother's Feelings

In general, women report that they have more mood swings, are more open about their feelings, are more aware of the cycle of life, and seem to have increased emotional reactions to events. Probably the most common feeling at this time is ambivalence about being pregnant, no matter if the pregnancy was planned or not. "Is this really the best time to be pregnant?" "I wonder if I can really be a good mother?" "Will the baby love me?" "What will happen to my career?" It takes time to accept this new, very special, and exciting reality—you're going to be a mother.

Toward the end of the first trimester, pregnant women usually become more introspective, remembering the relationship they had with their own mothers. This is a step toward developing their own mothering roles.

The First and Second Trimesters

By the second trimester, most women have accepted the reality of their pregnancy. The thrill of hearing the baby's heartbeat and feeling him move in the uterus verifies his existence, and you may find yourself imagining your baby's personality, sex, and physical characteristics. The baby is now recognized as a separate person. At the same time, a woman often needs more affection and reassurance from her mate, and she may become more dependent on him and increasingly concerned over his safety.

The Father's Feelings

Fathers, too, must accept the reality of the coming event. Ambivalence is a common emotion—you are facing possible financial changes, the reality of "settling down," and the responsibilities of parenthood. Most men are proud of their virility. An increase in emotions usually occurs, with which some men are more comfortable than others. You may feel rivalry or resentment toward the baby if your mate is more introverted and giving you less attention. You may feel left out.

You will have reactions similar to those of the mother during the second trimester. When you feel your baby move, the emotions and realities of fatherhood begin. Your idea of the baby's looks, sex, and personality develops, although most men tend to imagine an older child rather than an infant. It is no wonder that at such an emotional time fathers often experience increased creativity, some at work, some at home, and others in artistic outlets.

As a pregnant couple you are sharing many emotions, doubts, needs, and joys. Because you are unique, your reactions to pregnancy may differ from one another and other couples. It is important to be aware of and to talk about your needs and to offer each other support and love.

SEXUAL RELATIONS

Most women need more tenderness, reassurance, and intimacy from their partner during pregnancy. This emotional nourishment is important —the mother-to-be thrives on it, and it is necessary for her to develop maternal love.

Sexual relations during pregnancy can help meet this need for attention and affection. Oftentimes, though, pregnancy alters a couple's sexual desires and intimacy and can cause concern or anxiety unless they understand the reasons for the change. There are no data to support a general theory about when couples feel more or less sexual desire. The phases of pregnancy can affect each woman in a different way. Some couples experience a decline in sexual desires and frequency of intercourse, others feel a new surge of interest.

Generally, however, there are some factors during the first trimester that can influence sexual desires, and it is helpful for couples to realize that some of these may alter their sexual relationship.

1. There is a relief that contraception is no longer necessary. This freedom can have a positive effect on a sexual relationship. Some couples feel relaxed and comfortable during the months in which they are trying to conceive, whereas others with infertility problems can be frustrated and tense. Unless it was unplanned, most couples feel a great deal of satisfaction once conception has been confirmed.

2. After conception, hormonal changes begin to affect the woman's body. Many women are overwhelmingly fatigued during the first trimester, and all they want to do is sleep. Nausea and vomiting can affect a woman's sexual desires, and real or imagined fears of miscarriage may make couples avoid intercourse or orgasm. The physician can advise couples about whether intercourse and/or orgasm would be a threat to the pregnancy. In most cases it is not. A changing body with enlarged, sensitive breasts may create pride in some women and enhance their sense of sexuality. Thus the woman's changing body and the fact that she is now carrying a baby may enhance the couple's sexual life.

Many couples report an increase in sexual desire and lovemaking during the second trimester. Nausea, fatigue, and the fear of miscarriage are usually over. The uterus is enlarging but is not yet much of an obstacle. Although the baby is beginning to move, it is not yet kicking vigorously.

Many women feel that the second trimester is the time of greatest physical comfort during pregnancy. An enlarged uterus and movements of the baby help make the pregnancy a reality to both mother and father. Together these can enhance a couple's lovemaking.

COMMON PHYSICAL CHANGES OF PREGNANCY

In addition to emotional changes during pregnancy, there are many physical ones, which may be easier to tolerate if you understand the reasons for their occurrence. Women vary in their reactions to them. Some of you will be bothered by going to the bathroom quite frequently and others will simply accept it as part of having a baby.

The following is a list of the more common changes or complaints of pregnancy and suggestions to help make them more tolerable.

- *Nausea and vomiting:* Morning sickness
  Cause: Believed to be caused by adaptation of the body to pregnancy, allowing the stomach to become empty, and changes in

carbohydrate metabolism; aversions to certain foods and odors can also cause nausea. Usually only occurs during the first trimester.
Suggestions:
Eat smaller amounts of food five to six times per day.
Eat dry toast or crackers before rising in the morning.
If these conditions are severe, your doctor may prescribe medication.

- *Breast changes*
1. Breast sensitivity or tenderness (tingling, throbbing sensation); enlargement of breasts; prominence of veins.
   Cause: Hormonal changes and increased blood supply to the breasts.
   Suggestions: Wear a bra that fits well and gives good support.
2. Darkening of areola (dark skin around nipple).
   Cause: Increased hormones during pregnancy; disappears following pregnancy.
   Suggestions: None.
3. Colostrum: Precursor to milk; can be manually expressed by third month of pregnancy.
   Cause: Hormonal changes.
   Suggestions: None.

- *Constipation*
   Cause: Increased pressure of the uterus causes crowding of the digestive organs.
   Suggestions:
   Drink a glass of warm water before breakfast.
   Watch your diet. Drink plenty of fluids, especially water and juices.
   Eat adequate roughage—bran, whole wheat products, fruits, and vegetables. Try an occasional natural laxative such as figs, prune juice, raisins.
   Get adequate exercise.
   Use only doctor-recommended stool softeners and laxatives, and only if diet doesn't help.

- *Hemorrhoids:* Varicose veins of the rectal area.
   Cause: Pressure of the uterus on the rectum interferes with venous return; aggravated by constipation.
   Suggestions:
   Watch your diet to avoid constipation.
   Apply ice packs, or doctor-recommended medication.

- *Heartburn:* Mild to severe "burning" behind the sternum or breastbone.
   Cause: The pregnancy hormone, progesterone, may cause relaxation of the stomach's cardiac sphincter, allowing the stomach's contents to spill back into the esophagus.
   Suggestions:
   Eat smaller amounts more frequently. Eat slowly.
   Sleep with your head elevated on several pillows.
   Avoid spicy foods.

Use only doctor-recommended alkaline medication, and only if these suggestions don't help.

Do not use baking soda because the sodium content is too high.

- *Varicose veins:* Enlarged veins whose walls have thinned and stretched.

  Cause: Progesterone may contribute to the problem by causing muscle relaxation. Return of blood from the legs is poor because of uterine pressure on blood vessels.

  Suggestions:

  Avoid prolonged standing if at all possible. When standing, shift your weight from one foot to the other. Elevate one leg on a stool if possible.

  Lie with your legs elevated higher than your heart or hips so that the blood pooling in your legs is relieved. Try to do this for five minutes every hour. Do the sand-digging exercise (see the prenatal exercises in Chapter 3).

  Avoid constricting clothing: tight pants, knee-high hose, girdles. Elevate the end of your bed or sleep on your left side with your legs elevated on several pillows.

  If your doctor recommends it, put on support hose first thing in the morning.

  Do not sit with your feet or legs crossed.

- *Calf cramps*

  Cause: Pressure of the uterus on the nerves supplying the lower extremities; fatigue, chilling, or tension in legs; an imbalance in the amount of calcium and phosphorus in your body (too much phosphorus).

  Suggestions:

  Avoid pointing your toes like a ballet dancer.

  If the calf cramps, pull your toes up toward your face and stretch the calf muscle or stand on the cramped leg and bend your knee while keeping your heel on the floor.

  Your doctor may prescribe pills to increase your calcium intake.

- *Edema:* Swelling of hands, feet, sometimes face.

  Cause: Retention of fluids in the body.

  Suggestions:

  Sleep on your left side with legs elevated; rest frequently in this position during the day.

  Headaches are possible because edema can occur in your head, which cannot enlarge because of the skull bones. However, if headaches continue, call your doctor.

  Use moderation in your salt intake. Do not eliminate salt completely. Avoid those foods high in sodium: carbonated beverages, salad dressings, and the like. Use salt when you cook, but watch your use of table salt.

  Increase your fluid consumption.

  Follow the suggestions for varicose veins.

  Call your doctor if swelling is extreme. Fluid retention, especially in your face and hands, can be a symptom of toxemia.

- *Backache:* Universal complaint of pregnancy.

  Cause: Increased sway in your lower back caused by the weight of the enlarging uterus; relaxation of the pelvic joints because of the ovarian hormone, relaxin; stress on the uterosacral ligaments which attach to the back of the uterus and the sacrum, or backbone. Stress on these ligaments increases as the baby's size increases.

  Suggestions:

  Make an effort to maintain good posture at all times (see Chapter 3).

  Wear shoes with a slight heel and good support. Avoid high-heeled shoes; they increase the curve in your spine.

  If backache occurs, do pelvic tilts and have your mate rub your back (see the discussions on prenatal exercises in Chapter 3 and massage in Chapter 8).

- *Skin changes*
  1. *Striae Gravidarum:* Stretch marks on the abdomen, breasts, hips, buttocks, and thighs.

     Cause: Breakdown of skin tissue as it stretches to accommodate the growing fetus.

     Suggestions: Stretch marks cannot be prevented or removed once they appear. From their original red appearance they will fade to a less noticeable silvery white mark. If they itch, a body lotion may be soothing.

  2. *Linea Nigra:* Dark line from umbilicus (navel) to the genital area.

     Cause: Hormonal changes causing increased pigmentation of the skin.

     Suggestions: None. The line usually remains after pregnancy, although it is not as noticeable.

  3. *Chloasma:* "Mask of pregnancy"—irregular blotches of brown on a woman's face.

     Cause: Hormonal changes.

     Suggestions: It will disappear after pregnancy, and can be camouflaged with makeup.

- *Urinary frequency*

  Cause: Pressure of the uterus on the bladder, especially noticeable during the first and third trimesters.

  Suggestions:

  Relief in the first trimester occurs as your uterus continues to grow up and out of the pelvis, relieving pressure on the bladder. Relief in the last trimester occurs only with delivery of your baby.

- *Round ligament pain:* Sharp, sudden pain in the groin area.

  Cause: Sudden movement which puts pressure on the already greatly stretched ligaments supporting the uterus.

  Suggestions:

  Move carefully and avoid sudden movements. Turn over carefully when you're in bed or getting up.

- *Bleeding gums*

  Cause: Insufficient Vitamin C.

  Suggestions:

  Eat more foods rich in Vitamin C. Be sure to brush and floss your teeth daily (see the discussion on nutrition later in this chapter).

- *Shortness of breath*

    Cause: Expanding uterus applies upward pressure on the diaphragm, especially in the last trimester.

    Suggestions: Maintain good posture. Sleep with your head elevated on pillows. Avoid lying flat on your back. This condition is alleviated as your baby moves lower in your pelvis near the end of pregnancy.

FETAL GROWTH AND DEVELOPMENT

Although much fetal development occurred before pregnancy was confirmed, it is included here because it is such an intriguing subject. These highlights of fetal development are thoroughly discussed and illustrated in Geraldine Flanagan's excellent book, *The First Nine Months of Life.*

Most fetal *development* occurs during the first trimester of pregnancy. Most *growth* occurs during the second and third trimesters.

Conception occurs when an egg released by the woman's ovary is *fertilized* or penetrated by a sperm from the man. The result is a single cell—the beginning of your baby.

The egg is round and much larger than the sperm, which resembles a dot with a tail, only much smaller. Only one egg is released each month by the woman's ovaries. Twenty to 500 million sperm are present in a single ejaculation of semen. Neither the egg nor the sperm can survive longer than a day or so. Thus, conception can only occur on one or two days of the woman's menstrual cycle. The sperm carries the man's genes, including the sex of the baby; the egg carries the woman's genes.

The sperm released during intercourse may pass through the cervical mucous during the proper phase of the woman's menstrual cycle. The sperm travels through the uterus into the Fallopian tube where fertilization usually occurs. The fertilized egg continues its two- or three-day journey down to the uterus. It has now become 36 cells. The fertilized egg continues to divide into many cells so that by seven days there are about 150 cells. These cells are different from one another—some are programmed to become blood, others brain tissue, and so on.

The egg implants, or "nests," on the uterine wall about one week following conception and becomes the site of the placenta. It may implant high in the uterus and remain there during pregnancy or implant low in the uterus and move up later.

The cells continue to increase—great changes are taking place day by day—so that by the end of a month, the whole *embryo* has been formed. Only a quarter of an inch long, the tiny body has arm and leg buds and a head. Although a very simple organism, the embryo has eyes, ears, mouth, brain, kidneys, liver, and a blood stream. Your baby's heart began beating around the twenty-fifth day.

"By the end of the month the embryo completes the period of relatively greatest size increase and greatest physical change of a lifetime. The month old embryo is ten thousand times larger than the fertilized egg was."[1]

By the seventh week, all the baby's internal organs are present. She is only one inch long, but her heart, liver, and kidneys are functioning. During the third month she begins to move, although the mother is probably not aware of her movements. The baby swallows amniotic fluid. She is about three inches long, weighs an ounce, and has human features.

By about six months your baby has grown to approximately a foot in length and weighs around one and one-half pounds. Her eyes open and she moves about in a quart of amniotic fluid. Her body systems and organs are still immature. During the third trimester, growth and maturation of these systems will be completed.

At the beginning of the eighth month your baby, weighing about two and a quarter pounds, is viable—that is, capable of surviving outside of the uterus—but if born at this time, would require intensive medical care.

During the last three months, some of the mother's immunities are transferred to the baby. These antibodies will help protect the baby during her first six months of life. The placenta produces gamma globulin which helps protect the baby and makes the mother more resistant to disease during this last trimester.

At birth your baby will have grown to be more than 200 million cells—all from her beginning as a single cell.

NUTRITION

Nutrition has long been an unglamorous subject, yet one that is extremely important to the pregnant woman. The quality of the food you eat before and during pregnancy affects your unborn child.

Eating nutritious foods that supply the requirements your body and baby need can contribute to a healthier baby. Faulty intake reduces the available building material necessary for the development of fetal cells.

The development of sound eating habits now will carry over to the diet you offer your child once he begins to eat solids, and in general, your entire family will benefit.

Some Facts about Weight

1. "The Committee on Maternal Nutrition of the National Academy of Sciences recommends an average weight gain of 24 pounds during

[1]Geraldine Lux Flanagan, *The First Nine Months of Life* (New York: Pocket Books, 1965), pp. 58-59.

Before you read the pages on nutrition, keep track of your diet for two days. Write down everything you eat, including the amount.

DAY 1

Breakfast

Lunch

Dinner

Morning Snack

Afternoon Snack

Evening Snack

DAY 2

Breakfast

Lunch

Dinner

Morning Snack

Afternoon Snack

Evening Snack

9

pregnancy. This is commensurate with a better than average course and outcome of pregnancy."[2]

2. A weight gain of more than 40 pounds is generally discouraged.
3. During the first trimester you should gain 1½ to 3 pounds.
4. During the remainder of your pregnancy you should gain a little less than 1 pound per week.
5. You should not attempt to lose weight at any time during pregnancy.

Although sources vary about the distribution of weight gain, the following is an approximate breakdown:

Fetus	7 to 8 pounds
Placenta	1 pound
Fluid	2 pounds
Breast tissue	3 pounds
Uterus	2 pounds
Protein storage	4 pounds
Blood volume	4 pounds
	23 to 24 pounds

Calories and Nutrients

During pregnancy calories provide energy to build the new tissue of the placenta and fetus and to sustain the mother's body during a time when it is working overtime.

1. The 25-to-30-year-old woman, weighing 128 pounds and being 5'5'' tall, requires approximately 2,000 calories per day to maintain good health.
2. During the latter half of pregnancy, the pregnant woman needs approximately 300 more calories per day than the nonpregnant woman.
3. The woman who is breast feeding (lactating) needs approximately 500 more calories per day for milk production.

A woman has an increased need for many different nutrients during pregnancy and lactation. The suggested daily requirements of the following nutrients are from the *Food and Nutrition Board, National Academy of Sciences-National Research Council Recommended Daily Dietary Allowances.*

Protein is essential for (1) production and maintenance of cells, muscles, and tissue in the baby; and (2) repair and maintenance of cells, muscles, and tissue in the mother's body.

[2]Joy Clausen *et al., Maternity Nursing Today* (New York: McGraw-Hill Book Company, 1973), p. 337.

The nonpregnant woman needs 46 grams of protein per day. The pregnant woman needs 76 grams, and the lactating woman needs 66 grams. (See also a discussion of protein sources later in this chapter.)

Iron is an essential part of hemoglobin, which enables red blood cells to carry oxygen through the mother's body and to the baby. Iron is needed for (1) fetal growth and development—the formation of fetal blood supply; (2) storage by the fetal liver for use during the first few months of life; (3) reserve for the mother following delivery; and (4) maintenance of hemoglobin levels in the increased maternal blood supply.

The nonpregnant woman needs 18 milligrams of iron daily. During pregnancy and lactation the need remains the same. Many physicians prefer that their pregnant patients have a higher intake of iron.

Your doctor will check your iron level during pregnancy by a simple blood test, which measure the amount of hemoglobin in your red blood cells. A low hemoglobin reading indicates low iron, or *anemia*.

Good sources of iron include liver, cooked dry beans, lean beef, spinach and other dark green leafy vegetables, raisins, prunes, dried peaches and apricots, and eggs.

Five milligrams of iron is supplied by 2 ounces of liver or 1 cup of beans. It is difficult to get sufficient iron from diet alone, so during pregnancy a supplement of 30 to 60 milligrams of iron daily is often recommended during the second and third trimesters.

Folic acid is a B vitamin that is essential for (1) normal growth and development of fetal cells, and (2) development of red blood cells.

The nonpregnant woman requires 400 micrograms of folic acid daily. During pregnancy the need increases to 800 micrograms, and during lactation to 600 micrograms.

Sources of folic acid include beef and chicken liver as well as dark green leafy vegetables and brewer's yeast. Because it is difficult to get sufficient folic acid from diet alone, it is usual to prescribe folic acid as a vitamin supplement during pregnancy.

Vitamin C (ascorbic acid) is essential for (1) resistance to infection; (2) formation of bones and teeth; (3) the healing process; (4) healthy gums and teeth; and (5) maintenance of cartilage, bones, muscles, and tissues.

The nonpregnant woman needs 45 milligrams of vitamin C daily. During pregnancy the need increases to 60 mg, and during lactation to 80 mg. (See also sources of ascorbic acid later in this chapter.

Vitamin D is essential for (1) the utilization of calcium and phosphorus by bones, teeth, and blood; (2) the formation of strong bones and teeth in the fetus.

The nonpregnant woman does not require vitamin D if she is over 22, but during pregnancy and lactation she needs 400 International Units of vitamin D daily.

Vitamin D can be acquired through foods or exposure to the sun. Good sources include fortified milk, fish, egg yolks, and yeast. One quart of fortified milk daily provides the necessary vitamin D. If you have an intolerance for milk, vitamin D can be supplied by yogurt, cheese, or vitamin supplements.

Vitamin A is essential for (1) healthy skin, hair, and fingernails; (2) cell growth and development; (3) tooth formation; (4) bone growth; and (5) proper functioning of the thyroid gland.

The nonpregnant woman needs 4,000 International Units of vitamin A daily. During pregnancy the need increases to 5,000 International Units, and during lactation to 6,000 International Units.

Beef and chicken liver, sweet potato, greens, cantaloupe, and squash are good sources, as are leafy green vegetables and yellow fruits and vegetables.

Vitamin B₁ (thiamine) is essential for (1) the use of carbohydrates by the body, and (2) appetite and digestion.

A nonpregnant woman requires 1 milligram of thiamine daily. During pregnancy and lactation the need increases to 1.3 milligrams because of the increased number of calories needed at this time.

Good sources of thiamine include pork, green peas, liver, oatmeal, orange juice, milk, potato, and whole wheat bread.

Vitamin B₂ (riboflavin) is essential for (1) maintenance of tissue function, (2) use of protein by the body, and (3) growth of the fetus.

The nonpregnant woman requires 1.2 milligrams of vitamin B₂ daily. During pregnancy the need increases to 1.5 milligrams, and during lactation to 1.7 milligrams.

Good sources of riboflavin include liver, milk, cottage cheese, spinach, winter squash, beef, and pork.

Vitamin K is essential for the production of prothrombin, which is necessary for blood coagulation, or clotting.

Good sources are green leafy vegetables, cauliflower, carrots, and liver.

Calcium, a mineral, is essential for (1) the formation and calcification of fetal bones and teeth, especially during the third trimester; (2) maintenance of the mother's bones and teeth.

The nonpregnant woman needs 800 milligrams of calcium daily; during pregnancy and lactation the need increases to 1,200.

Good sources of calcium include milk and cheese. The requirement is met by one quart of nonfat or lowfat milk per day.

In addition to the specific nutrients mentioned, you need to have adequate *liquids* in your diet, including water. The pregnant or nonpregnant woman needs four servings of liquids daily. During lactation, the need rises to six servings to help with milk production.

We have included only the main nutrients essential to good health during pregnancy and lactation. An excellent resource for more extensive reading is Phyllis Williams' *Nourishing Your Unborn Child.*

The "Daily Food Guide" contains protein foods, vegetables, fruits, milk products, and grain products. The following lists of foods, which will help you plan nutritious meals, are adapted from *Nutrition During Pregnancy and Lactation.*[3]

Proteins. If you are pregnant or breast feeding, eat four servings of the following:

- *Animal Protein (complete protein):* A serving is 2 to 3 ounces, cooked and boneless, unless otherwise specified.
  Beef, poultry, pork, fish, veal, lamb
  Tuna, salmon, crab, lobster—½ cup
  Shrimp, scallops—6 medium
  Sausage links—4
  Cottage cheese—½ cup
  Cheese—2 ounces
  Eggs—2
  Milk—1 cup
- *Vegetable Protein (incomplete protein):* A serving is 1 cup cooked, unless otherwise specified. *Note:* These alone will not supply the requirement. See the discussion that follows.
  Garbanzo, lima, or kidney beans
  Dried beans or peas
  Lentils
  Nuts—½ cup
  Sunflower seeds—½ cup
  Peanut butter—2 tablespoons (without sugar, not hydrogenated)
  Rice—¾ cup

Protein is supplied by both animal and vegetable sources. It is either complete or incomplete depending on the number of essential amino acids it contains. Complete protein (milk, cheese, eggs, fish, and meat) contains the essential amino acids in the proper proportions to meet the body's requirements. Incomplete protein (legumes, grains, seeds, nuts) is missing one or more essential amino acids. By serving the incomplete protein with complete protein (cereal and milk, peanut butter and whole wheat bread) or by combining two incomplete proteins (beans and corn), you can have all the essential amino acids. A very good resource on protein is *Diet for a Small Planet* by Frances Moore Lappé. A protein deficiency can cause problems for both the mother and baby.

[3]California Department of Health, *Nutrition During Pregnancy and Lactation* (1975), pp. 37-41.

The following chart is a guide to help you plan your daily menus.

DAILY FOOD GUIDE			
FOOD GROUP	NUMBER OF SERVINGS		
	NON-PREGNANT	PREGNANT	BREAST-FEEDING
PROTEIN GROUP (Animal and Vegetable)	3	4	4
MILK AND MILK PRODUCTS GROUP	3	4	5
GRAIN PRODUCTS GROUP	3	3	3
VITAMIN C FRUITS AND VEGETABLES GROUP	1	1	1
LEAFY GREEN VEGETABLES GROUP	2	2	2
OTHER YELLOW FRUITS AND VEGETABLES GROUP	1	1	1

This chart appeared in *Nutrition During Pregnancy and Lactation.* Credit is given to the California Department of Health, Maternal and Child Health Unit. Revised 1974.

Milk and Milk Products. If you are pregnant, eat 3 to 4 servings of the following. If you are breast feeding, eat 4 to 5 servings.

- *Milk Products:* A serving is 1 cup or 8 ounces, unless otherwise specified.
    Cheeses—1½ ounces
    Cottage cheese—1⅓ cups
    Milk—whole, nonfat, lowfat, nonfat dry reconstituted, or buttermilk
    Creamed soup—12 ounces or 1½ cups
    Ice cream—1½ cups
    Ice milk
    Milk shake
    Pudding
    Yogurt
    Dry milk—3 to 4 tablespoons

1. Buy only fresh dairy products. Bacteria multiply rapidly when milk is left at room temperature, so refrigeration is essential.
2. Natural cheeses are preferable to processed cheeses and spreads which contain many additives. Read the labels.
3. Flavored yogurts contain sugar. Plain yogurt can be flavored with fresh fruit.
4. A quart of milk daily provides excellent protein as well as one-fourth of your daily energy needs. There are many ways to incorporate milk into the diet; for example, dried milk may be added to meat loaf, puddings, soups and sauces.

Grain Products. If you are pregnant or breast feeding, eat three of the following daily.

- *Whole grain products:*
    Brown rice—½ cup
    Cereals (hot): oatmeal, rolled wheat, cracked wheat, malted barley —½ cup
    Cereals (cold): puffed oats, shredded wheat, wheat flakes, granola —¾ cup (read label to note amount of sugar and additives)
    Cracked and whole wheat bread—1 slice
    Wheat germ—1 tablespoon

1. Whole grain products are often more nutritious and provide more fiber than enriched products. It is possible to buy lasagna, spaghetti, noodles, pancake mix, and so on made with whole wheat flour.
2. When you bake use whole wheat or unbleached white flours since they are more nutritious. Use part soy flour when baking for extra nutrition.
3. When baking, use the Cornell Triple Rich Flour Formula.[4] In the bottom of a measuring cup place: 1 tablespoon soy flour, 1 tablespoon dry milk, 1 teaspoon wheat germ. Add flour to make one cup.

[4]Vicki Lansky, *Feed Me I'm Yours* (Wayzata, Minn.: Meadowbrook Press, 1975), p. 58.

- *Enriched grain products:*
    Bread—1 slice
    Hot cereals: cream of wheat or rice—½ cup
    Cornbread—2-inch square
    Crackers—4
    Macaroni, spaghetti, noodles—½ cup cooked
    Muffin, biscuit, or bagel—1
    Pancake or waffle—1
    Rice—½ cup
    Corn tortilla—2
    Flour tortilla—1

Fruits and Vegetables with Vitamin C.   If you are pregnant or breast feeding, eat one of the following daily.

- *Juices:*
    Orange or grapefruit—½ cup
    Tomato—1½ cups
    Fruit juices enriched with vitamin C—¾ cup

- *Fruits:*
    Cantaloupe—½   Strawberries—¾ cup
    Grapefruit—½   Tangerines—2 small
    Orange—1 medium

- *Vegetables:*
    Broccoli—1 stalk or ½ cup   Raw cabbage—¾ cup
    Brussels sprouts—3-4   Green peppers—½ medium
    Cooked cabbage—1⅓ cups   Tomatoes—2 medium

1. Unless enriched with Vitamin C, canned fruits and juices are lower in Vitamin C content than fresh or frozen.

2. Ascorbic acid is extremely perishable. Exposure to bright light, air, prolonged cooking, preparation in blenders, or soaking in water destroys it.

Leafy Green Vegetables with Vitamin A, Folic Acid, and Iron. Choose two of these each day if you are pregnant or breast feeding.

- *Leafy Green Vegetables:* A serving is 1 cup raw or ¾ cup cooked.
    Asparagus

    Broccoli   Dark leafy lettuce (endive, escarole,
                                  red leaf, romaine)

    Brussels sprouts   Greens (beet, collard, kale, spinach,
    Cabbage   swiss chard, turnip, scallions)

Yellow Fruits and Vegetables with Vitamin A. Choose one of these each day if you are pregnant or breast feeding.

- *Yellow Fruits:* A serving is ½ cup unless otherwise specified.

  Apricot—1
  Nectarines—2
  Peach—1
  Prunes—4
  Apple—1
  Banana—1
  Berries
  Dates—5
  Figs—2
  Grapes
  Pear—1
  Pineapple
  Plums—2
  Raisins
  Watermelon

- *Yellow Vegetables:* A serving is ½ cup unless otherwise specified.

  Artichoke
  Bean sprouts
  Beets
  Carrots
  Cauliflower
  Celery
  Corn
  Cucumber
  Eggplant
  Beans—green or waxed
  Lettuce
  Mushrooms
  Onions
  Peas
  Potatoes
  Squash
  Yams

Consider these suggestions:

1. Generally speaking, fresh is the best, frozen the second, and canned the least nutritious way to buy fruits and vegetables. When buying canned fruits, avoid those packed in syrups, choosing natural juices when available. Look in the diet foods section of your store for fruits packed in water or natural juice. Some major companies now produce lightly sweetened fruits. Be sure to read the label for other additives.

2. Eat raw vegetables or cook minimally, just until done.

3. Store foods in airtight containers. Wash vegetables just before cooking and avoid long exposure to air. Remember that most vitamins are near the skin so scrub lightly and pare only if necessary. After paring or slicing, cook immediately. Care in preparing vegetables will maximize the nutritional content.

4. Steaming is a preferable way to cook vegetables, and a perforated steamer is an excellent investment. Frying foods increases calories but not nutrition.

5. Another good investment is *The Joy of Cooking,* which describes how to purchase, store, prepare, and serve all kinds of vegetables.

A Few Other Comments about Food

Sugar. Sugar is fifty calories per tablespoon. It contains no vitamins, minerals, or protein. It is a known factor in tooth decay, obesity, and heart disease, yet it is present in most processed foods—even those that don't taste sweet. It should have a minimal part in your diet. Sweetness can be supplied by fresh fruits and unsweetened juices. Check your area for classes in sugarless cooking methods.

When your baby begins to eat foods, you might want to look at Vicki Lansky's *The Taming of the C.A.N.D.Y. Monster (Continuously Advertised Nutritionally Deficient Yummies).*

Additives. "The food industry puts more than 1 billion pounds of chemicals per year into the processed foods you and I eat. This averages out to about five pounds per person annually."[5]

Not all additives have been proven safe. The more fresh, unprocessed foods you eat, the better.

Labels. Read labels. The ingredients are listed in the order of their prevalence in the product: the ingredient listed first is found in the greatest quantity, and so on.

An excellent investment is *The Supermarket Handbook* by Nikki and David Goldbeck.

Feeding Your Baby

Although it is early to be thinking about your baby's diet, here are some points to consider now and again later.

To help prevent allergic reactions, many pediatricians recommend waiting six months before introducing solid foods. During the second six months of your baby's life, slowly introduce solids and continue to breast feed or formula feed your baby. It is often suggested that you delay switching to cow's milk until the child is one year old, especially if your family has a history of allergies.

When you do introduce solids, you will choose between the commercially prepared and home prepared foods. If you purchase the former, be sure to read the labels. Sugar, salt, tapioca, and other additives are unnecessary additions to baby food. There are now many commercially made baby foods that do not have additives and are high in vitamins and minerals.

You may want to make some or all of your own baby food. If so, make sure that you use fresh, quality produce and meats. Cook produce minimally so you retain most of the vitamins and minerals. Do not add sugar or salt. Make sure your utensils and pots are absolutely clean.

[5]Lewis A. Coffin, M.D., *The Grandmother Conspiracy Exposed* (Santa Barbara, Cal.: Capra Press, 1974), p. 36.

Now that you have completed the section on nutrition, see if you can plan two days of nutritious meals that meet the requirements suggested in the "Daily Food Guide." How do these menus compare with those you suggested before reading this section?

Day 1

Breakfast   Lunch   Dinner

Morning Snack   Afternoon Snack   Evening Snack

Day 2

Breakfast   Lunch   Dinner

Morning Snack   Afternoon Snack   Evening Snack

19

Prepare in quantity whenever possible. For instance, cook a two-pound bag of carrots and then grind or puree them. You can fill an ice tray with the carrot mixture. When frozen, put the carrot cubes in a plastic freezer bag and store in the freezer until you need them. Warm them in a baby food dish or in a pyrex dish in boiling water.

2

This chapter includes emotional changes and sexuality during the third trimester, warning signs during pregnancy, preparation for childbirth, breast feeding, and buying wisely for your baby.

CHANGES

The final three months of pregnancy, known as the third trimester, mark a shift toward active preparation for the birth of the baby. Couples take childbirth preparation classes, decorate the nursery, and choose names for their babies. They begin to think of themselves less as a pregnant couple and more as parents with new responsibilities.

The Mother's Emotional Reactions

The last trimester is usually the time of most physical discomfort. You will probably be very ready for the baby to be born, even though you are nostalgic about the end of this special time in your life. The heightened sensitivity and mood swings you had earlier in pregnancy continue.

Fears about childbirth are common. You are about to experience something totally new, and to fear the unknown is natural. You may wonder whether you can cope with labor and delivery, how you will act, whether there will be pain, and about the health of your baby.

Women are often engrossed in conversations about children and dreams of their babies. At the time of birth, the child you had imagined will have to be emotionally replaced with the real child. Sometimes it can be an adjustment, especially if a child of the opposite sex was expected or the baby's physical appearance is very different than imagined.

Because of your physical appearance—an enlarged abdomen, large breasts, clumsiness, and so on—your body image may change. You may

The Third Trimester

doubt your physical attractiveness, especially to your mate. On the other hand, some women feel beautiful throughout pregnancy.

The Father's Emotional Reactions

The father's emotions also become directed toward the reality of the baby and the end of pregnancy. Concerns over the safety of the baby and mother during labor and delivery are common. Your thoughts are often filled with questions about fatherhood. "What kind of father will I be?" "Will I be able to provide enough financial security?" It is a time of increased awareness of the meaning of family.

In addition to these concerns, you are also involved in those of the mother and in her increased emotional sensitivity. Now is an important time to offer reassurance that her changing shape is desirable and that together you can cope with labor, delivery, and parenthood.

Very crucial to this time in pregnancy is open communication or discussion of feelings and concerns between father and mother. Childbirth education classes are another source of reassurance to a couple. The information from class can decrease fears, increase knowledge, and provide positive tools to use in labor and delivery. Also, the social experience with other couples is invaluable; usually you learn that you are all having many of the same emotions and concerns.

SEXUAL RELATIONS

How couples feel about sex during the last three months of pregnancy can vary greatly. Some couples feel an interest in lovemaking and continue to have intercourse through these last months. They are able to overcome the obstacles of a larger, cumbersome uterus and the mother's awkward movements by experimenting with new positions and new forms of physical closeness. Positions may include facing each other while side-lying, rear entry, woman superior, and so on. Other couples experience a decline in sexual interest or may decide to limit or restrict intercourse during the last months. Sometimes physicians counsel against intercourse or lovemaking that results in maternal orgasm, perhaps because of vaginal bleeding, ruptured membranes, a deeply engaged presenting part, incompetent cervix, or pain during intercourse.

Women can have mixed feelings about their bodies. To some women, their enlarged, redefined bodies—swollen breasts, large abdomen, awkward movements, and increased vaginal secretions—are disturbing. They may feel embarrassed or dislike their bodies, which can influence how they feel about relations with their mate. Other women seem to blossom and take real delight in their womanliness. They may have a continued or even increased sexual desire.

Men can have equally varied feelings regarding their mate's changing body and the impending delivery of their baby. Some men take great interest in the enlarging body and fetal movements. The woman may take on special qualities to the man, and her fertility adds a special quality to their lovemaking. New positions, as well as new forms of sexual behavior, may appeal to some men and not to others. Some men feel uncomfortable with the physical appearance of their mate. They may be concerned about injuring the baby during intercourse or initiating labor.

Following are some of the physical facts regarding intercourse during the third trimester:

1. Before your baby's birth, there is little risk of infection unless the membranes are ruptured and bacteria from the vagina can enter the amniotic sac.
2. Masters and Johnson concluded from a study on pregnant women that orgasm can initiate labor if the mother is near term and conditions for labor are ripe.[1]
3. Toward the end of pregnancy, the increased size of the woman's abdomen may necessitate a change in position. Excessive pressure should not be put on the pregnant uterus. When the baby's head drops lower in the pelvis, an erect penis may be uncomfortable for the woman, but it is not likely that the penis can rupture the membranes. Questions about sexual relations as they pertain to your own medical condition can be discussed with your physician.

Whether the couple continues to have intercourse or whether there is a decline in sexual activity, it is important that the lines of communication be kept open. Being frank and honest in your discussions about how you feel can be beneficial to you as a couple. The way you feel is not wrong; feelings are legitimate. Many couples increasingly need affection, closeness, tenderness, kissing, and touching. These are other ways of expressing love and can make the last months of pregnancy a time of closeness—emotionally and physically. An excellent resource is *Making Love During Pregnancy* by Bing and Colman.

WARNING SIGNS DURING PREGNANCY

Call your doctor if any of these occur:

1. Pain or burning when you urinate, or a decrease in the amount of urine
2. Vaginal bleeding or spotting
3. Persistent headache
4. Swelling or puffiness (retention of fluid) in hands, feet, face

[1]William H. Masters and Virginia E. Johnson, *Human Sexual Response* (Boston: Little, Brown and Company, 1966), p. 166.

5. Sharp abdominal pain or severe cramping. Nausea or queasy feeling in stomach
6. Rupture or leakage of amniotic fluid
7. Fever of 100 degrees or higher
8. Dizziness
9. Blurred vision
10. Any illness you have

Toxemia

Toxemia is a condition of pregnancy with several different symptoms, including

- Hypertension—the mother's blood pressure rises. .
- Edema—fluid accumulates in the mother's body, especially in her hands and face.
- Proteinuria—protein or albumin is present in the mother's urine.

These symptoms are easily identifiable and should be checked at each prenatal visit.

Mild toxemia is termed pre-eclampsia. If the mother's blood pressure increases, she has protein in the urine, and/or edema, she is said to have pre-eclampsia. She may have had a sudden weight gain, headaches, blurred vision, nausea, vomiting, a decrease in the amount of urine, and emotional tension. When the condition becomes more severe it is called eclampsia.

The causes of toxemia are not completely understood. It occurs most often in women younger than 20 or older than 30 having their first babies, in multiple pregnancies, in women with more than five pregnancies, and in nonwhites.

Treatment for toxemia is very important, and women should watch for symptoms between prenatal visits. Treatment usually includes bed rest on one's left side with the feet elevated. A diet with adequate protein is encouraged. Excessive salt should be avoided, but the elimination of all salt is discouraged. Toxemia can often be controlled with these measures, but delivery is the only way to eliminate the disease.

PREPARATION FOR CHILDBIRTH

Everyone who comes to the experience of childbirth is prepared. The crux of the matter is whether the preparation is positive and realistic or negative and inaccurate.[2]

Unfortunately, many of us approach childbirth with negative expectations. For centuries most cultures have held that pain is inevitable

[2]Joy Clausen et al., Maternity Nursing Today (New York: McGraw-Hill Book Company, 1973), p. 367.

during childbirth. Rarely have television shows, books, or movies expounded on the thrill and excitement of childbirth; rather, they dwell on the pain, which seldom is portrayed as controllable. Your culture has influenced your mental attitude toward childbirth and will influence how you perceive your labor contractions. Stories told to you by your mother, friends, and relatives about their childbirths or your own observations and previous experience can also affect how you feel about childbirth, and consequently, how you will react to your labor and delivery.

During the third trimester, many expectant couples find themselves anticipating the impending childbirth experience with some apprehension. The purpose of childbirth education is to prepare couples to deal positively with the birth experience. They are educated about the process of labor and delivery, they are taught techniques to deal with the mother's discomfort and pain, and they are informed about the variations that can occur. Most couples begin childbirth preparation during their third trimester.

Lamaze

Lamaze is one method of childbirth preparation. It is a "man-made," not a "natural," method of dealing with labor contractions, and it prepares you emotionally, intellectually, and physically for childbirth. Its primary goal is to have a healthy mother deliver a healthy baby. It offers you psychological techniques, or tools, you can use during your labor to make it a more shared, enjoyable, and meaningful experience. Lamaze techniques have been proven to be beneficial in decreasing the mother's perception of pain during labor and delivery.[3]

The basis of Lamaze originated in Russia where women were conditioned or trained to respond to their contractions with relaxation. In the 1950s, Fernand Lamaze, a Frenchman, adapted the Russian techniques and introduced his method of prepared childbirth. The conditioned, or automatic, response is still the basis, but Lamaze added special breathing techniques to the Russian method. In the United States the method has been expanded to include fathers in a coaching role, allowing couples to share actively in the birth of their child. Today, Lamaze is a very popular method to control the pain of labor.

Causes of Pain during Childbirth

During childbirth the woman must deal with two different sources of pain—one during labor; the other during delivery. The anatomy of childbirth is thoroughly discussed later, but briefly the following is what occurs:

[3]Richard J. Stevens, "Psychological Strategies for Management of Pain in Prepared Childbirth, II: A Study of Psychoanalgesia in Prepared Childbirth," *Birth and the Family Journal,* Vol. 4, No. 1 (1977), 6.

Your baby is now securely inside a muscle called the uterus or womb, which looks like an upside-down pear with a small opening at the bottom. This lower portion of the uterus is your cervix. During labor the cervix has to open enough for your baby to pass through; it has to change from a very small opening to one about four inches across. This miraculous event occurs because the muscle fibers of your uterus are capable of contracting, or getting shorter, and then relaxing, or lengthening. These are the labor contractions about which you've probably heard. Contractions push the baby's head against the cervix, causing it to open. Pain during labor is primarily caused by the opening of your cervix. During the pushing or delivery stage, however, pain is mostly caused by the stretching and pressure which occur as the baby moves down the birth canal (or vagina).

Perception of Pain during Childbirth

Sensations (stimuli) during labor and delivery travel through nerve fibers up the spinal cord to the brain, which interprets them. You respond behaviorly depending on your interpretation. Unprepared women respond by tensing, screaming, and becoming frightened. Prepared women respond by using breathing and relaxation techniques.

How your brain perceives or interprets labor contractions or how much discomfort you actually feel depends on a number of factors:

1. *Fear:* How anxious or frightened are you about your labor and delivery? Your *level of anxiety* plays a large part in determining how you will interpret and respond to uterine contractions. Anxiety sets up a negative cycle, called the fear-tension-pain cycle, which is often seen in untrained laboring women. Their fear makes them become tense, which increases the pain, which in turn makes them more frightened, and the cycle repeats.
2. *Physical factors:* Are you healthy and well rested when you go into labor? How long since you last ate? How close together and strong are your contractions? How long have you been in labor?
3. *Emotional factors:* Are you highly motivated to use Lamaze techniques? Is your labor coach supportive? Do you feel comfortable where you're laboring and with the birth attendants caring for you?
4. *Focus of attention:* Are you attending to the intensity of the contractions or is your focus of attention elsewhere? Are you actively using the techniques taught in childbirth education classes?

Increasing Your Pain Threshold

Richard Stevens, a neurophysiologist, has presented research on psychological strategies, or techniques, which enable people to tolerate more pain, or increase their pain threshold.[4]

[4]Richard J. Stevens, "Psychological Strategies for Management of Pain in Prepared Childbirth, I: A Review of the Research," *Birth and the Family Journal,* Vol. 3, No. 4 (1976), 157-64.

1. *Active relaxation:* relaxing the muscles in your body except the uterus.
2. *Cognitive control:* using your mind to help deal with pain.
   a. *Disassociation:* concentrating on a nonpainful aspect of the stimulus, or contraction.
   b. *Focusing attention:* actively involving your mind with techniques, such as breathing patterns, instead of thinking about your contractions.
3. *Rehearsal:* becoming educated to reduce your fear of the unknown.
4. *Hawthorne effect:* someone important to the laboring mother giving her attention, namely, the coach, the staff, and the physician.

Using Psychological Strategies

Lamaze can help you use these psychological strategies to raise your pain threshold in the following ways.

1. *Active relaxation:* You will be trained to actively or consciously relax during labor contractions, and your coach will be trained to help you. Instead of reacting to a contraction with tension, you will be taught to relax your muscles.
2. *Disassociation:* In Lamaze we speak about labor contractions not labor pains. You will learn to think of a contraction as the mechanism causing your cervix to open so your baby can be born.
3. *Focusing attention:* Your mind will be occupied with the Lamaze techniques—breathing patterns, relaxation, massage, and focusing your eyes on an object in the room. For example, concentrating on the discomfort of a headache increases the pain, whereas engaging your mind elsewhere decreases your awareness of the headache. In the same manner, focusing your attention on Lamaze techniques will keep your mind so occupied that you will be less aware of the uterine contractions.
4. *Cognitive rehearsal:* One of the purposes of Lamaze classes and this book is to teach you about the childbirth process. This knowledge will enable you to mentally and physically rehearse what will occur during labor, eliminating many of the fears and anxieties you may have from misinformation or lack of information.
5. *Hawthorne effect:* Having a labor coach who practices with you before labor and is with you throughout labor and delivery insures that you have help and attention. Your coach should be someone to whom you are close emotionally. A study on the effect of a husband or coach on the perception of pain determined that practical help was more effective than only moral support.[5] Lamaze teaches your coach specific ways to assist you. Another positive influence is the time your nurse and doctor spend with you, helping with techniques or keeping you informed about your labor.

[5]Carolyn Block and Richard Block, "The Effect of Support of the Husband and Obstetrician on Pain Perception and Control in Childbirth," *Birth and the Family Journal,* Vol. 2, No. 2 (1975), 43-50.

In summary, you can psychologically or physiologically manage the pain of childbirth. Your mind interprets sensations from your body. You can block your awareness of the sensations coming from the uterine contractions by occupying your mind with the psychological strategies just listed. You can also block or decrease painful stimuli by using physical means, such as light massage (effleurage), on the surface of your body.

Your goal is to make the Lamaze techniques become automatic responses to uterine contractions. Instead of becoming tense and frightened you will automatically relax and use special breathing patterns. This change in behavior occurs through practice. Just as riding a bicycle becomes automatic after practice, so will your Lamaze techniques.

It is important for both you and your coach to rehearse your labor roles daily. You need to learn to respond to your coach's touch, voice, and presence. At the same time, the coach learns how to help you relax and what techniques work best for you. You will become a labor team. Stevens reports that the more time you practice your techniques, the more effective they become.[6] In addition to the technical reasons, the time you devote to practice illustrates your emotional support for each other in the preparation for the birth of your child.

During your third trimester you will need to make some decisions regarding the care of your baby, for example, the method of feeding and what clothes and equipment to purchase. Here are a few facts that you may want to consider.

BREAST FEEDING

Until modern times and in less industrialized and affluent societies, breast feeding has been the accepted method of feeding babies. With affluence came the prestige of being able to afford to bottle feed babies. Breast feeding also diminished in popularity as a woman's breasts began to be seen as more of a sex symbol.

However, in recent years there has been a renewed interest in breast feeding, especially among couples taking childbirth preparation classes. If you haven't already, you should begin now to decide how you will feed your baby. This decision deserves consideration from both parents. After you have an intellectual understanding of breast feeding, sit down and discuss how each of you feels about it emotionally.

Benefits

1. *Nutrition:* Breast milk is perfectly suited to an infant, and it is more easily digested than cow's milk. Breast-fed babies usually don't require additional sources of nutrition until 4 to 6 months of age.

[6]Stevens, "Psychological Strategies, II," p. 6.

2. *Immunities:* Immunities are passed to the baby through colostrum, the substance produced by the breast during pregnancy. The baby drinks colostrum until the mother's milk comes in.

3. *Convenience:* Breast milk is always ready, the right temperature, and easily transported on trips.

4. *Emotional gratification:* Breast feeding fosters a close physical and emotional relationship between a mother and her nursing baby. It is gratifying to be able to supply your baby with the nourishment she needs.

5. *Economics:* Breast feeding requires that the mother consume an extra five hundred calories per day. This food and perhaps supplemental vitamins are your only extra expenses. Bottle feeding can be an obvious addition to the family food bill.

6. *Time:* No preparations are necessary for breast feeding other than a nutritious diet and rest when you're trying to establish your milk supply those first few weeks. You need the rest to recover from childbirth anyway. Preparing bottles and formula takes time, which would be more fun to spend with your baby. There's also no heating bottles at 2:00 A.M. while your baby cries, waiting to be fed.

7. *Allergies:* Breast-fed babies are less likely to develop allergies to milk. The sooner cow's milk and solids are introduced, the more likely a child is to develop an allergic reaction.

8. *Obesity:* Breast-fed babies are usually not overfed. If the baby has frequent wet diapers you can assume he is getting enough to eat. The baby simply nurses until satisfied. Bottle-fed babies are sometimes encouraged to finish the bottle, and consequently, are overfed. Recent studies are beginning to show that the extra fat cells we acquire as babies stay with us and contribute to weight problems later on.

9. *Dental development:* The sucking action at the breast fosters good jaw and facial muscle development.

10. *Bowel movements:* The stools of a breast-fed baby are loose and the odor is mild. Constipation is rarely a problem.

Breast Function

There are two main things you need to understand about your milk supply. First, milk is produced as a result of a hormone called *prolactin* and the sucking of your baby. How much the baby nurses determines how much milk the breast produces. It stands to reason, then, that a newborn will want to eat frequently to build up your milk supply. Second, when your baby begins to nurse, the sucking stimulates your pituitary gland to release a hormone called *oxytocin.* This reaction causes the milk to be let down from the milk ducts so the baby can get it. Your let-down reflex is strongly affected by emotions. If you are tense, worried, or in some way emotionally upset, you will not relax enough for the milk to let down. Then you end up with a frustrated mother and a hungry baby. This problem is bound to occur sometime to any nursing mother, so try to remedy the situation with some conscious relaxation, a hot shower, a little beer or wine, imagining the milk letting down, and removing the source of anxiety, if possible.

Preparing the Nipples

The value of this preparation during pregnancy seems to lend itself to controversy. Many women never have sore nipples from breast feeding, but others do. It is generally believed that fair-complexioned people are more susceptible. Many women believe it was beneficial for them to have done some or all of the following during the last few weeks of pregnancy to toughen their nipples.

1. Pull the nipples out slightly and roll them between thumb and finger. This exercise will make the nipple more erect and easier for your baby to grasp.
2. Discontinue using soap on your nipples because it tends to dry the skin, making them more susceptible to cracking.
3. Rub the nipples with a terry towel and expose them to the air and your clothing, by occasionally not wearing a bra.
4. Hand express colostrum. It is believed by some to open the milk ducts and possibly decrease engorgement.

Beginning to Breast Feed

First, you need to realize that it takes time to establish a milk supply and time for you and the baby to learn to breast feed. Some babies nurse right away and others lick the nipple and seem initially disinterested. They need time to learn. Also, it is easier for some mothers than it is for others.

When should you start? Some women are comfortable nursing in the delivery room. Others prefer to wait until they get to recovery and can adjust their position more easily. Be sure to ask for help if you need it. The nurse can show you how to get the nipple in the baby's mouth and how to position yourself for comfort. No one expects you to know how to nurse if you've never done it before.

At first your baby will be getting colostrum, not milk. This substance is full of protein and immunities and is usually all your baby needs those first few days. Your milk will come in about 2 to 4 days after birth. Most women's breasts become engorged when their milk comes in; the breasts become sore and swollen because of the inelasticity of the milk ducts. This condition usually subsides as soon as the milk supply adjusts and the milk ducts become more elastic. Sometimes heat (a hot bath) or hand expressing some milk will relieve some of the soreness.

Nurse your baby as frequently as he seems hungry. If your hospital allows rooming-in, take advantage of it so your baby will be with you when he gets hungry. Start right away to drink plenty of fluids. It takes about 2 to 3 quarts of fluids a day for you to produce milk and maintain your own body's hydration.

Once you get home be sure to get plenty of rest and drink something each time you nurse. Ignore the housework temporarily and take advantage of relatives' or friends' offers to help with a meal or the house.

It might take four to six weeks before your milk supply is established and you and the baby are really comfortable nursing. During this time it is very important for you to have someone you can call on to answer your questions. This person might be a friend who has breast-fed, your Lamaze instructor, or a member of LaLeche League, an organization of nursing mothers available to help you. Select a doctor for your baby who supports breast feeding and can answer your questions.

Persevere. Soon you and the baby will be a happy breast feeding team.

If you're beginning to feel tied down, remember how easily your baby can go out with you. Short outings will be less tiring. You might have a friend baby-sit while you go out for an hour after feeding the baby.

Obstacles to Breast Feeding

Some women develop sore nipples when they begin to breast feed. Usually the discomfort is noticed most when the infant first starts to suck. Some of the following might help:

- Expose the nipple to air and sun (don't get burned).
- Use pure hydrous lanolin on the nipples after each feeding to keep them supple. (It can be purchased at a pharmacy.) Lanolin does not have to be wiped off before your baby nurses the next time.
- Don't wait so long between feedings that your breasts become full and the baby can't grasp the nipple easily.
- Change nursing positions for each feeding.
- Avoid nursing bras or nursing pads with plastic liners; they don't allow air to get to your nipples.

Mastitis, or a breast infection, sometimes occurs. Completely emptying your breasts of milk at each feeding allows for good drainage and usually insures against mastitis, but not always. If you notice a red spot on your breast or have a fever and feel like you're getting the flu, call your doctor immediately. If you treat an infection in the beginning, it usually does not become bothersome. The usual treatment includes (1) moist heat on the area of infection, (2) antibiotics, (3) rest, and (4) continued nursing on the affected breast (since the usual cause of the infection is incomplete emptying of the milk).

As a preventive measure, be sure to alternate the side on which you begin nursing. Nursing in different positions (sitting up, lying down) will also help to insure that the baby completely empties the milk ducts.

The attitudes of your friends and relatives who are negative about breast feeding can be difficult to deal with when you're first starting to nurse. The first time the baby fusses after you've fed him and your friend suggests you don't have enough milk, you wonder just a little if it's true.

Worrying about it *can* affect your milk supply, so be confident and ask your friend not to interfere.

Finally, life can be miserable if you feed your baby by the clock. Your baby is the best judge of when he's hungry. On the other hand, don't get into the routine of feeding him every hour round the clock, you'll both be exhausted.

Is it worth it? Ask any breast-feeding mother who's past the initial adjustment and she'll say yes. The close relationship with the baby and the confidence in being able to nurture your child are very gratifying.

Fathers Can Help

First and foremost, fathers can help by offering their encouragement and emotional support. Your mate needs to know that you want her to succeed and are willing to help her. You can help by insisting that she rest when the baby rests and reminding her to drink plenty of fluids. You can help initially by bringing her the baby at night, straightening the house, and fixing some of the meals. Be flexible. Your dinner may be late occasionally; babies always seem to eat right at the dinner hour.

Some fathers think that because they don't actually feed the baby they aren't needed. Nothing could be more incorrect. The baby needs your love just as much as the mother's. Enjoy your baby, learn to diaper and care for him, and help him get to know you. Relax and be confident that your baby is being well nourished in a very natural way.

Deciding to Bottle Feed

If you decide that bottle feeding is more suitable for you and your baby, have confidence in your decision and enjoy this experience with your baby. You can develop the same nurturing, close relationship as long as you hold and cuddle your baby while you feed him. *Please* don't prop the bottle.

Follow the advice of your baby's doctor about formulas and bottles. You can feed the baby on demand and let him eat as much as he wants; he might not need the last two ounces in the bottle. A real benefit of bottle feeding is that the father can enjoy feeding the baby too.

BUYING FOR YOUR BABY

You are about to embark on what is an expensive venture—the raising of a child. By careful planning before you shop, however, you can make or buy equipment, clothing, and toys of good quality and still be economical. One source calculates that raising one child is 15 to 17 percent of the yearly family income,[7] so careful shopping is important.

Make a list of the things you will need before you go shopping. Find out what is considered good quality for each item and what the safety requirements are. Your local Consumer Safety Commission office has free information, or you can write to the Washington office: U.S. Consumer Products Safety Commission, Washington, D.C. 21207. Another source of information is *Consumers Union Guide to Buying for Babies,* published by *Consumer Reports.* This book rates many baby articles: cribs, diapers, sleepers, carriages, bike seats, gates, vaporizers, pins, pacifiers, and so on.

The following discussion considers some major pieces of equipment.

Car Seats. A car seat is an important investment, and the purchase of a safe one should be high on your list of priorities. You should have one in which to bring your baby home from the hospital.

Two sources to consult are (1) *Consumer Reports Magazine,* June 1977 (or the latest article); and (2) "Don't Risk Your Child's Life" (1976), published by Physicians for Automotive Safety, 50 Union Avenue, Irvington, New Jersey 07111. Keep in mind that some companies make one car seat only for babies and a different model for an older child. Other companies make models that can be used for both ages. Follow the manufacturer's suggestions for installation to maximize safety.

Cribs and Highchairs. A safe crib and highchair are two other important, costly investments. To be sure that you understand the safety features of each, consult your local Consumer Safety Commission office, write to the national office requesting their pamphlets, or read *Consumer's Guide.* Most new products meet these requirements, but if you plan to refurbish an antique or accept a hand-me-down, do yourself and your baby a favor and find out how to make it safe.

Baby Carrier. Many new mothers and fathers find these a wonderful invention for getting out or for dealing with a fussy baby. The Snugli is a well-made corduroy or seersucker infant carrier, which allows you to carry the baby on your chest or back and leaves your arms free. Many stores carry them, they can sometimes be bought used or borrowed from friends; or you can write to Snugli Cottage Industries, Route 7, Box 685A, Evergreen, Colorado 80439. Check with a children's store about other types of baby carriers or packs.

[7]Sylvia Porter, *Sylvia Porter's Money Book* (1975), p. 704. Copyright © 1975 by Sylvia Porter. Reprinted by permission of Doubleday & Co., Inc.

Toys. For information on toy safety write to Toys, Washington, D.C. 20207; the toll-free number is (800) 638-2666. For an exhaustive description of age-appropriate, good-quality toys, books, and music, consult the appendix in *How To Parent* by Fitzhugh Dodson.

Diapers. Diapers are a major investment whether you buy cloth or disposable diapers or use a diaper service. Many parents use a combination of all three. Consult *Consumer's Guide* for information on each type of diaper.

A diaper service supplies you with a specific number of diapers in the size you request (ask for the newborn size initially). All you do is rinse the diapers; the company picks up soiled diapers and delivers clean ones. If your baby has very sensitive skin, this may be your best option. Call companies in your area to compare prices and service.

For cloth diapers, an initial investment is required in the purchase of five or six dozen diapers, after which there are maintenance costs—hot water, soap, dryer, and so on. You, of course, are responsible for rinsing, washing, drying, and folding diapers. Care must be taken to rinse the diapers thoroughly when laundering to avoid irritating the baby's sensitive skin.

Cloth diapers come in different sizes, weights, and quality. Invest in *good* diapers and a size that your child won't outgrow, you can always fold them smaller for a newborn. After your baby is through with the diapers, you can use them for your next child, and later you will have a large supply of dustcloths.

Disposable diapers are convenient but can be expensive and of questionable value environmentally. Also they irritate some babies' skin. They come in different sizes, depending on your baby's age and weight, and have different absorbencies, depending on the manufacturer and whether they are for the day or night. They vary considerably in quality and price.

Many parents choose to use a combination of the above. Ask for diaper service as a gift, or treat yourself during the immediate postpartum period. Buy your own diapers and use them most of the time. Use disposable diapers when you go out, or as a treat occasionally. Watch for sales.

Infants' Wear. A basic layette for a baby includes diapers, six to ten pairs of rubber pants, and a few crib sheets. A summer baby will probably do well in undershirts and a sun-shielding hat or bonnet. A few sunsuits are nice but not necessary. A winter infant requires more clothing: undershirts and six to twelve uncomplicated, front-opening stretch suits (one-piece stretch terry outfits). It's hard to have too many of these. They are so useful that the baby can wear them in the day and sleep in them at night; or you can invest in a few nightgowns (long gowns with string closing at the bottom) and a few heavier blanket sleepers.

Blankets are necessary. Lightweight ones are good for summer, but in the winter you'll also need some heavier ones. Square blankets are best. Consider making your own out of lightweight, 45-inch wide, flame-resistant flannel.

Be cautious about the three-month size. The garment may look big to you while you are pregnant, but babies are notorious for rapidly outgrowing those little sizes. Your baby will do nicely with *one* special outfit. Somehow those fancy little dresses and suits don't get used very much.

Even if you plan to use disposables or diaper service, buy a dozen diapers for your own use. They are drool pads, burp pads, changing pads, and have all kinds of other uses.

Be sure to follow the laundering directions on the labels of your baby's clothing to maintain their flame-resistant quality. For more information on laundering, read Brochure #24: *Laundering Procedures for Flame Resistant Fabrics, U.S. Consumer Products Safety Commission, Washington, D.C. 20207.*

THINGS TO DO BEFORE YOUR BABY'S BIRTHDAY

Things for the baby:

_____ 1. Make early arrangements for diaper service if you plan to use one, or watch newspapers for sales on disposable diapers.

_____ 2. Watch newspapers for sales on baby clothes and cloth diapers.

_____ 3. Launder and put away baby clothes.

_____ 4. If you plan to bottle feed, have formula and necessary equipment your doctor recommends on hand.

_____ 5. Have on hand nursery items, such as powder, soap, oil, cornstarch, etc. Discuss with your doctor what products he prefers. Some doctors are particular about what they want you to use.

_____ 6. If breast feeding, read a book on nursing and take it with you to the hospital.

_____ 7. Buy or borrow a car seat for an infant, and plan to use it from the very beginning. Try it in your car to make sure that it fits the car's seat belts.

Things for the parents:

_____ 1. Cook or bake several casseroles and freeze them. Solicit offers of meals from your friends.

_____ 2. Plan a week of menus, and stock your freezer and pantry for these meals. Fresh fruit, vegetables, and dairy products can be bought later.

_____ 3. Start looking for baby-sitter possibilities. An exchange of baby-sitting with some members of your childbirth preparation class is a good possibility.

_____ 4. Buy, address, and stamp birth announcements. You can fill in the vital statistics in the hospital. If you're planning to design an original birth announcement, have some ideas ready and a printer or copying place in mind.

_____ 5. Buy presents and cards for the birthdays and other occassions that occur around your due date.

_____ 6. Buy sanitary pads for the first weeks at home.

_____ 7. If you are breast feeding, buy nursing bras, two front-opening nightgowns, and nursing pads. You can make your own pads from soft, absorbent material or use handkerchiefs.

_____ 8. Do not prematurely pack away your maternity clothes. These or other loose-fitting clothing will be more comfortable for the first few weeks.

_____ 9. Have plenty of film on hand.

_____ 10. Pack your suitcase for the hospital.

Include here any other things you would like to accomplish before your baby is born.

_____

_____

CHOOSING A DOCTOR FOR YOUR BABY

The decision about who will care for your baby (whether a pediatrician or a family practitioner) is an important one. It should be made during your third trimester, long before your due date.

Try to think of yourself as a health consumer. You will want the best possible care for your new baby. Sometimes it is hard for those without children to really know what's important. One thing you can do is talk to friends who already have children and find out their priorities. Also, make a list of your concerns and needs. Then interview some doctors. A face-to-face meeting is usually more productive than a phone call. Ask the doctor how she sees her role as provider of health care for your baby. Go over your list of questions and concerns. Finally, evaluate your feelings about the doctor. Can you communicate? Is she reassuring? Try to think of her as more than just a baby doctor. Do you think you will feel comfortable discussing problems with her? Often the doctor cares for the parents as much as she cares for the baby during the first year.

In the space below, make a list of questions for discussion with prospective pediatricians or family practitioners. These topics may stimulate some questions: feeding theories, what to do in an emergency, availability by phone, knowledge and screening of developmental growth, knowledge and interest in helping parents deal with behavior problems, fees, and opinion regarding circumcision.

3

This chapter includes information to help you look and feel better during your pregnancy and to help you prepare for labor and delivery. Posture, comfort positions, prenatal exercises, and the pelvic floor are discussed.

POSTURE

Good posture maintained throughout your pregnancy and for the rest of your life will help you feel more energetic and more comfortable. Many of the common aches and pains associated with pregnancy can be prevented or alleviated if you stand and sit properly. By aligning your body correctly, you relieve stress on muscles, joints, and ligaments, and the uterus will maintain its proper position in the pelvic cavity.

Standing

Imagine that a string is attached to the crown of your head and is pulling you up, trying to make you stand straight.

1. You will find that your chin should be tucked in just a little, to align your head with your body. Many people walk around as if they are in a big hurry, with their heads preceding their bodies.
2. Your shoulders should be pulled back slightly. Rounded shoulders are a common postural defect.
3. Your pelvis should be tilted backward so your low back is straight, not swayed. To get your pelvis back, you need to tuck in your buttocks and pull in your stomach.
4. Your knees should be slightly flexed, or bent, and your feet should be pointed forward.
5. Most of your weight is on the outer borders of your feet.

Comfort and Exercise

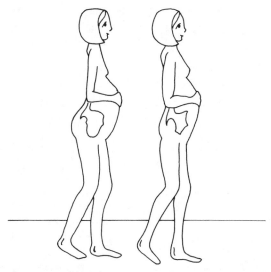

Incorrect Posture—Pelvis tilted forward—Back is swayed
Correct Posture—Pelvis tilted backward—Back is straight

Check your posture by leaning against a wall with your feet about five inches away. Tilt your pelvis backward so that your entire back is touching the wall. Now step away from the wall and see if you can maintain this posture while you walk. Do not walk stiffly, but simply make an effort to hold in your stomach and tuck in your buttocks. An occasional glance into the mirror can help you determine if your back is straight or swayed.

Poor posture stretches and weakens abdominal muscles while tightening back muscles, resulting in increased stress on joints, ligaments, and muscles. Backache is often the result of poor posture. If you need to stand for prolonged periods at work or perhaps waiting in line, you can prevent your pelvis from tipping forward by placing one foot on a step or stool. This position automatically tilts the pelvis back and reduces the sway in your back. Avoid wearing high-heeled shoes, as they throw your weight forward, and to compensate, you arch your back.

To prevent pooling of blood in your legs while standing, shift your weight from one foot to the other or rock back and forth on your heels and toes. This exercise helps the leg muscles force the blood up out of your legs. Excessive pooling of blood in your legs results in varicose veins and can reduce your blood pressure, causing a subsequent feeling of faintness or dizziness. Always sit down if you start to feel light-headed.

Sitting

Because many of us sit for prolonged periods of time at work or school, it is important to sit correctly. While sitting, elevate your legs when possible and get up as often as you can to stretch and walk around.

1. If you are sitting in an upright chair, tilt your pelvis back, moving your bottom slightly forward away from the back of the chair seat. Do not slump in your chair.

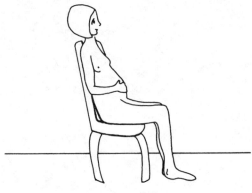

Correct Sitting Posture

2. If you are leaning forward in a chair, as in typing or writing, sit with your buttocks against the back of the chair, lean your body forward, and keep your back straight, not swayed. In other words, don't throw your shoulders back in order to sit up straight as this posture only increases the curve in your lower back.

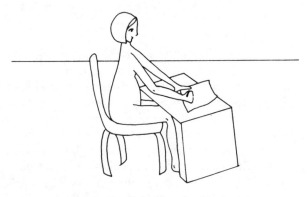

Correct Sitting Posture

COMFORT POSITIONS

The following positions are designed to help make your pregnancy more comfortable by relieving the pressure of the uterus on various parts of your body and by reducing the strain on some of the muscles and ligaments. None of the positions should be maintained for prolonged periods of time since they would not be good for your circulation. Also, when getting up from any of the positions, you should do so slowly, so you won't feel light-headed.

● *Tailor Sitting*
Purpose:
To allow air to circulate around the perineum
To shift the weight of the uterus from the back to the front of the pelvis
A comfortable position for pregnancy and labor
Position:
Sit on a carpeted floor or rug with your hips and knees flexed, but don't let one foot rest on top of the other since this position impedes the circulation in your legs. You may rest your arms on your legs.

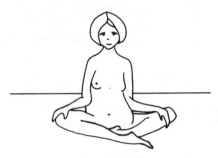

Tailor Sitting

● *Semireclining*
Purpose:
A comfortable position to assume for practicing relaxation
An excellent position to assume if you are having trouble lying on your back because of a light-headed feeling or backache
A comfortable position for labor
Position:
Lie in a semireclining position. Use pillows behind your head and back to prop you up to a 30 to 40 degree angle.

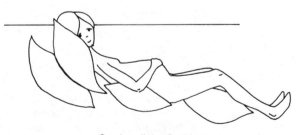

Semi-reclining Position

● *Side-lying*
Purpose:
A comfortable position to assume for sleeping or resting in pregnancy
A good position for labor

Position:

Version 1

Lie on your side with lower arm behind your back and the other arm in front of you. Place pillows under your head and shoulders, forward arm, chest, and uterus and one between your legs. Both knees should be drawn up slightly toward your chest with the top leg drawn up higher and ahead of the bottom leg. This is the "runner" position.

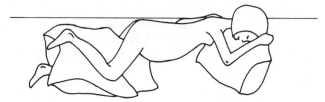

Sidelying in "Runner" Position

Version 2

Lie on your side. Place one pillow under your head and shoulders and several pillows under your lower legs to raise them higher than your hips.

Note: Lying on your side, especially on your left side, is a recommended position for pregnancy because it keeps pressure off the blood vessels behind the uterus while at the same time helping to drain excess fluid from your legs and feet.

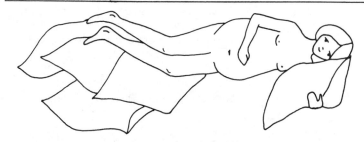

Sidelying Position with Legs Elevated

- *Back-lying*
  Purpose:
    For some, a comfortable position for sleeping, reading, or relaxing. This position is not recommended for labor because of the increased pressure of the uterus on the inferior vena cava (blood vessel behind the uterus), which can result in a drop in the woman's blood pressure (venous hypotension) and a subsequent faint feeling.

Position:
Lie on your back with a pillow under your head and one under your knees and thighs.
Note: Do not keep a pillow under your knees for prolonged periods of time as this can impede circulation in your legs.

● *Using Knee-Chest or All-Fours Position*
Purpose:
Takes the pressure of the uterus off the nerves and blood vessels that go to the legs and pelvic organs.
Can help relieve backache, cramps in the groin or legs, vaginal and rectal swelling.
Note: The knee-chest position should not be used in labor.
Positions:
Knee-Chest
Get on your knees on a bed or carpeted floor. Lean forward, placing a pillow under your head and chest. Do not maintain this position for more than two or three minutes. Get up slowly.

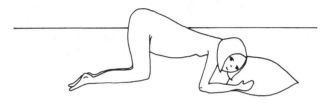

Knee-chest Position

All Fours
Get on your hands and knees with your arms directly under your shoulders and your legs under your hips. This position can be assumed when scrubbing the floor, gardening, or picking up after your children. *Don't let your back sag.*

● *Elevating Legs*
Purpose:
To relieve pressure on nerves and blood vessels as well as on pelvic organs.
To improve circulation and decrease leg swelling.
Position:
Version 1
Assume a leg-elevated, head-down position. Lie on the floor and put your feet up on the couch or low chair. Place pillows under your hips so your entire body is almost straight, not flexed. You should be at about a 30 degree angle. Do not stay in this position for more than 5 minutes at a time and get up slowly.

Position:

Version 2

To promote good circulation while sitting or lying, elevate your legs so they are higher than your heart. Do the sand-digging exercise.

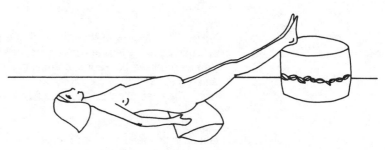

Body elevation—Backlying with feet up

- *Squatting*

Purpose:

The best alternative to bending over when opening drawers, or picking up things from the floor.

Stretches lower back muscles and loosens pelvic joints.

Position:

Unless your legs are strong and you feel stable, squat while holding onto a piece of furniture or other object.

Once down, you can continue to stabilize yourself by keeping your hands on the floor.

To get up, keep your back straight and lift by straightening your knees. Again use something stable to balance yourself as you rise. Do not straighten your knees and then lift up your back from the waist.

If squatting is difficult for you, don't worry about it. You can kneel instead.

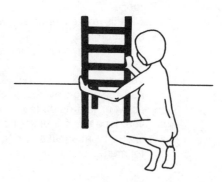

Squatting

BODY MECHANICS

Practicing proper body mechanics when rising from a bed, a chair, or the floor will prevent strain on muscles and unnecessary stress on your back.

- *Rising from a chair:* Slide to the edge of the seat, place your feet on the floor with one foot slightly in front of the other, lean forward, and push yourself up to standing by using your hands and leg muscles.
- *Rising from bed:* Roll over onto your side and swing your legs over the edge of the bed as you raise yourself up by using your arms. Once sitting, continue as above.
- *Rising from the floor:* Roll onto your side and use your arms to push yourself to a side sitting position. Then kneel. Put one knee in front with your foot on the floor. Bend forward over this knee and use your arms and legs to stand. Keep your back straight.

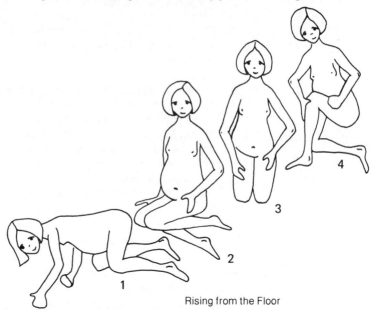

Rising from the Floor

PRENATAL PHYSICAL PREPARATION

Exercises should be an important part of your preparation for childbirth. If you have not begun prenatal exercises, it is not too late to start. Although you may not be able to build a great deal of strength late in your pregnancy, you can maintain tone and stretch muscles in preparation for birth.

Even though you may have been fairly active during your pregnancy, most sports and daily activities don't exercise muscles used during childbirth. An exercise program, as outlined in this chapter, will do the most to insure proper tone and elasticity for these muscles. You may continue to engage in sports you have previously enjoyed unless your doctor advises otherwise. Don't, however, take up a new sport that is strenuous or dangerous during your pregnancy. Walking, swimming, and bicycling are good forms of exercise.

YOU SHOULD EXERCISE DURING PREGNANCY FOR THE FOLLOWING REASONS:

1. To help your body withstand increased stress on muscles, joints, and ligaments.
2. To relieve back strain and improve your posture.
3. To maintain stability in your pelvis; hormonal changes during pregnancy soften fibrous tissue and ligaments in the pelvis to loosen the joints; strong muscles in the abdomen and in the pelvis are necessary to maintain good pelvic stability and good posture.
4. To increase circulation in your legs; pressure of the expanding uterus on blood vessels in the lower extremities decreases circulation.
5. To relieve pelvic and rectal pressure.
6. To stretch and strengthen the muscles needed for childbirth.
7. To renew energy and relieve nervous tension.
8. To strengthen the abdominal muscles so they can support the growing uterus and other abdominal organs; occasionally these muscles are pulled apart in the center of your abdomen during your pregnancy, leaving a gap. If muscles are strong, this problem is less likely to occur or to be severe.
9. To improve your self image and feeling of well being.

There are some muscles that stay relaxed during childbirth and some that contract, or work. During delivery, the upper abdominal muscles will contract to help move the baby down the birth canal, and the lower abdominal muscles and the pelvic floor must remain relaxed. Having exercised the appropriate muscles, you will have the strength and control necessary during childbirth. Your body will also be able to cope with the demands put upon it during labor and delivery if you are in good physical shape.

Having maintained some tone in the muscles, you will regain your strength much faster after delivery. You will also feel better because you are not extremely weak and fatigued. Because you have maintained flexibility in your back and tone in the abdominal muscles, you will be able to resume good posture without any difficulties.

Before beginning the exercise program, you should check with your physician to make sure the exercises are medically acceptable for you. You should try to exercise twice a day if possible, doing each exercise five times and gradually increasing the number of repetitions to ten. Don't exercise just before going to bed because the exercises may be stimulating enough to keep you awake. Also, do not exercise right after eating. Should the exercises result in painful muscles or joints, cut down on the number of repetitions. If any exercise is difficult or painful, eliminate it completely.

Exercise on a folded blanket or exercise mat on the floor in a well-ventilated room. Wear loose, comfortable clothing.

THE PRENATAL EXERCISES

Assume the position given for each exercise. Inhale during the first part of the exercise and exhale during the last part, except where otherwise stated. Do each exercise slowly, relaxing briefly between repetitions and a little longer before beginning a new exercise.

- *Pelvic Tilt*
  Purpose:
    To increase strength in your abdominal muscles.
    To maintain flexibility in your lower back muscles.
    To relieve pressure on the nerves and blood vessels of the uterus, rectum, pelvis, kidneys, and legs.
    To prevent or relieve bachache caused by increased strain on muscles and ligaments.
    To improve posture.
  Position:
    Version 1
    Lie on your back with your knees bent.
  Exercise
    Tilt your pelvis back by pulling in your abdomen and squeezing your buttocks together. Feel the small of your back flatten against the floor. Don't lift up with your feet. Relax. Repeat. (Arrows show tilt.)

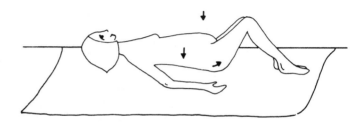

Pelvic Tilt—Backlying Position

Position:

Version 2

Get on the floor on your hands and knees, keeping your hands under your shoulders and your knees under your hips. Keep your back straight; don't let it sag.

Exercise:

Round your lower back by pulling in your abdominal muscles and tightening your buttocks. Your pelvis will tilt backwards as your back arches up. Return your back to a *neutral* position by relaxing the muscles.

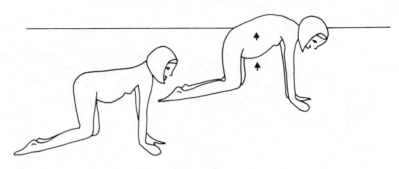

Pelvic Tilt—Hands and Knees Position

● *Bridging*

Purpose:

To strengthen the back muscles, which together with your abdominal muscles, keep your pelvis tilted back to avoid strain on your back.

Position:

Lie on your back with your knees bent.

Exercise:

Raise your hips off the floor, forming a "bridge." Keep your back straight. Return to the starting position, slowly lowering your back and buttocks. Repeat.

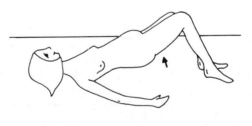

Bridging

● *Straight Leg Raising*

Purpose:

To increase abdominal and leg strength.

To maintain flexibility in your lower back.

To improve circulation in your legs.

Position:

Lie on your back. Bend one knee and keep the other straight. Tilt your pelvis back as in the preceding exercise (pelvic tilt, version 1). Maintain the pelvic tilt throughout the exercise.

Exercise:

Raise your straight leg up toward the ceiling until the muscles pull behind your knee. Slowly lower the leg, remembering to hold the pelvic tilt. Repeat, raising the opposite leg.

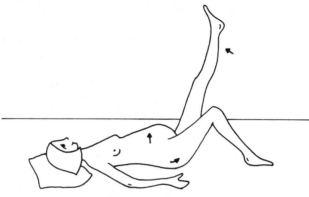

Straight Leg Raising

● *Partial Sit-up*

Purpose:

To increase abdominal strength.

Position:

Lie on your back with knees bent and pelvis tilted back. Maintain the pelvic tilt throughout the exercise.

Exercise:

Version 1

With your hands outstretched toward both knees, raise your head and shoulders up off the floor *as you breathe out.* You do not need to come up all the way. Do not grab your knees. Return to the starting position as you *breathe in.*

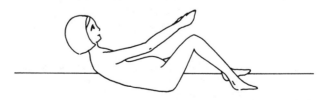

Partial Sit-up—Lifting head and shoulders

Exercise:

Version 2

With both hands outstretched and reaching outside the right knee, raise your head and shoulders up off the floor. (The oblique abdominal muscles are being exercised.) Repeat, reaching outside the left leg with both hands. Remember to breathe out as you rise and breathe in as you relax.

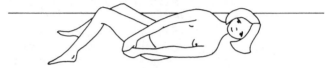

Partial Sit-up—Lifting head and shoulders diagonally

Note: If the abdominal muscles separate during the latter months of pregnancy, you will notice a bulge in the center of your abdomen, near the navel, when you raise your head and shoulders straight up (Version 1). Should this problem occur, support the muscles by crossing your hands across your abdomen and pushing the muscles together. Do not raise up very far and do not allow the bulge to appear. Do this a few times during the day to prevent further separation and to maintain tone. Do not do the oblique abdominal exercise (Version 2.)[1]

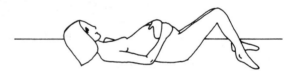

Partial Sit-up—Supporting abdomen with hands

● *Tailor Stretching*
Purpose:
To stretch the inner thigh muscles.
To circulate air around the perineum.
Position:
Sit with your knees bent and the soles of your feet touching. Wrap your arms around the outside of your legs and place your hands just below your knees on the front side of your lower leg.
Exercise:
Push your legs toward the floor, resisting the motion with your arms. Relax, let go of your knees, and use the outer thigh muscles to press your knees further toward the floor.[2]

[1]Elizabeth Noble, *Essential Exercises for the Childbearing Year* (Boston: Houghton Mifflin Company, 1976), pp. 60-61.
[2]*Ibid.*, pp. 100-101.

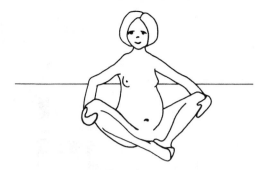

Tailor Stretch

- *Sand Digging*

    Purpose:

    To improve circulation in your legs.
    To help reduce swelling in your feet and legs.
    To reduce or prevent cramping and fatigue in your legs.

    Position:

    Lie on your back with your legs elevated or sit in a chair with your feet up.

    Exercise:

    Slowly make circles with your feet, stretching your ankles in both directions. Imagine that your feet are making circles in the sand at the beach.

- *Calf Stretching*

    Purpose:

    To relieve or prevent cramps in the calves.

    Position:

    Version 1

    Simply stretch the calf muscle by pulling your toes up toward your face. Do this before getting out of bed in the morning and during the day before getting up from a sitting or reclining position.

    Position:

    Version 2

    Stand, placing your hands on the back of a chair or on a counter. Bring the leg with the cramp backward, keeping your heel on the floor. Now bend that knee, getting a good stretch in the calf muscle. The opposite knee will bend too.

    Position:

    Version 3

    Another person can stretch your calf by placing his or her hand under your heel and with the forearm gently pushing your foot up. Your knee should be straight.

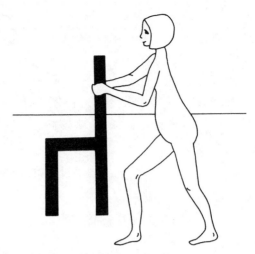

Calf Stretching—Supported by chair with one leg forward, other back

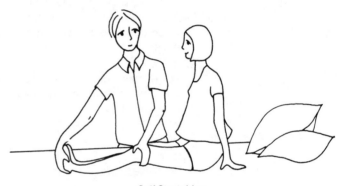

Calf Stretching

- *Shoulder Circling*
  Purpose:
  > To promote better posture by making you conscious of keeping
  > your shoulders back.
  > To stretch the chest muscles that can cause rounded shoulders
  > if they are tight.
  > To increase circulation in the postural muscles.
  > To stretch muscles that if tight can impinge on nerves, causing
  > tingling or numbness in your hands and fingers.

  Position:
  > Sit tailor fashion or stand.

  Exercise:
  > Shrug your shoulders up toward your ears; then pull your shoulders
  > back, pinching your shoulder blades together. Return to the start-
  > ing position and repeat.

- *Arm Stretching*

  Purpose:

    To expand the rib cage, reducing the discomfort caused by increased pressure in the chest area (helps decrease heartburn, indigestion, and shortness of breath).

    To stretch shoulder and back muscles, improving posture.

  Position:

    Sit tailor fashion or stand.

  Exercise:

    With both arms above your head, reach up toward the ceiling as far as you can with one arm and then the other. Continue alternating and stretching as far as possible.

- *Forearm Pressing*

  Purpose:

    To strengthen the muscles under your breasts, thus giving them better support.

    To increase circulation to the breasts.

  Position:

    Sit or stand with your arms at shoulder height; bend your elbows and grasp your forearms.

  Exercise:

    Push your arms in toward each other without letting go of your forearms. Only your skin will move a little. Push and hold to the count of five; repeat.

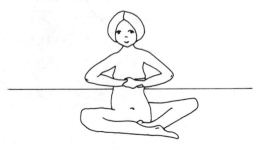

Forearm Press

THE PELVIC FLOOR

The pelvic floor consists of layers of muscles which form a sling across the bottom of the pelvis. The internal muscles act to support the pelvic organs and their contents, and the external, more superficial muscles act as sphincters to open and close the urethra, the vaginal outlet, and the rectum. The pubococcygeus is one of the most important internal muscles. It acts as the primary support for the uterus, vagina, bladder, and rectum. As its name implies, it extends from the pubic bone in front to the coccyx, or tailbone, in back. While you are pregnant, the pubococcygeus must bear the weight of the growing uterus. During the birth of your baby, it must totally relax to allow passage of the baby's head.

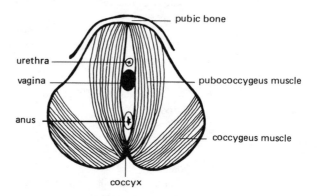

Internal Pelvic Floor Muscles

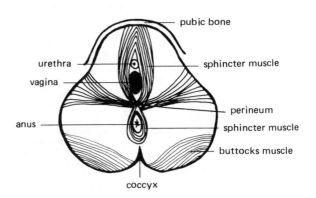

External Pelvic Floor Muscles

As was mentioned, the pelvic floor muscles support the internal organs, including the growing uterus. As it enlarges during pregnancy, more stress is placed on the pelvic floor, resulting in sagging muscles and loss of tone. Exercising the muscles during pregnancy will help keep them stronger so they can better support the uterus. The birth canal distends more easily and is less likely to be damaged during the birth if the muscles are supple and strong. Also, the pelvic floor exercises help relieve pelvic congestion or swelling during pregnancy and can alleviate or prevent hemorrhoids.

Passage of the baby through the birth canal stretches the pelvic floor muscles even further, resulting in more loss of tone despite your efforts to keep them strong during pregnancy. If you do not continue to exercise the muscles after the baby's birth, loss of tone can result in difficulties. Urinary incontinence is the most frequent problem, which is the inability to voluntarily retain urine when the bladder is full. Laughing, sneezing, coughing, or other stress on the bladder results in involuntary passage of urine. This loss of control can be very annoying or embarrassing if the problem is severe.

Another very important function of the pelvic floor is the tightening of the vaginal canal during intercourse. When the muscles are strong, better contact is made between the vagina and the penis. The resulting stimulation of nerves increases sexual satisfaction.

Doing the pelvic floor exercises immediately after the baby's birth will promote healing of the episiotomy (*see* Chapter Six). Contracting and relaxing the perineum (pelvic floor muscles between the anus and the vagina) helps bring oxygenated blood to the site of the incision and keeps the tissues healthy.

Exercising the pelvic floor after the birth will also prevent prolapse, or sagging, of the rectum, bladder, and uterus. If severe prolapse occurs, the organs may not function well and surgery may be required.

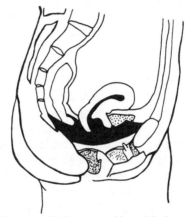

Pelvic Organs—Well-supported by pelvic floor muscles

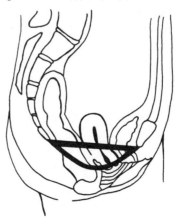

Pelvic Organs—Poorly-supported by pelvic floor muscles

- The easiest way to learn to contract the pelvic floor is to stop and start the flow of urine. Discontinue this exercise once you are familiar with the location of the muscles.
- Contract the pelvic floor, hold tight to the count of two, and relax. Repeat. One contraction only takes a few seconds.
- *Elevator exercise:* Remembering that the muscles are in layers, pretend that you are on an elevator going up. Start by tightening the superficial sphincter muscles on the ground floor. As you count to four, contract higher and higher, around the birth canal. Hold tight to the count of two, and then slowly come back down to the ground floor. Don't let go all at once. Your pelvic floor always maintains a certain amount of tone unless you are consciously relaxing it, as you will be during delivery.
- The strength of your pelvic floor can be determined by evaluating the pressure exerted on the penis during intercourse.

The pelvic floor exercises should be done before the birth of your baby and continued for several weeks or months until you regain good tone in the muscles. Since nobody is aware that you are exercising the pelvic floor, you can do the exercises anywhere. It will help you remember if you plan to do a few every time you engage in a particular activity— while you are doing dishes, talking on the phone, watching television, or feeding the baby. Immediately after the baby is born, it will be easier to do the exercises lying down because you will be eliminating the pull of gravity on the muscles.

The pelvic floor muscles are not strong like your thigh muscles, for example, and especially after childbirth, will not tolerate excessive exercise. Start by doing five or six repetitions at a time, and if you feel the muscles becoming tired even before then, stop, and next time decrease the number of repetitions. Do these exercises eight to ten times a day. Gradually increase the number of repetitions to ten or twenty. In six or eight weeks you should be able to do about thirty repetitions without difficulty. At this point your muscles are quite strong, and you can stop doing the exercises on such a regular basis. However, always check yourself to make sure you don't lose tone over a period of time.

PRACTICE GUIDE

We know that the more conditioned a mother becomes through practice, the better she will do in labor. Try to practice twice daily, at least once with your coach. Set a definite time to practice each day. Some people find it helpful to have a chart on which to check off practice sessions.

	Week 1							Week 2							Week 3							Week 4							Week 5						
	m	t	w	t	f	s	s	m	t	w	t	f	s	s	m	t	w	t	f	s	s	m	t	w	t	f	s	s	m	t	w	t	f	s	s
Prenatal Exercises																																			
Pelvic Floor Exercises																																			
Relaxation																																			
Drill 1																																			
Drill 2																																			
Drill 3																																			
Massage																																			
Breathing																																			
Level 1																																			
Level 2																																			
Level 3																																			
Expulsion Breathing Position																																			
Back Pressure																																			

	Week 6							Week 7							Week 8							Week 9							Week 10						
	m	t	w	t	f	s	s	m	t	w	t	f	s	s	m	t	w	t	f	s	s	m	t	w	t	f	s	s	m	t	w	t	f	s	s
Prenatal Exercises																																			
Pelvic Floor Exercises																																			
Relaxation																																			
Drill 1																																			
Drill 2																																			
Drill 3																																			
Massage																																			
Breathing																																			
Level 1																																			
Level 2																																			
Level 3																																			
Expulsion Breathing Position																																			
Back Pressure																																			

58

4

You will better understand the changes occurring in pregnancy and childbirth if you are familiar with the anatomy of the mother and baby. It will help you to communicate with your doctor and the hospital staff if you understand the process of childbirth and are familiar with some commonly used medical terms.

ANATOMY OF MOTHER AND BABY

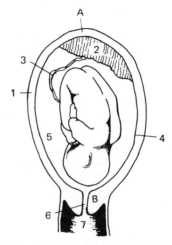

(1) uterus; (A) fundus; (B) cervix; (2) placenta; (3) umbilical cord; (4) amniotic sac; (5) amniotic fluid; (6) mucous plug; (7) vagina (birth canal).

Anatomy and Physiology of Childbirth

Uterus

The uterus (1) is a hollow, thick-walled muscle which receives the fertilized egg and houses the fetus as it grows. The uterus is capable of tremendous stretching to accommodate your baby's growth.

The uterus is composed of muscle fibers that are arranged in a length-wise and circular fashion. Because of this arrangement, the uterus is capable of very powerful contractions, which gradually open the cervix during labor.

The *cervix* (B) is the thick, closed, bottleneck-like opening to the uterus. During labor it must open enough for the baby to pass into the birth canal. The *fundus* (A) is the upper third of the uterus.

The uterine muscle is an *involuntary* muscle, which means that you cannot control its contractions.

Following delivery the uterus will *involute* or return to near prepregnant size in two to six weeks.

Placenta

About seven days after conception, the egg (now called an *ovum*) implants in the wall of the uterus and begins to develop into various organs. One of them is called the *placenta* (2). The placenta, or *afterbirth*, functions as an exchange station between the mother's and baby's bodies. Oxygen and nutrients are supplied by the mother's blood stream and pass through the blood vessels of the placenta to the baby. Carbon dioxide and waste materials from the baby pass back through the placenta to the mother's body to be eliminated. The mother's immunities will also pass to the baby through the placenta. The fetal and maternal bloods do not actually mix. The porous vessels are close to one another, allowing substances to absorb between them.

The placenta does not function as a barrier to keep out undesirable substances, but rather it is more like a sieve. For example, if medication or alcohol are in the mother's system, they also appear in the baby's system. Check with your doctor before taking any kind of medication, including over-the-counter drugs. Research indicates that there are harmful effects on the fetus from smoking, alcohol, and many over-the-counter drugs. *Be very careful what you put in your system when pregnant or trying to get pregnant.* At birth the placenta weighs one pound. Following its delivery, contraction of the uterus helps to control bleeding from its site of implantation. The uterus is very sensitive to touch following delivery.

Umbilical Cord

The umbilical cord (3) is attached at one end to the placenta and at the other end to the baby. It contains two arteries which carry fetal blood to the placenta and one vein carrying fetal blood back to the baby. The site where the cord attaches to the baby becomes the *umbilicus* (navel, or belly button) once the cord has been clamped and cut at birth.

At birth the cord is about two feet long, or the length of the baby. It is filled with a substance called *Wharton's jelly*, which surrounds and protects the cord's blood vessels. Because of the Wharton's jelly and the force with which the blood flows through the cord, it becomes very rigid, helping to keep the cord from knotting and tangling as the baby moves. It is similar to the way a garden hose cannot be knotted when the water is rushing through it.

Because of the length of the cord, it is possible for the baby to become tangled or for the cord to wrap about some part of the baby's body. During pregnancy this occurrence is not a problem. As the baby moves deeper in the pelvis during labor, there may be some strain if the cord is around the baby's neck. Your doctor or nurse would recognize this condition during labor from the pattern of your baby's heartbeat. It is not uncommon for a baby to be born with the cord around his neck, and it is usually not a problem. Once the head is born, the doctor slips her finger under the cord and pulls it over the baby's head.

Amniotic Sac and Fluid

The fetus is enclosed in tough, slightly elastic membranes called the amniotic sac (4). These are sometimes called the *membranes* or the *bag of waters*. All these terms mean the same thing. The sac acts as a seal to protect the baby from infection. Within this sac is a clear, colorless, watery substance called *amniotic fluid* (5), which serves many functions for the baby. It regulates temperature, is a medium for movement, and cushions the baby from blows. It is completely replaced every three hours. At birth there are usually one to two pints of fluid.

Sometimes during or just before labor the amniotic sac will rupture or tear. You may feel a trickle or gush of fluid and perhaps confuse it with accidental leakage of urine. *It is important that you call your doctor if you suspect that your membranes have broken.* If they are ruptured, it means that the protective seal around the baby is gone, and the baby and you are subject to infection. If the membranes do not rupture on their own, your doctor will probably rupture them either at the end or sometime during your labor. This is a painless procedure.

Mucous Plug

The mucous plug (6) is a protective mass of mucous filling the cervical canal. It helps to protect the baby from infection caused by bacteria in the vagina. As the cervix begins to change before labor, the mucous plug will often be discharged. It looks like a clump of mucous which is blood-tinged or pinkish. It is not a lot of bright red blood. Should you experience this kind of bleeding call your doctor. Sometimes women lose their mucous plug and don't notice it. Its loss is not considered a definite sign that labor is imminent, although it frequently precedes labor.

Vagina

The vagina (7), or birth canal, extends from the cervix to the vulva, or external opening to the vagina. After the cervix is open, the vagina is the canal through which the baby passes. The vagina is very elastic, made more so by the hormones of pregnancy. Because it can easily stretch to accommodate the baby, it does not require contractions to open it up as did the cervix. Toward the end of pregnancy you may notice an increase in vaginal secretions.

Ligaments

Three main ligaments maintain the position of the uterus: the broad, round, and uterosacral. The increase in size and weight of the uterus during pregnancy puts stress on these ligaments and can cause discomfort where they attach in the low back and groin areas.

UTERINE FUNCTION

If you were to look up "labor" in a medical text, you would read something like this:

The rhythmic contraction and relaxation
of the uterine muscle
with progressive effacement and dilatation
of the cervix
leading to delivery of your baby[1]

But what does it mean? Let's break it down into parts.

Contractions

If you have never had a baby, how do you know what contractions are? Maybe you have felt your abdomen getting tense or hard, then relaxing or softening; or perhaps you have experienced an intermittent backache or menstrual-like cramping above the pubic bone. These are contractions. More specifically, they're called *Braxton-Hicks contractions,* or warm-up contractions. Your uterine muscles have been contracting throughout pregnancy, but you become more aware of it during your

[1]Joy Clausen *et al., Maternity Nursing Today* (New York: McGraw-Hill Book Company, 1973), p. 433.

last trimester. Usually Braxton-Hicks contractions are not painful, but they may be uncomfortable. Often they occur when you're trying to rest or when you've been standing or walking for a while. Braxton-Hicks are useful because they are preparing the cervix for labor; that is, they are softening or *ripening* the cervix in preparation for the changes that will occur during labor.

Contractions begin at the fundus, or top of the uterus, and radiate over the body of the uterus toward the cervix.

Contractions should be called contractions. *They should not be referred to as labor pains.*

We can draw a picture of a contraction, like the following:

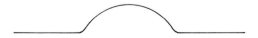

This is a contraction of early labor. It has a gradual buildup in *intensity,* or pressure, a period of greatest intensity called the *apex,* or *peak,* and then an easing off of pressure.

A series of contractions could be pictured as follows:

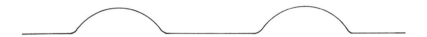

Here you see the rhythmic, wave-like quality of the contractions.

You need to know how to talk about contractions. One thing you're interested in is how long the contraction lasts, or its *duration.* You also want to know how often the contractions are occurring, or their *frequency.* The frequency of contractions is measured from the beginning of one to the beginning of the next one. The *interval* is the rest phase between them. For example:

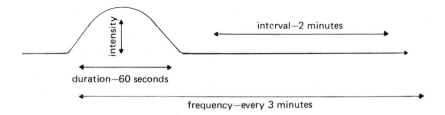

- The *interval* of this contraction is two minutes.
- The *duration* is sixty seconds.
- The *frequency* is every three minutes.
- The *intensity* is a personal evaluation of the strength of the contraction and can be measured with a monitoring device as milliliters of pressure.

As a woman progresses through labor, a pattern usually evolves and her contractions become progressively longer, stronger, and closer together. Because this pattern occurs gradually over a period of several hours, the woman is able to adjust to it.

As labor becomes more active, the quality of the contractions changes; that is, the buildup time shortens, the apex lengthens and seems to be consistently more intense, and the easing-off time shortens. This change could be illustrated as follows:

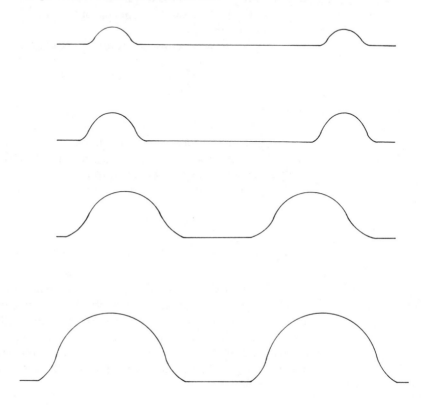

Effacement

The term refers to the thinning of the cervix. When you have a contraction, the lengthwise uterine fibers are *contracting*, or *shortening*, and pulling up the circular fibers around the cervix—which causes the two-inch-thick cervix to thin out, or efface, until it is paper thin.

Effacement is measured in percentages by your doctor or nurse during a pelvic exam. Complete effacement, or thinning, would be called 100 percent effaced.

If you are having your first baby, most cervical effacement occurs before much dilatation begins. If you are having a second or later baby, the cervix can efface and open at the same time. Sometimes effacement occurs before labor if a woman has a lot of Braxton-Hicks contractions.

Effacement for a primipara, or woman having her first baby, can be shown as follows:

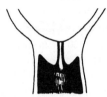 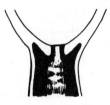 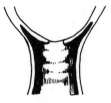

Before Labor—Cervix is thick and closed

Early Effacement—Cervix is partially effaced

Complete Effacement— Cervix is paper thin—Dilatation has begun

Dilatation

Dilatation is the opening of the cervix to allow the baby to pass out of the uterus and into the birth canal. It is caused by contractions and the pressure of the baby's presenting part—usually the head—on the cervix. As in the case of effacement, dilatation can sometimes begin before a woman actually goes into labor. Dilatation is measured in centimeters, or cm. Complete dilatation is 10 cm, or about 4 inches.

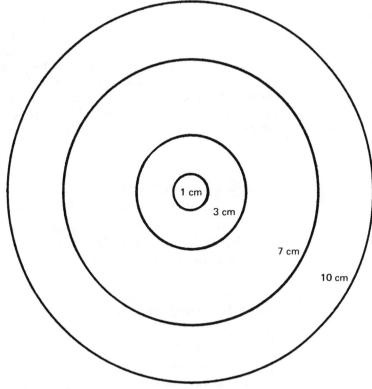

Cervical Dilatation

Dilatation can be determined by your doctor or nurse during a pelvic exam. It is a somewhat arbitrary measure, since each person may judge the distance the cervix has opened slightly differently. For this reason, the doctor often says, "You're one to two cm," or "You're five to six cm."

When doing a vaginal exam during labor, your birth attendant uses two fingers to periodically measure the dilatation of your cervix. You can spread your first two fingers to measure the opening in the chart above. Occasionally dilatation is described by fingers instead of centimeters—one finger equaling approximately 2 cm and five fingers meaning complete dilatation.

Dilatation can be illustrated as follows:

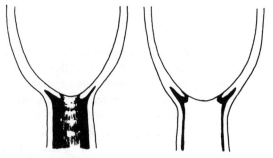

Partial Dilatation   Complete Dilatation to 10 cm

The time during which effacement and dilatation of the cervix take place is called *labor*. When the cervix is 100 percent effaced and 10 cm dilated, it is said to be *complete*. The cervix has opened and been incorporated into the uterus and a funnel-like structure now exists for the baby to make his exit. Labor is completed, and the delivery or expulsion stage begins.

STAGES OF CHILDBIRTH

Childbirth is divided into various stages. Labor, one of the stages, is divided into various phases. The chart on the opposite page illustrates the stages of childbirth.

THE MATERNAL PELVIS

The pelvis is made up of four bones—two hip bones, the sacrum, and the coccyx (tailbone)—united at four joints.

These bones are united by fibrocartilage and ligaments. In the front, the two hip bones meet each other to form the *symphysis pubis*. They meet the sacrum at the two *sacroiliac joints,* and the sacrum and coccyx unite to form the *sacrococcygeal joints.*

Early in your pregnancy, your baby is protected within the pelvic cavity, but as he grows, the uterus will grow up and out of the pelvic cavity and then descend again close to your due date or when you go into labor (see lightening and engagement, Chapter Five).

STAGES OF CHILDBIRTH

Stage 1—Labor	(Phases of Labor)
The cervix effaces and dilates.	*Latent or early labor* Effacement occurs and the cervix dilates 2 to 3 cm.
	Active labor Dilatation progresses from 3 to 7 cm.
	Transition Cervix dilates from 7 to 10 cm.

Stage 2—Expulsion
   The baby moves down the birth canal and is born.

Stage 3—Delivery of the Placenta
   Delivery of the placenta, or afterbirth, occurs shortly after the baby's birth.

Stage 4—Postpartum
   The mother's vital signs stabilize. She is carefully monitored during this recovery phase.

There are several things the doctor wants to know about the relationship of the baby to your pelvis. This relationship will have a direct influence on how you experience labor and delivery. It is important for you to understand what your doctor is looking for in your last few weeks of pregnancy. If you talk to your doctor, you will have a better understanding of what is happening to your body and what to expect about your labor and delivery. When your doctor or nurse does a pelvic examination, ask about the findings. Stay informed.

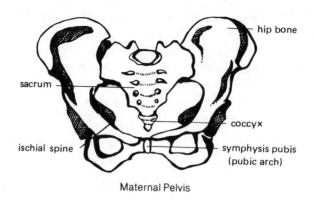

Maternal Pelvis

Size

Early in your pregnancy your doctor measured your pelvis by palpating, or feeling, the bones. He was checking to see that your pelvis can accommodate the average seven-pound baby.

Late in your pregnancy, your pelvic joints relax somewhat. The maternal hormone, *relaxin,* causes the ligaments of the pelvis to soften and become more mobile, allowing it to expand to accommodate the baby. In addition to some give in the mother's pelvis, there is also some in the baby's head. The skull bones of the baby are not yet solidly fused, allowing them to *mold* during the birth process. The give in the mother's pelvis and the give in the baby's head permit delivery of a normal-sized baby to a woman with a normal pelvis.

If in doubt about the fit, your doctor may request an *ultrasound* or *x-ray pelvimetry* (see Chapter Twelve) to measure your pelvis and the baby's head.

Presentation

Presentation can easily be remembered by asking, "What part presents itself first to the doctor?" About 97 percent of the time the baby's head comes first, giving a *cephalic,* or *vertex,* presentation.[2] In general, the baby's head makes the best dilator of the cervix and the best occupier of the pelvis.

When it is not a vertex presentation, it may be a *breech* presentation. The incidence is about 3 percent.[3] There are different types of breech presentations. In the *complete breech,* the buttocks and legs are born first, and the knees and hips are flexed.

[2]Harry Oxorn and William R. Foote, *Human Labor and Birth,* 3rd ed. (New York: Appleton-Century-Crofts, 1975), p. 48.
[3]*Ibid.,* p. 48.

68

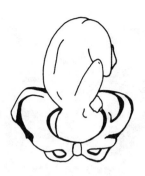

Cephalic or Vertex Presentation

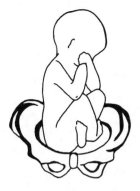

Complete Breech

In the *frank breech*, the buttocks are still first, but the legs are straight and the feet are up by the baby's head.

A *footling breech* can be single or double footling, depending on whether one or both feet are first.

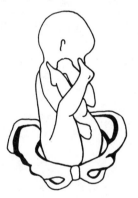

Frank Breech

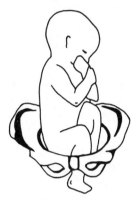

Footling Breech

In the *kneeling breech*, the baby is in a kneeling position.

A third way in which a baby may be presenting is called *transverse lie*, in which the baby is lying across the mother's pelvis. It is not possible for a baby in this position to be born vaginally, and unless the position changes, a Cesarean section will be performed. The incidence of transverse lie is rare.

Position

Position refers to which way the baby is facing in relation to the mother's back. Looking at the mother's pelvis we could label the following directions:

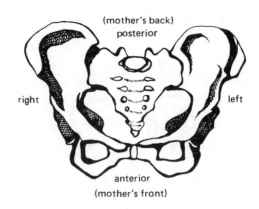

(mother's back)
posterior

right   left

anterior
(mother's front)

As the reference point on the baby's head, we use the *occiput* or crown. Let's say the baby is arranged in a vertex presentation. He can be anterior or posterior, to the right or to the left. Let's look at each of these positions in more detail to see how they can influence your labor and delivery.

Anterior. If the baby is head down with the occiput toward the mother's front (the baby is looking toward the mother's back), this is the *occiput anterior position*, either right or left. It would be labeled in this manner:

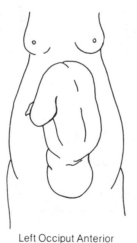

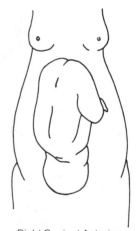

Left Occiput Anterior

The baby's occiput is toward the mother's abdomen and left side.

Right Occiput Anterior

The baby's occiput is toward the mother's abdomen and right side.

The left occiput anterior position is the most common and also the most preferable since it requires the least amount of rotation for the baby to be born. Position is important because of its influence on labor and delivery, and in anterior positions the following labor usually results:

1. The mother is able to lie comfortably on her back with the head of the bed elevated. She may complain of mild backache.
2. The contractions will probably be felt more in the abdominal area and have an equally long and strong pattern.[4]
3. The baby rotates and is born looking toward the mother's back.

Posterior. If the baby is head down with the occiput toward the mother's back (the baby is looking toward the mother's front), this is the *occiput posterior position*, either to the right or the left.

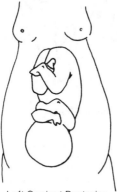

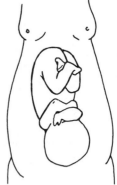

Left Occiput Posterior

The baby's occiput is toward the mother's back and left side.

Right Occiput Posterior

The baby's occiput is toward the mother's back and right side.

The incidence of posterior is about 15 to 30 percent, with ROP more common than LOP.[5]

The following labor usually results from posterior positions:

1. The mother is unable to lie comfortably on her back. She complains about persistent or intermittent backache (see Chapter Ten).
2. The contractions are often irregular—the length, interval, and intensity may vary. The contraction pattern is sometimes one longer, stronger contraction followed by one or two shorter, milder contractions.[6]
3. Contractions are felt mainly in the back rather than the abdomen.
4. There is a longer pushing stage if the baby fails to rotate.

Station

Station describes the vertical descent of the baby into the pelvis, or the amount of downward progress the baby has made. An imaginary line, called *zero station*, is drawn across the ischial spines of the pelvis.

[4]Clausen, *Maternity Nursing*, p. 472.
[5]Oxorn and Foote, *Human Labor*, p. 133.
[6]Clausen, *Maternity Nursing*, p. 473.

If the baby's head is above the ischial spines it is described as −1 cm, −2 cm, and so on. If the baby's head is below the ischial spines, it is described as +1 cm, +2 cm, and so on. You can remember this designation by thinking that you become positive as the baby moves deeper in the pelvis and you are closer to delivery.

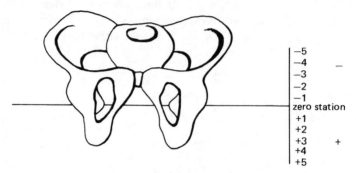

Pelvis Showing Station

When the widest diameter of the baby's head has reached the level of the ischial spines, or 0 station, it is said to be *engaged*. Once the head is engaged, it usually doesn't move up out of the pelvis. Before it is engaged the baby's head may be *floating* above the pelvic inlet or *dipping* into the inlet. Your doctor will be able to determine whether or not the baby's head is engaged and what station it has reached through a pelvic or abdominal exam.

When the baby has descended to the plus stations, the mother may feel the urge to push, the sensation that she needs to bear down to help deliver the baby (see Chapter Six).

5

This chapter discusses what happens prior to and during labor. The definition of labor is:

The rhythmic contraction and relaxation
of the uterine muscles
with progressive effacement and dilatation
of the cervix
leading to delivery of your baby.[1]

GOING INTO LABOR

Labor generally begins when the fetus is able to survive outside the uterus. *Term* refers to the time when the infant has reached the point of maximum intrauterine development, usually 38 to 42 weeks following the last menstrual period (abbreviated LMP). Labor optimally begins 266 or 267 days following conception, or 272 to 280 days following the LMP, or approximately 40 weeks. "Nine months" is misleading. One way to predict the due date is Naegele's Rule: To the first day of your LMP, add seven days and then subtract three months.

Most doctors would agree that it is not easy to predict accurately when labor will begin. Many babies are not born on their due date, or estimated date of confinement (EDC). At best your doctor can estimate whether the cervix appears favorable for labor to begin.

When labor begins before 37 weeks of gestation, the baby is said to be *premature.* There may be some concern about how well prepared the infant is to withstand the rigors of labor and delivery, and then to function independently of the mother.

When labor has not begun by 42 weeks of gestation, the baby is said to be *postmature.* Here, the main concern is whether the placenta is still functioning adequately and whether the baby's source of oxygen and nutrients is being compromised. Your doctor can perform estriol tests to determine placental functioning (see Chapter Ten).

[1]Joy Clausen *et al., Maternity Nursing Today* (New York: McGraw-Hill Book Company, 1973), p. 433.

Labor

Special precautions are sometimes taken when a laboring woman is giving birth to a premature or postmature infant, which may include decreased medication or anesthesia for the woman and special arrangements in the delivery room (equipment, pediatric personnel, and so on).

Many different theories exist regarding what causes labor to begin, such as ovarian hormones, placental hormones, volume of the uterus, size of the infant, strength of the cervix, or a signal from the fetus. To date, however, there is not a definitive answer to this intriguing, sometimes exasperating, question.

THE LENGTH OF LABOR

Both the mother and the labor coach are concerned about how long it will take to have the baby. Emanuel A. Friedman, a physician, has compiled statistics and arrived at average times for labor.[2] He has plotted these on a graph, which we have adapted below. The curve shows the progress of an average first labor. Keep in mind that the baby can be born much more quickly than this average, and also, that it can take longer.

Early (latent) labor dilatation to 3 cm	8	hours
Active labor dilatation from 3 to 7 cm	3	hours
Transition dilatation from 7 to 10 cm	2	hours
Delivery	14¼ hours	

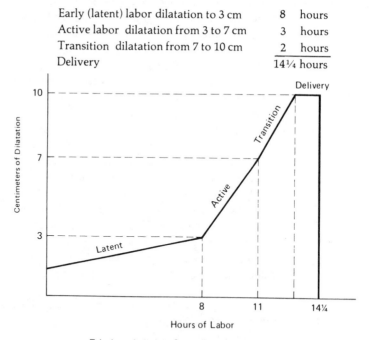

Friedman's Labor Curve for a Primapara

[2]From Emmanuel Friedman, M.D., *Labor: Clinical Evaluation and Management,* 2nd ed., p. 33. Copyright © 1978 by Appleton-Century-Crofts. Used courtesy of Appleton-Century-Crofts and the author.

Centimeters of dilatation are plotted vertically on the graph, and the number of hours of labor is plotted horizontally. The curved line represents the progress of the *average* labor for a first baby.

In general, your doctor likes to see a primipara dilate at least one centimeter per hour during the active and transition phases of labor.

PRELUDE PHASE

Sometimes women experience a prelude phase, which is an indefinite period—a couple of weeks or days—prior to labor. Many changes may occur during this time. You may feel excited, apprehensive, and irritable. You may be feeling uncomfortable because of the large size of your uterus, and you are feeling very *ready* to have your baby.

During these weeks *it is important for the mother to get plenty of rest*. She should make a concerted effort to be ready for labor. If she is well rested she will find that labor is easier to handle and recovery is more rapid. For a while, your new baby will be getting up for night feedings, so it will not be as easy to get the sleep you need once he is born.

The final weeks of pregnancy are sometimes hard on both the mother and father. It is helpful for the mother to have as much diversion as possible, without fatiguing herself. She may want to continue to work or spend time with her friends. Now is a good time to splurge on an evening out and doing some nice things: get a new haircut, go out for lunch with a friend, enjoy your baby showers, make something special for yourself or the baby.

Fathers can help by seeing that the mother gets extra rest, by helping her practice breathing and relaxation techniques, and by reassuring her. Try not to allow yourselves to get discouraged if the due date comes and goes. Massage and back rubs will be appreciated. Labor and those early postpartum days will also be easier for the father if he approaches them well rested.

It may seem as if you're going to be pregnant forever, but these last few days and weeks will pass.

Changes Prior to Labor

To help you recognize your progress during the last weeks of pregnancy, here is a summary of changes you *may* notice. Not all women will experience all of these.

1. *Lightening and engagement:* This is the process in which the baby moves deeper into the mother's pelvis. It occurs as the lower uterine segment begins to soften, allowing the baby to move lower in the uterus, and as relaxation of the pelvic ligaments allows more room for the baby.

This change can occur two to three weeks prior to labor for a primipara, and a few hours or days prior to or during labor for a multipara. You may know this change has occurred because it becomes easier to breathe but more difficult to walk gracefully. At the same time you may notice you need to urinate more frequently and urine may occasionally leak because of weak pelvic floor muscles. You may also notice pressure or discomfort where the uterine ligaments attach in the groin, as well as increased pressure in the lower abdomen.

2. *Ripening of the cervix:* The cervix softens and begins to swing forward to an anterior position. During a vaginal exam, the cervix is much easier to reach than previously.

3. *Loss of the mucous plug:* This is a blood-tinged mucous discharge sometimes called "bloody show." It sometimes occurs but may go unnoticed by the woman.

4. *Increased vaginal secretions.*

5. *Backache:* There may be occasional backache because of the increased weight of the uterus pulling on uterine ligaments attached to the lower back and relaxation of the pelvic joints.

6. *Braxton-Hicks contractions:* Warm-up contractions or episodes of false labor may occur and may help begin effacement and dilatation of the cervix.

7. *Weight:* There may be stabilization of weight or loss of one to three pounds.

8. *Diarrhea:* Softer stools or diarrhea are sometimes noted a few days prior to labor.

9. *Rupture of membranes:* A leaking or gush of amniotic fluid may occur if the membranes rupture. This clear, odorless fluid is sometimes difficult to distinguish from urine. Call your doctor if you suspect your membranes are leaking, and be sure to report the color of the fluid. Testing with Nitrazine (litmus) paper can determine whether the fluid is urine or amniotic fluid. The vagina is usually acidic and becomes neutral or alkaline when amniotic fluid is present.

10. *Spurt of energy:* This change is meant for labor, *not* for spring housecleaning.

11. *Nesting instinct:* The woman may become involved in getting everything ready for the baby.

True and False Labor

One question that usually causes anxiety for the pregnant couple is how to know when true labor begins. A common fear is to arrive at the hospital only to find that the labor has stopped; everyone worries about being sent home to wait for true labor to start. Another fear is that delay of the hospital trip might result in delivery in the car or at home. *Many* couples worry about whether they can tell true labor from false labor.

Your doctor and the hospital staff have seen a lot of false labor. Even women who have already had children can go to the hospital in false labor, because it is sometimes very difficult to tell the difference until after the fact, when cervical dilatation has occurred. One woman can be in true labor and only moderately aware of the contractions, whereas another can be in false labor and find contractions quite strong. If you go to your doctor's office or the hospital in false labor, don't be embarrassed or upset, and try not to be too discouraged.

The following are a few guidelines for distinguishing true from false labor:

TRUE LABOR	FALSE LABOR
The contractions: 1. Regular pattern 2. Become closer, stronger, longer 3. Walking increases intensity 4. Early contractions rarely exceed 60 sec. duration 5. Often accompanied by backache 6. Hot bath, heating pad, or alcoholic drink will not stop them	The contractions: 1. Often irregular pattern 2. Can vary 3. Changing position may stop them 4. May last 35-45 sec., or longer than a minute 5. May have backache 6. Heat or alcohol may stop them
The cervix: Ripens, effaces, dilates	The cervix: May ripen and show minimal effacement and dilatation
The baby: Starts to descend in the pelvis	The baby: May or may not descend in the pelvis

STAGE 1: THE LABOR PROCESS

We have already given an overview of the childbirth process. We now need to look at each of the phases of labor in more detail.

EARLY OR LATENT LABOR

This is usually a lengthy phase with slow progress. Uterine contractions are generally manageable.

- *Progress of cervix*
  Effacement of the cervix.
  Dilatation of the cervix to 3 cm.
- *Contractions*
  Length: A range of 20 to 60 seconds, but usually 30 to 45 seconds long.
  Interval: Every 20 minutes, working their way down to every 5 minutes, is usual. However, it is possible that your contractions may not start out at 20-minute intervals but may be either further apart or closer together.
  Time: 6 to 8 hours is common for the first labor; however, it may be shorter or longer.
  Intensity: Short, mild contractions, with a generally mild apex—gradual increase in pressure and gradual easing off of pressure. Long rest phase between contractions. Contractions get progressively longer, stronger, and closer together.

PHYSICAL SIGNS THAT *MAY* OCCUR:

- Loss of the mucous plug.
- Rupture of the membranes or continued leaking of the membranes.
- Contractions may be felt in the lower back or in the abdomen.
- Increased frequency of urination because of the engagement of the baby's head.
- Constipation because of the slowing of digestion.
- Increased vaginal discharge.
- Increased pelvic pressure because of the descent of the baby.
- Menstrual-like cramping.
- Cramps in hips or legs.

EMOTIONAL SIGNS THAT *MAY* OCCUR:

The mother's behavior reflects the energy and excitement she feels about being in labor.

- Ambivalent and anxious until the question of true versus false labor is settled.
- Excited, energetic—relief that labor has begun.
- Very optimistic and confident—assured of her ability to handle labor. Seems to be very independent and self-motivated.
- Talkative, vivacious, spontaneous.
- Feels that things are progressing faster than they really are.

THE MOTHER'S ROLE

1. Maintain your activity. If labor starts at night, try to get more rest. If labor starts in the day, engage in a light, relaxing activity. In other words, don't go to bed, but don't decide to go grocery shopping, clean the refrigerator, or work overtime.
2. Take a shower *if* someone is home with you. Don't take a bath (your membranes may be ruptured) unless your doctor says you may.
3. Use distraction to get through these early hours of labor; watch television, go to a movie (if your doctor agrees), or play cards.
4. Urinate frequently. A full bladder is uncomfortable and can impede the descent of the baby's head.
5. Don't eat anything hard to digest because labor causes digestion to stop. If your doctor approves, have a light diet, similar to what you would have after stomach flu; Jello, bouillon, tea with honey, ginger ale, toast, and so on. Do not eat any milk products.
6. Call your doctor according to his instructions.
7. Use this initial phase as a time to assess your own particular kind of labor: Where do you feel the contractions? Are they regular? How are they affecting you? Experiment with the techniques and positions you've learned.
8. Begin active relaxation if you feel the need.
9. Begin the first level breathing only when you feel the need.

THE COACH'S ROLE

1. If labor starts in the night, try to get some more sleep. Conserve your energy. You'll need it for the harder, later stages of labor.
2. Early labor is the time for you to take care of such things as eating a good meal, making arrangements to miss work, getting some rest. Later, it will be too hard on the mother if you have to leave her for these reasons.
3. Assess the situation and stay calm. Evaluate how the contractions are affecting the mother. Note what positions she seems to prefer and what techniques seem to help. Note any physical symptoms you want her to report to the doctor. Keep track of the frequency, duration, and intensity of the contractions.
4. Help the mother conserve energy, become comfortable, and stay relaxed. Massage may be helpful. Help her with breathing patterns, and stay with her while she showers or gets ready for the hospital.
5. Enjoy this early phase of labor. Share her excitement that labor has begun and your baby will soon be born.
6. If rupture of the membranes occurs, reassure her; she may feel embarrassed.
7. Prepare for the trip to the hospital. Extra pillows for comfort and a large waterproof pad or bath towels are helpful in case the membranes rupture.
8. Work together to make decisions about the mother's care.

ACTIVE LABOR

The speed of cervical dilation increases. Contractions, which are more intense, more frequent, and last longer, require more control by the mother.

- *Progress of cervix*
  Dilatation of the cervix from 3 to 7 cm
  100 percent effacement.
- *Contractions*
  Length: Usually 45 to 60 seconds.
  Interval: May start as far apart as 7 minutes. Toward the end of this phase, may be every 2 minutes. Every 3 to 5 minutes is usual.
  Time: 2 to 3 hours is common for a first labor; however, this time can vary.
  Intensity: Longer, more intense contractions with longer, stronger apex. Shorter rest phase. Contractions get progressively longer, stronger, and closer.

PHYSICAL SIGNS THAT *MAY* OCCUR:

- If your membranes are still intact, they *may* rupture spontaneously or be ruptured by your physician. Remember that contractions can be irregular following rupture and then will usually fall into a pattern of longer, stronger, closer contractions than before. Ask the doctor if your membranes need to be ruptured for medical reasons or if they can be left intact; laboring with intact membranes is usually more manageable.
- Contractions may be irregular and more intense following a pelvic exam.
- There may be discomfort or pressure in your hips and legs due to the pressure of the baby descending deeper into the pelvis.
- There may be nausea and/or vomiting.
- There may be backache.
- Involuntary reactions to stress may appear, such as an increase in respirations, heart rate, and perspiration.
- There may be muscle tension.

EMOTIONAL SIGNS THAT *MAY* OCCUR

The mother's behavior reflects the increased intensity of the contractions and her fatigue from dealing with them.

- Less talkative and sociable.
- Less aware of environment; more serious; more involved in the labor and dealing with the contractions. Needs to concentrate.
- Still interested in medical details concerning her progress—results of pelvic exams, observing contraction pattern on monitor tracing, if a monitor is used, and fetal heart tones.
- More dependent on her coach, doctor, and medical staff. Loses feeling of independence.

- Needs frequent encouragement.
- Begins to need strong coaching.
- Toward the end of this phase she may become worried about her ability to handle contractions.

THE MOTHER'S ROLE

1. Be sure to catch each contraction at the beginning. Avoid dozing or napping between contractions; you may be caught unaware.
2. Use intervals between contractions for maximum relief and rest.
3. Change position frequently; avoid lying on your back. Try lying on your left side or sitting propped in a bed or chair.
4. Use first-level breathing as long as possible, changing to second-level breathing only when you must. Use second-level breathing when apex of contraction becomes more difficult.

THE COACH'S ROLE

1. Coaching becomes increasingly important to the mother. Assess how labor is affecting her and try to help where she is having a problem. Actively coaching her through a contraction by breathing with her may be important at times. She will benefit more from being reminded about techniques rather than having to recall them. Remind her to have a focal point, stay relaxed, and use the appropriate breathing pattern.
2. Breathing pattern should be rhythmic, consistent in speed, and as slow as possible. Watch for signs of hyperventilation and help her correct her breathing pattern if necessary.
3. Watch or *gently* touch all body parts to check for signs of tension. Use touch and massage to relax specific body parts.
4. Use all available techniques for comfort:
   ice chips or popsicles
   cold cloth for neck or brow
   position change
   effleurage and petrissage
   back massage
   fresh gown, pad, or sheets
   blanket
   warm socks
   straightened bed sheets
   extra pillows
5. Sit down sometimes during her labor so that you don't become too fatigued.
6. Keep her informed of her progress.
7. Help minimize the distractions around her—glaring lights, noise from the hall, loud voices, and so on.
8. Encourage, encourage, encourage; praise, praise, praise.
9. Get ready for the transition phase of labor. If you must leave your mate, be sure to ask the nurse to coach her.
   a. Change into delivery (scrub) clothes.
   b. Get a bite to eat if hungry.
   c. Go to the bathroom.

TRANSITION

Transition is a difficult period before complete dilatation of the cervix. Progress is usually rapid, but there may be a slowing down around nine cm. You may be checked and told that there is still a "rim" of the cervix remaining. Because of the strength and frequency of contractions and some accompanying physiologic and emotional symptoms, transition is usually described as the hardest part of labor; but it is usually the shortest.

- *Progress of cervix*
  Dilatation of the cervix from 7 or 8 cm to 10 cm.
- *Contractions*
  Length: 60 to 90 seconds.
  Interval: Variable, usually 30 to 90 second rest period between contractions.
  Time: For average first labor, 30 minutes to 2 hours. The time can vary.
  Intensity: Contractions seem to consist mainly of apex with little buildup or easing off. There may be more than one apex.

PHYSICAL SIGNS THAT *MAY* OCCUR:

- Increased rectal pressure due to descent of the baby; may feel pressure or discomfort in hips, legs, and buttocks.
- Nausea and possible vomiting, especially near 10 cm.
- Shaking, trembling legs.
- Urge to push as the baby moves deeper in the pelvis; may occur before cervix is completely dilated.
- Fatigue and drowsiness.
- Cold feet caused by poor circulation as the baby moves deeper in the pelvis.
- Backache or feeling of pressure in the back.
- Leg cramps.
- Chills, shivers, or a feeling of being overheated; alternately hot and cold; perspiring.
- Continued leaking of membranes and bloody show.
- Loud, long burping.
- Restless; unable to find a comfortable position.

EMOTIONAL SIGNS THAT *MAY* OCCUR:

The mother's behavior reflects the very stressful contractions and her fatigue.

- Uncooperative and demanding; may verbally express these feelings. You may be ungrateful, despite your coach's attempts to help you.
- Panicky, especially if you lose control during a contraction and feel you won't be able to get through it.
- Discouraged—may cry; may say you can't continue.
- Very inward—totally involved with yourself and what's happening

to your body; loss of interest in progress of labor and baby. May not be interested in participating in decisions about your care.

- Confused, disoriented; not as aware of environment and things happening around you. May have to be told something several times before you really hear it. Unable to concentrate.
- Very dependent on the coach and staff. You may panic if your coach leaves the side of the bed to stretch his legs between contractions or lets go of your hand. May get upset if your doctor or nurse leaves the room, even momentarily.
- May feel trapped by the relentless quality of the contractions and the feeling that you aren't in control of your body. May say you've had enough and want to go home.
- May project some of the feelings you have to those around you, coach or staff. May verbally snap at them.
- Extremely sensitive to touch; external fetal monitoring belts, effleurage, back massage, wrinkles in the bed sheets, and so on may really irritate you.
- May question the reason for certain medical procedures and feel that nobody understands what you're experiencing.
- Loss of inhibition; personal modesty decreases; less cautious about what you say.

After reading this list of possible symptoms, you may wish that you did not have to go through transition.

Keep in mind that these are possibilities for all women in labor, and that no one woman will experience everything mentioned.

Transition is hard, but it is the shortest phase of labor for most women; and soon you will begin pushing and the baby will be born.

THE MOTHER'S ROLE

1. Concentrate on getting through one contraction at a time. With strong coaching and encouragement from those around you, you can work through each contraction and handle this phase of labor. Transition is hard work, but it can be managed.
2. Transition contractions are very strong and may no longer fit into the pattern established earlier in labor. Don't be upset or alarmed by their strength, frequency, or irregularity. These contractions are normal for transition. Don't be afraid that something has gone wrong with you or the baby. Strong contractions in transition are good; they are dilating your cervix.
3. Try to express any needs you have with which the coach or staff can help you, for instance, if you're cold or hot or want to change your position.
4. Relaxation is most difficult during transition but should be one of your main tasks. Don't think that you're doing the techniques incorrectly because you're having trouble getting through the con-

tractions. Labor, especially transition, is hard work; these techniques help *control* contractions but do not eliminate them.

5. Try not to give in to any panicky feelings about the contractions but to accept them as the mechanism that is causing your cervix to open enough to allow the baby to pass through. Visualize the cervix opening up more and more with each contraction.

THE COACH'S ROLE

1. Don't leave her. Be sensitive to how dependent she is and to how much she needs you.
2. Strong coaching is helpful; use simple directions and declarative statements. Be firm, quiet, and assured. Don't ask questions that require more than a yes or no. Take one contraction at a time. Help her stay alert between contractions. Make sure she's ready for each contraction and starts the breathing pattern right away. Remind her to relax and keep her focal point.
3. Adopt a thick-skinned attitude. Do not react to any "abuse" you may receive. Don't take it personally, even if she says it's all your fault. Some of the things she gets angry about may not seem to be rational, but don't argue with her.
4. Do not react to any panic or discouragement she shows. Be reassuring and supportive. Don't *you* panic. She's looking to you for support and encouragement, not sympathy.
5. Do not react negatively to anything she may do, such as crying or vomiting, or if she doesn't act as you thought she would. Don't have expectations about how your mate will react to labor before it happens. Transition is really hard, and she's never been through it before. No one knows ahead of time how it will be and how one will react.
6. When she's voicing discouragement or saying that she can't continue she's really asking for encouragement and support. *Saying* she can't do it doesn't necessarily mean that she wants you to agree with her. Tell her she's doing a good job; help her with the breathing; tell her the baby's almost here and soon she can start pushing. Do anything that seems to relieve her anxiety.
7. Be affectionate; praise her; give her lots of encouragement.
8. Stay close to her. She may want to use your face as her focal point. Be ready to breathe with her through a difficult contraction. Though she may be very sensitive to touch, she may still want you to hold her hand or be near her so that she feels you're physically helping her through the contractions and won't leave her alone. Continue to encourage relaxation, especially in her shoulders.
9. Be a screen from any disturbing things going on in the labor room. Remember she may be supersensitive to strong stimuli—lights, noise, conversation, someone bumping into her bed. Try to correct any of these situations if they seem to be bothering her.
10. Don't be embarrassed or intimidated in front of hospital staff about being a good coach. If you need assistance or suggestions, the staff is there to help you.

WHAT YOU SHOULD TAKE TO THE HOSPITAL

You will want to have things ready to take to the hospital a few weeks before your due date. You don't need to take the clothes you and the baby will wear home from the hospital, but put them where your mate can find them easily to bring to you.

SUITCASE

When you are admitted to the hospital, you will be taken to a labor room. Find out beforehand whether or not your suitcase goes with you or if it is put in your postpartum room. You may want to pack a bag of things you will need in the labor room and leave your suitcase locked in the trunk of your car until you are in your postpartum room.

ARTICLES NEEDED FOR LABOR

_____ Chapstick or other lubricant for your lips

> Once admitted to the hospital you probably will not be given anything to eat or drink, and your lips can become quite dry. Some doctors allow their patients to have ice chips or popsicles.

_____ Unscented powder, cornstarch, or lotion for back rubs and effleurage
Massage will be much more effective with some lubrication.

_____ Warm socks

> A must, even in July. Toward the end of labor the circulation in your legs may be impaired as the baby moves deeper in the pelvis. Cold feet can be quite uncomfortable.

_____ Hard candy

> If you want to take along hard candy, get the sour, not the sweet, version. Candy on a stick can be easily taken out of your mouth before a contraction begins. Ask if your doctor approves of hard candy for energy and to wet your mouth during labor.

_____ Paper bag

> This is to breathe in if you should hyperventilate, though a surgical mask is as effective and much less cumbersome. Tell your nurse if you need one. Take the bag in case you can't get a mask right away.

_____ Small hot water bottle

> For backache. Find out if your hospital provides one if you need it.

_____ Watch with a second hand

> In case there is no clock in the labor room. Check on this during your tour. Is it where you can see it?

_____ Camera and film

> A flash may not be acceptable in the delivery room if combustible gases are stored there. Check when you go on your hospital tour. If you cannot use a flash, you will need to use high speed film such as Kodak's Kodacolor 400 CG 135.

_____ This book and a pen
         You may want to refer to the labor section.

_____ Names and phone numbers of family and friends you want to call.
         Bring dimes, too.

_____ Lunch or snack for the labor coach
         The hospital cafeteria is probably not open all night long, but most hospitals have snack and drink machines. Bringing a lunch means the coach does not have to leave the mother to get something to eat, but the smell of the food may bother her. The father may have to eat the snack in the waiting room.

List phone numbers of people to call about the baby!

_____ _____ _____ _____

_____ _____ _____ _____

_____ _____ _____ _____

ARTICLES NEEDED FOR YOUR HOSPITAL STAY

_____ Nightgowns (two or three)
         Long, fancy nightgowns are pretty, but remember your lochia flow will be quite heavy the first few days, so shorter gowns are easier to manage. If you are breast feeding, gowns that open in front will be easier.

_____ Bras (two or three)
         Even if you are not breast feeding

_____ Robe and slippers

_____ Toilet articles
         Toothbrush, toothpaste, deodorant, shampoo, comb, brush, hair blower, make-up, and so on. Sanitary belts and pads are usually supplied by the hospital.

_____ Baby announcements and writing materials

_____ Addresses and phone numbers of family and friends

_____ Small amount of money for magazines, newspapers, television rental, and so on. You should leave your valuables at home.

_____ Transistor radio

_____ Baby book and your book(s) on breast feeding, so the nursery can put your baby's footprints in your book.

ARTICLES NEEDED FOR YOUR TRIP HOME FROM THE HOSPITAL

Mother: Loose fitting clothes such as something you wore when you were four or five months pregnant.

Baby: The baby will need a receiving blanket and a quilt (or heavier blanket, depending upon the weather), the outfit you have selected for her to wear home, a car seat, and a disposable diaper that the hospital will probably supply.

HOSPITAL FEES

This information can be obtained from the admitting or business office of your hospital and from your doctor.

Where can you cut costs if you have incomplete or no insurance coverage?

	3 days	4 days	5-7 days (Cesarean)

ROOM AND CARE $_____ $_____ $_____

What kind of rooms are available (private, semi-private, ward)?

What are the variations in cost?

Are there special room requirements if you want rooming-in?

How much of the room fee does your insurance pay?

What would a private room cost above your insurance coverage?

Can you go home after 12 to 24 hours?

NURSERY $_____ $_____ $_____

Is the nursery charge standard even if you have rooming-in?

Is the normal newborn placed in an intensive care or observation unit the first 12 to 24 hours? Does this service cost more?

If your baby requires phototherapy (being placed under lights for treatment of jaundice), what is the fee?

DELIVERY ROOM $_____ (Standard fee)

$_____ (Operating room fee for Cesarean)

Is there an alternative to using a delivery room, such as delivering in a labor or birthing room? Does it change the fee?

ANESTHESIA $_____

Is it a standard inclusion?

Does your obstetrician administer the medication or does an anesthesiologist? Is the fee different?

Is there a difference in charge depending on the type of anesthesia used for a Cesarean birth?

CENTRAL SUPPLY $_____ $_____ $_____

Items such as your admission pack, sanitary pads, tissues, nursing pads, and so on, are included here. How do costs compare to buying your own?

PHARMACY $_____ $_____ $_____

What medications might be used during labor, delivery, and postpartum? Is an IV standard?

LABORATORY $_____ $_____ $_____

What are the normal lab tests performed when you are admitted to the hospital?

What are the normal tests performed during your postpartum stay?

What laboratory tests will the baby receive?

CIRCUMCISION $_____

Will your obstetrician or your pediatrician perform the circumcision?

Is there a standard fee? When is it done?

TELEPHONE & TELEVISION $_____ $_____ $_____

6

Delivery, or stage 2 of the birth process, is the culmination of pregnancy and your hours of work during labor. At last the baby is soon to be born and you'll know its gender and appearance and the special feeling of having shared this experience together. The actual birth is an emotional time for both of you—experience it; allow your emotions to be expressed. This is *your* moment, not to be repeated many times in a lifetime.

THE PUSHING STAGE

The second stage of labor, or *expulsion*, begins when the cervix is dilated enough for the baby's head to pass through and ends with the birth of the baby. The mother pushes the baby down the birth, or vaginal, canal.

Two forces work together to help expel your baby:

- *Uterine contractions:* The contractions continue and their strength helps push the baby down.
- *Intra-abdominal pressure exerted by the mother:* This "bearing down" during a contraction helps move the baby down the birth canal.

The force necessary to expel the baby is 80 to 110 pounds.[1] The uterus exerts 50 to 55 pounds of pressure during a contraction, and the rest must be supplied by the mother.

The intra-abdominal pressure exerted by the mother may be in response to the *urge to push.* This urge is a reflex that women sometimes have as the baby's head reaches the pelvic floor. If you do not have this sensation, you will be instructed to push during a contraction, even though you may not feel the need. After you have pushed for a while, the pressure from the baby will cause some numbing of the vaginal and perineal tissues.

[1]John J. Bonica, "An Atlas on Mechanisms and Pathways of Pain in Labor," *What's New*, No. 217 (Spring 1960) (North Chicago, Ill.: Abbott Laboratories).

Delivery

Women usually describe pushing either as gratifying or difficult. For some women, the sensation of the baby moving through the birth canal is very pleasant. Most of the symptoms of transition have disappeared, and the mother begins to feel more in control. For some women, however, the pushing stage is difficult, perhaps because of the size or position of the baby as she comes down the birth canal. The sensations may include stretching, burning, or tremendous pressure and this can be uncomfortable.

Most women having their first baby push in the labor room until the baby's head has moved down the birth canal and is beginning to *crown*. True crowning is when the largest diameter of the baby's head reaches the vaginal outlet. You will probably be moved to the delivery room when a quarter-sized portion of the baby's head is visible to the doctor.

Some women may be able to labor and deliver in the same room, often called a *birthing room*. This option might be available to you, depending on your hospital's facilities, your labor, use of anesthetics, and your doctor's preference. In this case, the labor bed will be prepared for its delivery function, and you would not be taken to the delivery room.

THE PUSHING TECHNIQUE

In order to push effectively you must coordinate four different actions during the time of a contraction:

- Assume a proper pushing position.
- Do the proper breathing pattern.
- Relax your perineum.
- Use your abdominal muscles to bear down.

Pushing Position

Many positions may be used for pushing, but the one most commonly used in hospital labor or birthing rooms is *semireclining*. Raise the head of your labor or delivery bed to about 30 degrees. Your pelvis is flat on the bed. Do not sit on your tailbone to push because this position is uncomfortable and increases the angle of the vagina, making it difficult for your baby to deliver. Bend your knees, place the soles of your feet together and gently let your knees fall outward. The soles of your feet do not have to stay together but should rest on the bed. Your legs should be supported by pillows. During a contraction you will think of making your body into a "C" position by raising or tucking your head forward slightly and rounding your back. You may let your arms rest at your side or grasp your legs.

For added leverage you may pull your legs toward your chest as you push, but don't do so if the baby is low or crowning because it will make the perineum tight.

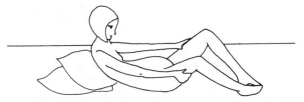

Semi-reclining Pushing Position

The side-lying pushing position is used in the labor or birthing room by a mother having back labor because it gets the baby's weight off her backbone.

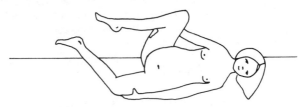

Slidelying Pushing Position

In this position, the upper leg may be supported by someone while you bear down during a contraction. The lower leg is bent slightly, and you still think of making your body into a C position. Your upper arm may grasp your upper leg.

Other less frequently used pushing positions include *squatting, kneeling, hands-and-knees,* and reclining in a bean bag chair. Some of these have the advantage of adding gravity to your pushing efforts and decreasing back pressure. Be sure to ask for help in assuming these positions. It is reassuring to have the side rails on the bed raised.

In the delivery room you will be in the *lithotomy position,* unless otherwise arranged with your physician.

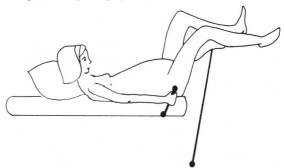

Lithotomy Position—Backlying with legs in stirrups

In this position your legs are in stirrups and you are lying on your back. You can modify the position by raising the head of the bed or using a wedge or pillows under your shoulders. On the delivery table, you can use the hand grips instead of holding your legs for more leverage while pushing. Your coach can help you assume the C position by reaching under your pillow and raising your shoulders.

Correct Breathing Pattern

In order to expend the least amount of energy, and yet have your pushing efforts be effective, you will push only from the peak to the end of the contraction.

1. When the contraction begins, take two deep chest breaths, as in first-level breathing. Inhale a third time and assume your pushing position with your perineum relaxed. While still holding this third breath, bear down as long as you can. Then exhale quickly. Take another breath by bringing your head slightly back to open the air passage. Breathe in deeply, hold your breath, and continue to bear down.
2. Continue breathing and pushing in this manner until the contraction is over or until you have been directed to stop by your nurse or doctor.
3. When the contraction is over, gently lie back and relax. Take a few deep breaths and resume normal breathing until the next contraction.

The pattern look like this:

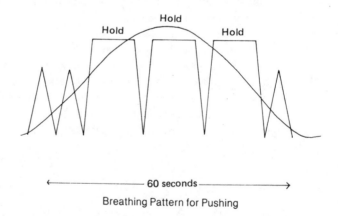

Breathing Pattern for Pushing

4. A variation to this pattern is to inhale and bear down while *very slowly* exhaling instead of holding your breath. When you run out of air, take another deep breath and repeat the pattern. Continue in this manner until the end of the contraction. This is especially effective if delivery is fast.

5. When the baby's head crowns, the doctor may ask you not to push, allowing the uterine contraction to do the final work of expelling your baby. If you have the urge to push lie back and pant (see Chapter Nine).

Relaxed Perineum

The perineum should be completely relaxed so that the baby's head meets with less resistance on its way out. You should concentrate on making the perineum bulge and think about pushing the baby out toward a particular place in the room. It may help you not to tense the pelvic floor if you are thinking about pushing down and out.

It may help you to review the Elevator exercise. Contract the pelvic floor muscles up; then relax down slowly. Go one "floor" lower, going to the "basement." You are bulging your perineum. Return to ground floor. Another way to understand the feeling of pushing is to think about urinating and trying to force the urine out quickly. These exercises are only a means of learning how to relax and bulge the perineum and should not be done regularly, nor during delivery.

Bearing Down

While you push, the upper abdominal muscles are contracting but the lower ones are not. To see if you are pushing correctly, place your hand over your abdominal muscles just above the pubic bone. If your hand moves up, away from the bone when you bear down, you are doing it correctly. If your hand moves in, you are contracting the lower abdominal muscles as you do when having a bowel movement. You are pushing incorrectly. You do not push as if you were having a bowel movement, but you push through the vagina. Different muscles are involved in each action.

HOW DO YOU PRACTICE PUSHING?

During practice, you are to assume the pushing positions but *not* to bear down. Your practice goals are

1. To practice the pushing positions.
2. To practice relaxing your perineum while in the pushing positions.
3. To learn to hold your breath at least 10 seconds during the pushing, and preferably longer.
4. For the coach to learn how and where to support your position and to help with breathing techniques.

STAGE 2: DELIVERY

- *Contractions*
    Length: 60 seconds is usual; however, this time can vary.
    Interval: 2 to 5 minutes.
    Time: 30 minutes to 2 hours. Average is 1¼ hours.
    Intensity: Usually easier to deal with than transition contractions since they are shorter, have a longer rest phase, and the mother is pushing during them.

PHYSICAL SIGNS THAT *MAY* OCCUR:

- Rectal pressure or sensation that you need to have a bowel movement. Urge to push caused by pressure from the baby's presenting part.
- Pressure as the baby moves through the vagina.
- Stretching, stinging, or burning and pressure on the perineum.
- Fatigue, but usually a return of energy for pushing.
- Backache.

EMOTIONAL SIGNS THAT *MAY* OCCUR:

- Decreased confusion, although you may forget the pushing techniques the first few times.
- Excited.
- More talkative and happier between contractions.

THE MOTHER'S ROLE

1. Push with each contraction.
2. Rest between contractions; you'll need your energy for pushing.
3. Make your needs known; ask for more pillows or help with positioning.
4. Try different pushing positions if possible; one might be more comfortable and effective for you than another.
5. Be sure you can see in the mirror when lying back on the delivery table, or if possible, look down and watch your baby being born.
6. Keep your eyes open so you don't miss the birth.
7. Hold, breast feed, and enjoy your baby as soon as possible.

THE COACH'S ROLE

1. Tell her how to push if she has forgotten. Suggest pushing in another position if she's not comfortable or pushing isn't effective.
2. Place your arms under the pillows behind her neck and shoulders. Help her get into and maintain the pushing position. Avoid straining your back. Ask for extra pillows or a wedge to help her into position. Gently ease her back down after the contraction.
3. Help her with the breathing pattern.
4. Remind her to relax her perineum and face while pushing.
5. Reassure her that pressure from the baby is normal.
6. Help her relax between contractions.

7. Have the mirror adjusted so both of you can see, or ask if you can sit at your mate's side so you can actually see the baby while still helping her push. Remind her to keep her eyes open so she can see the delivery.
8. Have your camera ready.
9. Hold and enjoy your baby as soon as possible.

THE DELIVERY ROOM

On the delivery table, you will move to the end much as you would for a pelvic exam in the doctor's office. Your legs will be placed in stirrups, unless you and your doctor have agreed that you will push without them. Be sure the stirrups are adjusted until you are comfortable. Sterile drapes are placed over your legs and abdomen. The doctor or nurse tells you where to place your hands on the hand grips and where not to place your hands because of the sterile drapes. The father is usually seated on a stool by your head. The mirror will be adjusted so that the mother and father will be able to see the birth of the baby together. The nurse will cleanse the perineal area with a warm, antiseptic solution that will feel slightly cold to you. Be sure to ask the staff and your mate for assistance in getting comfortable.

During these preparations for delivery, you may have more contractions, and preparations will usually be stopped while you bear down. If the baby is ready to be born, you may be asked not to push until preparations are complete.

While you are being moved to the delivery room and prepared for the delivery, the physician will be scrubbing his hands and putting on a sterile gown and gloves. Before entering the delivery room, the father will be given a mask, hat, and shoe covers.

The Baby

The baby is making his way through his mother's pelvis, accommodating himself to its shape. There are several movements that he goes through in order to be born. The following are the movements of an anterior, vertex baby:

Descent. The baby moves down in the pelvis. This movement begins with the engagement of the baby's head and continues through labor and delivery. Descent occurs because of the downward pressure of contractions, and during expulsion, because of the additional pushing of the mother. See the illustration on the next page.

Flexion. The baby's chin comes to rest on his chest, and then a smaller diameter of the baby's head is moving through the pelvis.

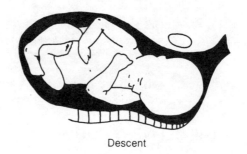

Descent

Internal Rotation. The baby turns his head because of the shape of the mother's pelvis.

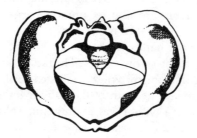
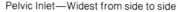

Pelvic Inlet—Widest from side to side

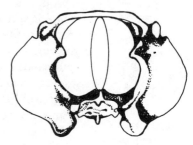

Pelvic Outlet—Widest from front to back

The pelvic inlet is widest from side to side. Since the baby's head is widest from front to back, he usually enters the pelvis looking toward the mother's right or left side. The outlet of the mother's pelvis is widest from front to back, so the baby's head adapts—it rotates internally. He is now looking toward the mother's back.

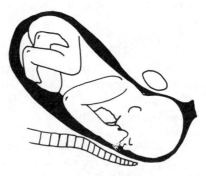

Internal Rotation

Extension. The baby extends, or arches his head back, and the occiput, or crown of the baby's head, is born. The nape of his neck passes under the mother's pubic bone, and the baby extends his head. The forehead, nose, mouth, and finally chin are born.

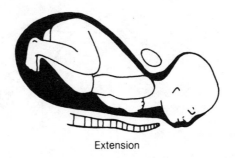

Extension

Restitution and External Rotation. The baby is usually born looking toward the mother's back. Once the head is born, he automatically rotates back to his original position. The baby's passage through the tight birth canal has put pressure on his chest and helped rid the lungs of mucous.

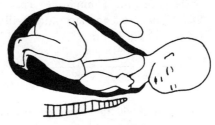

External Rotation

The doctor gently supports the baby's head, and with the next contraction she will pull down slightly on the head to facilitate delivery of the upper shoulder. A slight upward pull will allow the lower shoulder to slip through. The rest of the baby's body is born quite easily.

Episiotomy

Because the perineum may tear during delivery, an episiotomy is often routinely performed. This is a small incision made from the vaginal outlet toward the anus, enlarging the vaginal opening to allow for delivery of the baby's head. The length and direction of the episiotomy depend on the size and position of the baby and the elasticity of the perineum. Usually a *midline episiotomy* is performed—a straight incision toward the anus. If more room is needed, a *mediolateral* episiotomy may be performed—a diagonal incision, to the right or left toward the anus.

If you have been pushing hard for some time, the perineum will be numb from the pressure of the baby's head and you will not feel the episiotomy. However, many women prefer to be given a local anesthetic in the perineum before the episiotomy is performed so it will be in effect for the stitches. This injection would be given while you're in the delivery or birthing room once the head has crowned.

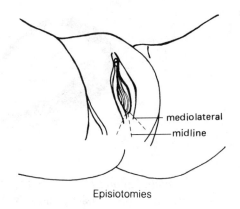

mediolateral

midline

Episiotomies

Rather than the doctor routinely performing an episiotomy, ask him to evaluate the need at the time of delivery. Another technique for enlarging the vaginal opening for the baby's head is a stretching massage of the perineum to thin it out. This technique requires time and patience. Occasionally a small laceration will occur, which is repaired in the same way as the episiotomy.

FOR YOUR EPISIOTOMY

1. Do pelvic floor exercises frequently to increase circulation to the perineum.
2. Ask for an ice pack in recovery room to decrease perineal swelling.
3. Make frequent use of sitz baths (hot-water baths); moist heat will promote healing.
4. To sit down following an episiotomy, first squeeze your buttocks together; then sit down squarely and relax your buttocks.

Forceps

If the force of uterine contractions and the mother's pushing efforts don't seem to be enough, forceps may be used to help deliver the baby. Forceps are two spoon-shaped metal instruments designed to help deliver the baby's head. At one end they are curved to accommodate the baby's head and the mother's pelvis. The other end is a handle which the doctor grasps. Each blade is applied individually, and then they are locked together at the handle so that they don't squeeze the head.

"Outlet," or low forceps, is the application of forceps when the baby's head has reached the perineum and can be seen at the vaginal outlet. "Mid-forceps" delivery of the baby occurs when the head is slightly above the perineum but still low in the pelvis. This delivery is not as common.

Your doctor may decide to use forceps if the second stage (expulsion) is long. Despite your pushing efforts, the baby may not be descending. You may be tired, the uterine contractions may not be of good quality, the baby may be presenting in an unusual way, he may have a large head, or there may be too much resistance in the birth canal or perineum. Forceps also enable the doctor to control the speed of delivery of the head. Forceps deliveries are safe in the hands of a competent doctor.

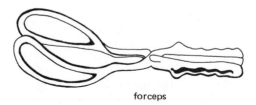

forceps

After the Baby Is Born

Sometimes the doctor will gently lay the baby on your abdomen so you may see and touch her. He clamps the cord in two places near the baby's abdomen and cuts between the clamps. The time may vary, but usually it is done very soon after the baby's birth. The doctor grasps the end of the umbilical cord and waits for the placenta to separate from the wall of the uterus. Some times the baby is placed in a heated crib and pushed near the delivery table so the parents can observe while the nurse or doctor cares for her (see Chapter Seven). This crib is normally stored in a corner of the delivery room. You may ask to have it moved over to the delivery area so you can see your baby.

Some couples elect to incorporate some of Leboyer's gentle birth techniques into their deliveries. Leboyer, a French obstetrician, advocates such measures as dim lights, warm delivery room, massage of the newborn, and allowing the baby to remain in his spine-flexed fetal position on the mother's abdomen for a time following birth. His techniques are meant for use in normal, uncomplicated births. If you should choose to use some of Leboyer's method you should consult your doctor about her normal delivery procedures and beliefs regarding this method. Some hospitals routinely use some LeBoyer techniques.

STAGE 3: EXPULSION OR DELIVERY OF THE PLACENTA

In the excitement of the birth you may forget about the placenta. It will detach from the uterine wall, your uterus will continue to contract, and your doctor will ask you to bear down to expel the placenta. Usually taking a deep breath, holding it, and bearing down is sufficient.

Your doctor will carefully examine the placenta to make sure it is intact and that no fragments have remained in your uterus. Fragments make it impossible for the uterus to successfully clamp down, or contract, to stop the bleeding. The placenta is a fascinating organ that sustained your baby's life while she was in the uterus. You may want to ask your doctor to show it to you, pointing out the maternal and fetal sides and the umbilical cord and blood vessels.

STAGE 4: IMMEDIATE POSTPARTUM

Immediate postpartum is your first hour of recovery after the birth. Part of this time will probably be spent in the delivery room. Your uterus, cervix, vagina, and perineum will be checked, and if necessary, any repairs made.

Following expulsion of the placenta, it is the task of the uterus to clamp down strongly to prevent hemorrhage. Your doctor will probably check your uterus to be sure it is contracted and that no placental fragments remain. If you nurse your baby, a hormone called *oxytocin* will be released, causing uterine contractions. Many doctors give an injection of an oxytocic drug such as Pitocin, Ergotrate, or Methergine following delivery to further encourage contraction. External urterine massage by your nurse or doctor will help keep the uterus contracted after delivery. You may find this massage uncomfortable because your uterus is very sensitive to touch at this time.

Your doctor will also check your cervix and vagina to make sure there were no tears during the birth process. If you had an episiotomy, he will repair your incision with stitches. Your local anesthetic will take care of this sensation in nearly all cases. You may feel an occasional prick if the local did not infiltrate all the nerves. Your doctor will carefully check your perineum for tears, repairing or stitching any he finds.

Depending on the amount of repair necessary, you may be in the delivery room 15 to 30 minutes more.

Chills are a common occurrence following delivery, often accompanied by shaking or trembling. The causes are uncertain and may be both psychological and physiological. The chills, although disconcerting, are common and last only a short time. An extra blanket may help until they subside.

The Recovery Room

You complete your immediate postpartum recovery in the recovery room, labor room, or birthing room. During this time, your nurse will further check your recovery from the birth process. Approximately every fifteen minutes for an hour your nurse will check:

1. To see if the uterus remains firmly contracted, massaging it if it is not. She will also check the height of the fundus.
2. To see that the vaginal bleeding doesn't become excessive and that you're not passing large clots. She will change your perineal pads (sanitary napkins) as needed. She will check your episiotomy site and condition of your perineum.
3. To be sure your blood pressure, pulse, and respirations have stabilized. She may also check your temperature.
4. To make sure that you have recovered from any medications used during the birth process.
5. To check for dehydration, perhaps offering fluids.

Hospital procedures vary, but you should all be together as a family in the recovery room—mother, father, and baby. Occasionally, a baby will need some immediate care and will go directly to the nursery, but if there are no problems, most families want to be together after the birth. This is an ideal time for mother, father, and baby to get to know each other.

Emotions Following the Delivery

Reactions can vary tremendously. Sometimes mothers and fathers are exuberant, completely revitalized following the labor process and anxious to hold and care for their new baby. Some mothers want to hold and breast feed their new infant on the delivery table or in the recovery room. This is a matter to discuss with your doctor before you deliver.

Other times both mother and father are exhausted, and it may take them a while to recover before they feel able to hold and deal with their tiny infant. Sometimes only the mother feels this way, and she urges the father to hold the baby in the delivery room. Labor is an inward time and it can take a while for parents to be able to focus on the end result of their efforts. Chills or the narrow delivery table may deter some mothers from holding the baby in the delivery room. Fathers are sometimes torn between attention to the mother and the new baby. They want to hold and comfort the mother, but they also want to count the toes and fingers on their new daughter or son.

Sometimes parents feel most comfortable observing their new baby as she rests in the crib pushed over beside the delivery table. Other times both parents may want to immediately hold and touch their new baby, which is usually possible once the baby has been suctioned, dried off, and wrapped warmly in a blanket.

Once in the recovery room, most parents feel able to hold their new child. Providing the mother and baby are doing well, the best situation is one that allows the parents and their new baby the opportunity to become acquainted in the manner in which they feel comfortable.

Right after your baby's birth, a very special relationship begins to develop among the three of you. The interaction between the parents and child is called "attachment," or "bonding." Klaus and Kennell have referred to this period following birth as the "sensitive period," during which "interactions between mother and infant help lock them together."[2] There is a similar action between the father and his infant.

These bonding interactions among mother and father and baby begin in the delivery room and carry over into the recovery room if the parents and baby remain together. They can include the following behaviors: stroking, holding, smiling, gazing, kissing, talking, touching, and nursing. Since your baby will probably be awake and alert for an hour or so following delivery, before going to sleep for a few hours, it is an ideal time to get to know one another.

Bonding is a continuing process, which is *enhanced by early, frequent contact between the parents and their baby.* "The power of this attachment is so great that it enables the mother or father to make the unusual sacrifices necessary for the care of their infant day after day, night after night." . . . [3]

Studies by Klaus and Kennell indicate that this early bonding or attachment can have long-lasting effects on later behavior between parents and child and between the child and other people with whom he forms relationships.[4]

Hospital personnel in many areas have become aware of this very important time between parents and their new child and routinely keep the family together through the first few hours of the baby's life. They also encourage postpartum rooming-in so there is much opportunity for contact between parents and baby. If your hospital does not routinely follow these practices, be sure to ask if you may be permitted to have them.

Birthing Centers

An alternative to a traditional hospital delivery is available in some cities. Birthing centers affiliated with hospitals provide care for low-risk deliveries. Birth attendants such as doctors and midwives provide patient care. Often the costs are lower, but medical facilities, equipment, and staff are nearby should an emergency arise.

---

[2]Marshall H. Klaus and John H. Kennell, *Maternal-infant Bonding* (St. Louis, Mo.: C. V. Mosby Company, 1976), p. 51.
[3]*Ibid.*, p. 1.
[4]*Ibid.*, p. 52

EMERGENCY HOME (OR CAR) DELIVERY

It is common for couples to worry about whether they will make it to the hospital. Most do, but occasionally a woman's labor will progress unexpectedly fast or with only minimal discomfort. She may find herself en route to the hospital or still at home and about to deliver. If you have time, call for assistance. Here are some procedures to follow until help arrives.

1. Assume a position that's comfortable for you. (The back seat of the car is better than the front.) Place clean towels or pads under your buttocks.
2. Do not push as the baby's head delivers. Lie back and pant, allowing the force of contractions to deliver your baby.
3. Slip the umbilical cord over the head if it is around the baby's neck.
4. Allow the baby to rotate on its own.
5. The top shoulder will deliver first; then the lower. The rest of the baby may deliver very quickly and is slippery.
6. Hold the baby so his head is slightly downward to facilitate drainage of mucous; do not hang your baby upside down by his heels. The baby should cry or be breathing. You can gently massage his back to stimulate breathing. If the sac is still around the baby, rupture it. Clear any remnants of the membranes from his nose or mouth.
7. *Quickly* dry your baby off and place him next to your skin or at the breast if the cord is long enough. Cover him with a clean blanket or your clothing.
8. Allow the baby to nurse or to lick the nipple, this will help contract the uterus and minimize bleeding.
9. Do not cut, clamp or pull on the cord. Use a clean strip of material or shoelace to tie the umbilical cord about six to eight inches from the baby. The placenta may detach and deliver. If so, wrap it in a blanket and put it next to the baby to keep the infant warm.
10. If delivery occurred in the car, proceed to the nearest hospital. If delivery occurred at home, again call your doctor for instructions or call the nearest rescue squad.
11. Both infant and mother need to be examined following delivery. Do not delay in getting to a medical facility or calling for assistance.

THINGS TO CONTEMPLATE . . .

1. Have you selected and interviewed a physician for your baby?
2. Will the father be allowed to remain in the labor room during the admitting procedures (history, enema, prep, and so on)? Would it be helpful if he was?
3. Is there a birthing room available for your use? What are the prerequisites for using it? How does your doctor feel about it?
4. Have you thought about, read about, and accepted Cesarean birth, in case it should be necessary? Do you understand the options involved?
5. What feelings do you have about using medication during your labor and delivery? What criteria determines whether you will use analgesia or anesthesia?
6. If it becomes necessary to use medication, what does your doctor prefer to use and why?

MEDICATION

1. What is it?
2. Why would I need it?
3. How long will it last?
4. How will it affect me?
5. How will it affect my baby?
6. Is it safe?

---

7. What are your options in terms of delivery positions? In the labor room? In the delivery room? In the birthing room?
8. How do you feel about the episiotomy? Do you have any options?
9. Do you want to include any of the Leboyer techniques for gentle birth in your delivery? Have you discussed this subject with your doctor?
10. What kind of early contact do you want with your baby? Do you want to hold your baby in the delivery room? Do you want to breast feed in the delivery room? Have you discussed this subject with your doctor?
11. Will you be together as a family in the recovery room? Can you keep your baby in the recovery room?
12. Do you want rooming-in? Partial, complete? What, if any, are the requirements for rooming-in? When does it begin? Can you vary it, once you decide?

104

BIRTH DAY PROCEDURES

1. Find out when you are to call your doctor.

   You are to call your doctor when your membranes rupture, or you think they may be ruptured, and when your contractions are lasting _____ seconds and occurring every _____ minutes.

   Example:

   Doctor, this is _____ . (I think I am) or (I'm sure I am) in labor. My contractions are (regular) or (irregular). They are _____ seconds long, every _____ minutes. This has been going on for (amount of time) _____ . My membranes (are) (are not) (might be) ruptured or leaking. My due date is _____ . I feel (state how contractions are affecting you) _____

   _____

2. Find out about admitting procedures.

   Are you preadmitted? Yes _____   No _____ .
   How do you get preadmission forms?

   When you are in labor, you will go to _____ if it is daytime. After _____ P.M. you will go to _____ . This is reached from (street) _____ . Parking is available (where) _____ and costs _____ . You will be taken to _____

3. Preparation procedures:

   Your labor nurse may or may not perform the following:

   _____   Check your weight
   _____   Give you a hospital gown
   _____   Take your temperature
   _____   Take your blood pressure
   _____   Listen to fetal heart tones
   _____   Use a fetal monitor (why used? when used?)
   _____   Order a blood specimen drawn
   _____   Give you an enema (any options?)
   _____   Prep you (how much? any options?)
   _____   Give you an IV (any options? is it standard? what does it contain?)

For the Father or Coach:

During this time you may be allowed to remain with your mate, or you may be asked to leave.

If you leave, a reasonable amount of time to complete the admission procedures is _____ minutes. If you are not called at the end of this time, you should check (where) _____

You should change from your street clothes into surgical clothes before your mate reaches transition. Where do you change?_____ . (Initially, you may be asked to wear a gown over your street clothes.)

4. Working together in the labor room.

During labor, mothers should express their needs. Coaches must try to be perceptive to unspoken needs. What can you expect to happen and how will you deal with the following common situations that may arise during labor?

Early labor:

a. The mother is having early labor contractions and is comfortable. Her membranes have not ruptured. What could she be doing?

b. At 3 to 4 cm the doctor may artificially rupture the mother's membranes. What can she expect to happen?

c. The doctor or nurse does a pelvic exam. Why? What can the mother expect to happen following the exam?

Active labor:

a. The mother has an aching sensation above the pubic bone. What might be done to help relieve it?

b. The mother is having difficulty relaxing during contractions. What can she and her coach do?

c. The mother's mouth is dry and she's thirsty. What may help?

d. The mother is discouraged by lack of progress despite strong contractions. How might she react and what can the coach do?

e. The doctor decides to speed up labor by administering pitocin intravenously. What can the mother expect to happen?

f. The mother is tired and dozing between contractions. What should the coach do?

g. The mother is having trouble staying in control of her contractions, begins to get tense, and loses the rhythm of the breathing pattern. What can the coach do to help?

h. The mother is dizzy, feeling numbness around her lips, and cramping and tingling in her fingers. What happened? What should she do?

106

Transition:

a. The mother is nauseated and may vomit. What can she and her coach do?

b. The mother is shivering and feeling chilled. What can be done?

c. The mother is complaining of backache. What can be done?

d. The mother is warm and perspiring. What can the coach do?

e. The mother wants to call it quits and give up. How can the coach help?

f. The mother suddenly doesn't appreciate anything the coach is doing to help. How should he react?

g. The mother has the urge to push during the peak of a contraction. What should the coach do? What should the mother do?

h. The mother is having trouble controlling the urge to push. What can be done?

Delivery:

1. Does your hospital have the option of allowing the mother to labor and deliver in a labor or birthing room provided there are no complications?
Yes _____ No _____ Under what circumstances?

2. Does your hospital have the option of a labor-delivery bed?
Yes _____ No _____ Under what circumstances could you use it?

3. The mother will begin pushing down _____ .
If this is your first baby, most of your pushing will be done in the (where)
_____ . You will be moved to the delivery room when
_____ .

4. Requirements for photography in the delivery room are:

5. Requirements for sound recording in the delivery room are:

Recovery Room:

1. Will mother, father, and baby be together?
Is it what you want? If not, what can be done?

2. When may the mother begin breast feeding? Have you discussed this subject with your physician beforehand?

Visitors:

1. Father and grandparents may visit _____ .

2. Other visitors may visit _____ .

3. Siblings may visit _____ .

7

This chapter includes information on the newborn—what happens to him immediately after birth, what his appearance and behavior are, and what procedures are commonly used to evaluate his health.

AT BIRTH

While in the uterus, your baby is supplied with oxygen from the mother's blood passing through the placenta. As soon as the baby is born, though, his whole system of circulation changes.

1. When the umbilical cord is exposed to air, the circulation is cut off. Air causes the Wharton's jelly in the cord to expand, compressing the vein and two arteries. Blood can no longer pass through, and the baby receives no more oxygen from this source.
2. The infant must begin to breathe on his own. The doctor gently suctions the baby's nose and mouth to clear out the mucous. These first breaths are thought to be the hardest, requiring five times the effort normally needed to breathe.[1] The baby must draw in air and expand thousands of tiny uninflated air sacs called *alveoli*. His immediate efforts at breathing will be irregular, he may gasp, choke, sneeze, and sputter. As the mucous clears out over the next several days, breathing will become easier for him.
3. With the first breaths, the baby's heart begins to pump blood through the lungs to pick up the oxygen the baby has inhaled. At this point, a major valve in the heart must close in order to separate freshly oxygenated blood from that already circulated through the body.

Two of the main concerns with a newborn are a clear air passageway and warm environment.

[1] Geraldine Lux Flanagan, *The First Nine Months of Life* (New York: Pocket Books, 1965), p. 134.

The Newborn

The doctor or nurse will continue to suction mucous from the baby's airway. To facilitate mucous drainage, the baby is usually placed on her side with her head tilted slightly downward. She may be placed on your abdomen or in the heated crib in this position. Sometimes she is given extra oxygen through a mask or a tiny tube inserted in her nostril.

The baby has emerged from the warmth of the mother's body to a delivery room that is sometimes as much as 25 degrees cooler than the mother's normal temperature. Chilling of the baby is a very real concern. The nurse will carefully dry your baby off and wrap him in a blanket. She may also place him in the heated crib. A chilled baby has more trouble breathing, so warmth is important. When the baby is given to the mother, the warmth of her body as she holds him close will help maintain his temperature. Skin-to-skin contact is especially effective in keeping the baby warm while you're holding him. Sometimes portable heating units are placed over the mother and baby.

While in the delivery room, the nurse will footprint the baby and fingerprint the mother. She will attach tiny identification bracelets around the baby's ankle and wrist and place a matching one on the mother's wrist.

At one and five minutes of age the baby will be given an Apgar score. This test evaluates how he fared through labor and delivery and predicts how he will do postpartum. Developed by Dr. Virginia Apgar, it rates the baby 0, 1, or 2 on each of five newborn characteristics. A score of 7 to 10 out of a possible 10 points is considered good. Be sure to ask your baby's Apgar scores.

APGAR SCORING SYSTEM			
Characteristic	0	1	2
Color	blue, pale	body pink, extremities blue	body completely pink
Respiratory Effort	absent	slow, irregular, weak cry	strong cry
Heart rate	absent	less than 100	more than 100
Muscle tone	limp	some flexing of extremities	active motion
Reflex irritability	absent	grimace	cry

Three other procedures are sometimes followed in the delivery room or soon afterward in the recovery room or nursery.

1. State laws require that a broad spectrum antibiotic be placed in the baby's eyes to prevent blindness caused by maternal vaginal infections. This substance will temporarily impair the baby's vision. It is now known that the newborn can see and discriminate patterns at birth, and for this reason, some hospitals delay administration of the antibiotic. They allow the family to be together in the delivery and recovery rooms to visually become acquainted. Once the baby is taken to the nursery, the antibiotic is put in her eyes. You can request this delay even if it is not routinely practiced at your hospital.

2. The baby will receive an injection of vitamin K. Vitamin K is synthesized by bacteria in the intestines, but since the new infant's body initially has no bacteria, he is not immediately able to produce vitamin K. This vitamin is needed by the liver to help with blood coagulation, so the injection is given to prevent any bleeding problems. It is often given when the baby goes to the nursery rather than in the delivery room.

3. Dextrostix is a blood test usually made within one to two hours after birth. It measures the level of glucose in your baby's blood. The blood is usually obtained by a "heel stick," or pricking of the baby's heel. If your baby is low in glucose, or hypoglycemic, you will probably be asked to feed her either glucose water or formula to raise the level. If the level is too low, further laboratory tests follow, and glucose can be administered through an IV.

Other tests your baby may have during his hospital stay include the following:

1. *PKU,* or phenylketonuria, is a disorder of metabolism in which an amino acid called phenylalanine cannot be metabolized because the body lacks the necessary liver enzyme. Failure to identify this metabolic error can lead to mental retardation. Screening programs have been established to diagnose PKU from blood samples. For accurate results, this test must be done after the child has digested colostrum, breast milk, or formula for at least 48 hours.[2] The treatment for PKU is a strict diet limiting the child's intake of proteins containing phenylalanine. When this diet is followed, mental retardation can be avoided.

2. *Hypothyroidism* (cretinism) is a condition that can result in mental retardation if it is not diagnosed and treated early. Since it is four to five times more prevalent than PKU, researchers have developed a test to detect it by using a sample of umbilical cord blood. Although the testing program is still being refined, it may become standard procedure. If you want your child tested, you should discuss this test with your baby's doctor.

3. In some hospitals, there is routine screening of the infant's hearing.

[2]Margaret Duncan Jensen, Ralph C. Benson, and Irene M. Bobak, *Maternity Care: The Nurse and the Family* (St. Louis, Mo.: C. V. Mosby Company, 1977), p. 480.

CHARACTERISTICS OF THE NEWBORN

When a couple learns that the woman is pregnant, one of the first things they may wonder about is whether the baby will be a boy or girl. Will the baby look like the mother or the father? What color eyes? What kind of hair? How tall? Lots of people will tell you that all babies look alike, but nothing could be further from the truth. They are all unique and special and no other human being will look like or be like your baby.

Originally it was thought that a newborn was capable of little more than eating, sleeping, crying, and filling her diapers. Research has shown, however, that she is more aware of her surroundings than was previously thought.

Since most of us haven't seen many newborns, we're often surprised at the baby's appearance. The following are some common traits and characteristics.

Appearance

Newborns seldom have beautiful skin. Immediately after birth it may be blue or mottled. As the baby's lungs fill with air, the oxygen will cause his skin to turn pink, though his hands and feet may still be bluish. The skin may be wrinkled, loose, or scaly. He may be covered with a cheesy, white substance, called *vernix caseosa,* or may have it in the creases of his arms and legs. It protected his skin *in utero.* If the baby is post-mature you may not see much vernix.

His cheeks, ears, shoulders, and back may be covered with *lanugo,* a fine downy hair. The younger the gestational age of your baby, the more hair he will have on his body. It will disappear within a few weeks in a full-term baby.

Your baby will probably weigh between 5 and 10 pounds and be 18 to 23 inches long. The average baby is about 7 to 7½ pounds and 20 to 21 inches. Most babies lose a few ounces the first few days and then regain their birth weight the first or second week.

Your baby may show signs of his long birth process. His head, which is large compared to his body, will probably be *molded.* The baby's head is not a solid skull, like that of adults, because the five bone plates in his head have not fused. During birth, they can overlap slightly without damage to his brain, making his head smaller for the tight squeeze through the birth canal. Areas where the bones are not solidly fused are called *sutures,* or *fontanels.* Because of this movable quality to your baby's head, it will probably not be nicely rounded at birth. Usually the head is elongated at the crown or is banana-shaped, and there may be some swollen areas. This molding usually disappears within the first week. The best-known fontanel is the one in front, the "soft spot." This area remains soft for about 18 to 24 months. The rear fontanel closes within the first few months. Don't worry about gently touching these fontanels.

Gestational Age

Within the first few hours after the baby's birth, an evaluation of his gestational age is usually performed by the nursery staff or your doctor. Since due dates are not always accurate, the baby is assessed to determine its age, that is, whether it is term, premature, or postmature.

Gestational age is one way to identify babies who might have complications or need additional observation and those who are term and low risk. It is difficult to tell the baby's age by his weight. Some premature babies can have normal birth weight, and some term babies can be large (large for gestational age, or LGA) or small (small for gestational age, or SGA).

By assessing the amount, shape, or stage of development of the following characteristics and comparing them to established criteria for gestational ages from 24 to 44 weeks, your baby's clinical gestational age can be accurately determined.

Vernix	Hair on head
Breast tissue	Skin texture
Nipples	Skin color and opacity
Sole creases	Skull firmness
Ear cartilage	Posture
Ear form	Tone
Genitalia	Reflexes

Be sure to discuss the results of this estimate with the doctor caring for your baby. It is interesting to know whether your dates were correct or not.

Other Characteristics

For most babies, presenting head first can produce some unusual facial features. The baby's nose can be slightly out of line, his face puffy, and his ears bent. These features will soon disappear and your baby's face will look normal.

Some little white nodules, called *milia,* may be on the baby's nose, chin, and cheeks. These are clogged oil glands, which disappear in a few weeks. A pinkish birthmark is sometimes seen across the bridge of the nose, over the upper lip, or behind the neck. These marks frequently disappear.

High maternal hormone levels in the baby may *temporarily* affect the appearance:

- In a female baby, the genital area may protrude a little and there may be a vaginal discharge, which is whitish with occasional spots of blood.
- In the male baby, the scrotum may be swollen.
- In both boys and girls, there may be engorgement, or swelling, of the breasts with a secretion of a substance called "witches' milk."

Your baby's breathing will be irregular and sometimes quite rapid and noisy. He may hiccough, even when sleeping, and not be disturbed. Babies sneeze fairly often too, not because they are catching cold, but because they are clearing their sensitive respiratory passages of lint and other small particles in the air.

Your baby's first bowel movements consist of a substance called *meconium.* This is a sticky, greenish-black collection of secretions from the intestinal tract. The stools will gradually become yellowish-green and then progress to the normal yellowish stool. Sometimes a baby will pass some meconium during labor, which *can* be a sign of fetal distress.

Your baby's arms and legs will be tucked in close to the body and will recoil if stretched. When turned on her stomach, your baby can lift her head and turn it from one side to the other.

All together, your newborn is very different from you. For instance:

His heart beats twice as fast as a grownup's, 120 beats a minute, and he breathes twice as fast as you do, about thirty-three times a minute. He may urinate as many as eighteen times and move his bowels from four to seven times in twenty-four hours. He sleeps fourteen to eighteen hours of his twenty-four hour day. On the average, he is alert and comfortable for only thirty minutes in a four-hour period.[3]

Jaundice

A common newborn problem is physiologic *jaundice.* Many babies develop a yellowish coloration of their skin and the whites of their eyes between 24 to 36 hours after birth. The condition worsens for two to three days and then starts to get better. After babies are born, some of their red blood cells break down. The by-product of this breakdown is *bilirubin,* which is then broken down by the liver for elimination. Some babies have immature livers and cannot assimilate these waste products fast enough, resulting in yellow-tinted skin. Generally, the jaundice will resolve itself. If the bilirubin level becomes too high, your baby's physician may have him placed under lights, which will chemically reduce the jaundice. Physiologic jaundice is distinguished from breast-milk jaundice, which can occur at two to three weeks and is caused by a substance in the milk that inhibits liver function.

Reflexes

Many of your baby's body movements are reflexes rather than voluntary movements.

1. *The startle, or Moro, reflex:* A sudden change in position, loud noise, bright light, or rough handling will elicit this reflex. The baby

[3]From *The First Twelve Months of Life* by Frank Caplan. Copyright © 1971, 1972, 1973 by Edcom Systems, Inc. By permission of Bantam Books, Inc. All rights reserved.

will arch his back, throw back his head, and fling out his arms and legs. He may then cry and pull his arms and legs back toward the center of his body.

2. *The rooting reflex:* If you stroke your baby's cheek or around his mouth, he will turn and root or search for the breast or bottle. This rooting reflex is followed by the sucking reflex, once he grasps the nipple. The sucking reflex is then followed by the swallowing reflex.

3. *The gag reflex:* We all have this reflex, which prevents food and liquid from entering the breathing passageway. If the baby gets too much in his mouth at one time, the gag reflex will help him get rid of some of it.

4. *The grasp reflex:* The baby will grasp anything that touches the palm of his hand. This grasp is especially strong in a newborn. He also has a grasp reflex with his toes if you stroke the sole of his foot.

5. *The stepping reflex:* The newborn will alternately lift his legs if he is held so that the soles of his feet touch the bed.

SPECIAL BABIES

Sometimes babies are born with problems that require extra medical care. These special babies could include those born with immature body systems because of prematurity (especially the lungs), ill babies, or those having any condition needing specialized treatment. The length of treatment varies from one baby to another, as does the severity of the problem.

The parents of these infants have many emotional adjustments to make. The ill baby may not look or act like the one they imagined, and attachment to him may occur more slowly. Mothers sometimes feel guilty that their babies weren't carried to term or that they "failed" to deliver a healthy infant. They wonder if they did something wrong during pregnancy. By seeking good prenatal guidance and following the recommended care, you have done the best you can for your child. There are circumstances that cannot be controlled.

If a child is quite ill, parents can be reluctant to get too close to the baby emotionally and find themselves grieving for his possible loss. This is a natural reaction. Once the baby's condition improves, parents can begin to accept and relate to their baby.

There are several things parents can do to make their adjustment easier and to help develop their relationship with the baby:

1. Many hospitals have intensive-care or special-care nurseries which can handle all but very severe problems. The ideal situation is for parents and special-care babies to be in the same hospital during the mother's postpartum stay, if it is medically possible and if the nursery staff welcomes parents and lets them help with their baby.

2. Have frequent and close contact with your baby; help care for him. Your baby needs you near and you need to know that you can help your child.

3. Communicate frequently with the medical staff about your baby's condition. Make frequent calls to the nursery to check on him.
4. Ask about your baby's treatment and the special equipment being used. If you understand *why* things are being done and the purpose of the equipment, it is easier to get used to it and to comfort your child during medical procedures.
5. Interact with your baby—talk to him, *touch* him, love him, stroke him, pat him, hold him, and rock him when possible. In their book, *Maternal-Infant Bonding,* Klaus and Kennell have noted that touch is extremely important to the premature baby. Studies note that daily stroking, rocking, and fondling can have beneficial results on the health of the newborn: increased weight gain, intellectual stimulation, and decreased breathing problems.[4]

Finally, communication between parents can be both reassuring and provide strength to meet the extra demands on you during your baby's illness and hospital stay.

THINGS TO ASK FOR AS BABY GIFTS

An evening or afternoon of baby-sitting by a trusted friend

A casserole (or complete dinner) you can just heat and serve

A Snugli or other type of baby carrier

Lunch out with a friend

Diaper service for a month (ask for newborn-sized diapers)

An outing or baby-sitting for your older child, so you can have some time alone with your baby

Clothes *not* in newborn sizes; things that will fit in 6 to 18 months (the special things are nice, especially if they are personalized with the baby's name, but so are the basics)

A baby-food grinder

A baby swing

A handmade baby quilt

A bike seat (you'll be able to use it before long)

A tree to plant in your yard—the "baby's tree"

A new haircut or hairdo

A car seat (make sure it's safe)

Some candid shots of the baby and *both* parents by a photographer friend

Picture frames or albums for all those baby pictures

A special nightgown which opens in front or has hidden slits for the nursing mother

Film

A copy of Caplan's *The First Twelve Months of Life* or Brazelton's *Mothers and Infants*

---

[4]Marshall H. Klaus and John H. Kennell, *Maternal-infant Bonding* (St. Louis, Mo.: C.V. Mosby Company, 1972), pp. 116-17.

8

The Lamaze method is based on the ability of the woman to actively or consciously relax her body while the uterus functions during labor. This ability is a conditioned response, learned by the couple through daily practice. Eventually, active relaxation becomes automatic behavior. This chapter includes exercises and massage techniques to help the mother learn active relaxation and to help the coach promote relaxation in his mate during practice and labor.

ACTIVE RELAXATION

Active, or conscious, relaxation is a physical state during which voluntary muscles (for example, arm and leg muscles) are totally relaxed, or passive, and the mind is awake and active. It is an art which can help you feel healthy, less tense and nervous, and more energetic. The Lamaze method utilizes active relaxation during labor contractions to attain a more comfortable, controlled labor.

Relaxation can help during labor in the following ways:

1. *Breaks the fear-tension-pain cycle.* It is known that pain increases fear and tension, and that tension only intensifies the pain. In labor, consciously relaxing your entire body while the involuntary uterine muscle contracts will help break this cycle.
2. *Conserves energy.* Contracting muscles unnecessary to labor uses excess energy, causing you to become more fatigued and less able to meet the physical demands of labor.
3. *Increases oxygen to the uterus.* Muscles utilize oxygen when they contract. If you are tense during contractions, you deprive the uterine muscle of oxygen. It will become more sensitive, more painful, and less efficient.
4. *Prevents increased adrenalin production.* Tension increases adren-

Relaxation and Massage

alin in your system, which inhibits the production of oxytocin, the hormone stimulating the uterus to contract. This reaction can prolong your labor by decreasing the efficiency of the uterine contractions. Adrenalin also decreases blood flow by constricting blood vessels. Since blood carries oxygen to the uterus, a decrease in flow can lessen the oxygen to the uterus and the baby.

5. *Provides a focus of attention.* Relaxation requires mental activity and will act as a focus of attention during contractions.

It is helpful to keep in mind that relaxation itself is passive; it is inactivity; it is absence of effort. It is not necessary to *do* anything when you are relaxing except think about letting your muscles "go negative."

There are three levels, or degrees, of relaxation. The first level is one in which the body parts feel *light* and airy. By practicing, you will achieve a deeper level, during which gravity begins to tug on your muscles, and you will have a *heavy*, or sinking, feeling. During the last and deepest state of relaxation, you will feel a sense of *detachment.* Your arms and legs may feel as if they are not attached to your body. To attain the deepest level takes patience and practice and requires that you release every thread of tension in your muscles.

Biofeedback is helpful in assessing muscle tension. If you have access to a biofeedback machine you might like to see how you are progressing in your relaxation.

Techniques

1. The mother should learn to *recognize tension and relaxation* in her own body. The coach should also learn to recognize tension and relaxation in the mother's body by observing and touching her muscles.
2. The mother should learn to use words, or *verbal cues,* that she says to herself or that her coach says to her to help her relax. Such words as melt, loose, heavy, warm, let go, sinking, and release are all good verbal cues.
3. The mother and coach should learn to use *visual imagery* to increase relaxation. Picture pleasant scenes that will promote relaxation: sitting under a tree in a grassy meadow on a warm spring day, lying in warm sand, sinking into a bed of feathers.
4. The mother should learn to *breathe slowly and deeply* as she concentrates on relaxing. Try to release, or let go, of tension each time you exhale or breathe out.
5. The coach should learn to use *massage* or gentle touch to reduce tension and provide reassurance and support.

Practice

To be able to reach a deep level of relaxation rapidly, as you will want to do during labor contractions, you should try to practice relaxation twice daily, at least one of these times with your coach. Choose a time during the day when you won't be interrupted. Remember your mind has to stay active and alert. If you have never consciously relaxed, don't spend more than 10 to 15 minutes at a practice session. As you improve you will be able to increase your practice time to 20 to 30 minutes. Use the suggested exercises in this chapter and other methods of relaxation with which you are familiar, such as yoga, meditation, or hypnosis.

Practice in a warm, dimly lit room. Relax in a semireclining position, well supported with pillows under your head, shoulders, back, arms, and knees.

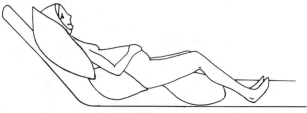

Semi-reclining Position for Relaxation

As you improve, practice in different positions—lying on your side, sitting tailor fashion, and sitting in a chair. (Recliner chairs are good for practicing.) Use pillows where needed, and don't allow one body part to bear the weight of another (see Chapter Three). Wear loose, comfortable clothing or very little clothing so the massage and stroking will be more effective.

Focal Point

One thing that helps you concentrate is a *focal point*, or any object upon which you focus your eyes. A focal point should be colorful and eye-catching. You can use something already in your labor or practice room or you can take a picture or object that you have used in practice sessions to the hospital. The focal point should be movable, as your labor position changes, or you can take several to put around the room. Avoid staring at the object, because this will cause it to blur.

Occasionally, a woman will say that it is easier to relax if her eyes are closed. In this case, she should practice both ways. However, it is preferable to keep your eyes open during labor so that you don't fall asleep and wake up at the peak of a contraction.

LEARNING ACTIVE RELAXATION

Your *goals* in practicing relaxation for use in labor are:

● To recognize how a muscle looks and feels when it is contracted or relaxed.

- To learn to release the tension or relax muscles that are tense.
- To learn to relax your voluntary muscles while your uterus is contracting during labor.

*Objective 1: Your first objective is to recognize how a muscle looks
and feels when it is contracted or relaxed.*

These exercises are for use in practice sessions. Apply what you
learn about relaxation to your own labor.

Contraction/Relaxation—Drill 1

*The coach's task is to begin to notice how the mother's body looks
when a muscle is contracted or relaxed.*

Ask the mother to contract or tighten individual body parts one at
a time, starting with her feet and ending with her face. Give her time to
accomplish each contraction. When her body is completely tense or contracted, reverse the order and have her relax each part of her body, starting
with her face and ending with her feet. Suggested body parts are:

> feet
> calves
> thighs
> buttocks
> stomach
> hands
> arms
> shoulders
> neck
> face

*The mother's task is to begin to recognize how a muscle feels when
it is contracted or relaxed.*

Following your coach's directions, contract individual body parts
until your whole body is tense. While your coach is talking about each
body part, concentrate on that part. Notice the sensations: the hard muscle,
the pull at the joints, and the dull ache if you contract too long. Now, as
your coach cues you to release the tension, concentrate on "letting go"
and notice how the muscles feel when they are relaxed: the heavy, limp
feeling and the comfortable looseness in the joints.

*Objective 2: Your second objective is to learn to release the tension
or relax muscles that are tense.*

Conscious Relaxation—Drill 2

*The coach's task is to help your mate relax muscles by talking
soothingly (verbal cues) and gently stroking (tactile cues).*

Direct the mother to inhale slowly while contracting the body part. Tell her to hold for a few seconds, then exhale and relax. Gently massage, stroke, or touch the tense body part as you tell her to release the tension. (See Massage later in this chapter.)

Forehead	Inhale and raise your eyebrows	Exhale and release
Jaw	Inhale and clench your teeth	Exhale and release
Neck	Inhale and push your head into the pillow	Exhale and release
Upper back	Inhale and pinch your shoulder blades together	Exhale and release
Shoulders	Inhale and shrug shoulders	Exhale and release
Right arm	Inhale and make a fist and straighten elbow	Exhale and release
Left arm	Inhale and make a fist and straighten elbow	Exhale and release
Abdomen	Inhale and pull in stomach muscles	Exhale and release
Buttocks	Inhale and tighten together	Exhale and release
Right leg	Inhale and tense your leg	Exhale and release
Left leg	Inhale and tense your leg	Exhale and release

Give her time to relax one body part totally before asking her to contract the next one. Give her verbal cues to help her relax deeper and deeper.

The mother's task is to become conditioned to respond to her coach's voice and touch with automatic relaxation and to condition herself to relax when she exhales.

When you contract a body part as your coach directs, think about how the muscles feel when they are tense. As you release the tension, notice the comfortable warmth of a relaxed muscle. Concentrate on letting it get heavier and heavier.

After repeated practice you should be able to respond immediately to your coach's touch and verbal cues.

As your ability to relax improves, contract the muscles a little less each time. Eventually, you will not need to contract the body part first but will focus your attention on that part and release residual tension.

Learning to Check for Relaxation

To instill confidence and help her relax, the coach should be *gentle* and considerate when checking the mother's relaxation. Try to develop your skill in observation so you can see tension in your mate as well as feel tension in her muscles.

- *Arms*
    1. Gently pick up her arm, supporting it at the elbow and wrist.

2. Slowly move her arm from side to side to see that it swings freely from the shoulder.

3. Maintaining the same gentle support of her arm, bend and straighten her elbow and wrist.

4. The joints should feel loose and relaxed and the arm should feel heavy.

5. Picking up her arm may make it difficult for her to relax, so instead, gently roll it back and forth.

- *Shoulders and neck*

   1. Feel for tension in the shoulders, upper back, and neck by placing your hands over the muscles in these areas and kneading gently.

   2. If tense, the muscles feel hard; if relaxed, they feel mushy.

- *Legs*

   1. Place one hand under the knee and the other hand under the calf, just above the ankle. Slowly raise the leg up just enough to gently move the leg at the hip and knee. Her leg should feel heavy and not offer any resistance. Place her leg back on the pillow and check her ankle for relaxation by moving her foot in a circle.

   2. Picking up her leg may make it difficult for the mother to relax, so instead, gently roll the leg back and forth at the thigh.

   3. Gently, but firmly, knead the upper thigh muscles and the calf to check for tension. If the muscles are not relaxed they will feel hard; if relaxed they feel mushy.

Objective 3: Your third objective is to learn to relax your voluntary muscles while your uterus is contracting during labor.

Lamaze Disassociation—Drill 3

The coach's task is to check for relaxation and to help the mother relax tense muscles.

Ask the mother to totally and consciously relax her body. Check her for relaxation. Then tell her to contract, or tighten, a part of her body, simulating the contracting uterus. Check the rest of her body for tension. Do not touch the contracted body part because your voice and touch are associated with relaxation. If she is tense, use verbal and tactile cues as well as massage to help her relax.

Use the following sequence:

1. Contract your right arm	Check relaxation	Release
2. Contract your left arm	Check relaxation	Release
3. Contract your right leg	Check relaxation	Release
4. Contract your left leg	Check relaxation	Release
5. Contract your right side	Check relaxation	Release
6. Contract your left side	Check relaxation	Release

7. Contract both arms	Check relaxation	Release
8. Contract both legs	Check relaxation	Release
9. Contract your right arm and left leg	Check relaxation	Release
10. Contract your left arm and right leg	Check relaxation	Release

The mother's task is to ignore the contracted body part and concentrate all her attention on total relaxation of the rest of her body. She will substitute another muscle for the contracting uterus during practice. In labor she will relax her entire body while her uterus contracts.

Find a focal point, contract one body part or parts as your coach directs, and concentrate on relaxing the rest of your body. If you or your coach notice tension in a body part, respond to your own cues to relax or to his coaching techniques.

Variation 1.

As your ability to relax improves, you can contract smaller body parts. Suggestions are:

1. Make a fist while keeping your upper arm relaxed.
2. Bend your elbow while keeping your wrist relaxed.
3. Tense your lower leg and ankles while keeping your buttocks relaxed.
4. Tense your forehead and eyes while keeping your mouth and jaw relaxed.

Variation 2.

To give the coach practice in locating tension, which he will be doing during labor, the mother should discretely contract a body part. The coach should try to locate the area of tension and coach her to relax.

SUMMARY OF THE COACH'S ROLE

1. To help the mother learn to relax.
2. To *develop techniques* that are effective in relaxing the mother—stroking, massage, verbal direction.
3. To check for and encourage relaxation during labor contractions.
4. To *practice daily* with the mother so she becomes conditioned to respond to your coaching.

LEARNING TO USE MASSAGE

Massage can be defined as the rhythmic stroking, kneading, tapping, or chopping of the body to cause either a sedative or stimulating effect on the underlying muscles.

Massage can be a pleasurable sensation for both partners, so the roles can be reversed occasionally, allowing the mother to massage her coach. This reversal can help the coach appreciate how difficult it can be to consciously relax and to realize that he is performing a pleasurable, helpful function during practice and labor.

Massage is to be used during practice sessions to increase relaxation and to assure that you'll know how to use it during labor. Used either during or between labor contractions, massage can help release muscle tension, increase circulation in the muscles, and give a pleasurable tactile sensation. It is usually reassuring to the mother, instilling confidence in her ability to control her labor as well as distracting her attention from the contracting uterus. Occasionally a woman will prefer not to be touched by her coach during contractions, but massage may still be helpful between contractions.

It is important for the coach and the mother to assume comfortable positions. The coach should be in a position that will avoid back strain.

Always massage bare skin by using some type of lubrication, such as powder, oil, or a nongreasy lotion. Your hands should glide, not bounce, across the skin. You should not massage the legs if the mother has varicose veins. However, if she has swelling in the ankles and legs, stroking the elevated leg muscles from the toes toward the body may help decrease the swelling.

Massage can be most successful if the mother tells the coach what feels good and helps her relax.

Effleurage, or Stroking

1. *On arms and legs:* Use your palms and fingers, molding your hands to fit the shape of the arm or leg. Stroke up and down, using long, smooth, rhythmic strokes, applying firm but gentle pressure. Do not lift your hands off the part you are massaging until you are finished. Repeat until the mother's muscles feel relaxed.

2. *On the back:* With your fingers spread apart and your thumbs on either side of the spinal column, start at the base of the mother's back and stroke up toward her shoulders, applying firm but gentle pressure.

When you reach her shoulders, go up and around them and come back down with lighter pressure. Repeat this pattern several times.

The mother should be lying on her side for this massage, unless she can still lie on her stomach supported by pillows under her head, chest, and hips.

3. *On the abdomen:* Do not apply deep pressure on the abdomen; stroke lightly, using your fingertips.

Start with both hands at the pubic bone. Bring them slowly and rhythmically up and out to both sides. Then stroke toward the middle and down the center to the pubic bone. You are making circles with each hand on either side of the abdomen.

Effleurage can be done in a semicircular motion with one hand in the area over the pubic bone.

Abdominal effleurage can be very effective when paired with a breathing pattern during contractions.

4. *On the lower back:* If the mother has mild lower back pain during labor, massage can be helpful.

Strokes are circular rather than in one direction. Using the heel and palm of your hand, make circular motions, moving slowly around the area. Pressure is firm but gentle, and you should not stay in one spot too long.

Petrissage, or Kneading

Petrissage is a gently squeezing, lifting, rolling motion over the muscles with firm, gentle pressure. It may be most useful between contractions, since it could be too distracting to use during them.

Use palms and fingers, molding your hands to fit the arm or leg. Start on either side of the lower leg or arm and knead the muscles, slowly moving upward toward the upper thigh or shoulder. Repeat until the mother's muscles feel mushy and relaxed.

A PATTERN FOR MASSAGE

1. Start by using effleurage; stroke in a downward direction with light pressure.
2. Go back up by kneading (petrissage).
3. Return in a downward direction, using lighter effleurage.

Remember: Effleurage can be used alternately with petrissage. Massaging too long, too fast, in an irregular pattern, or without lubrication can be stimulating rather than relaxing, resulting in muscle tension. It is important to make sure that you are not hurting the mother or producing tension. Communicate. Use these techniques postpartum, too.

9

Often when in pain or feeling uncomfortable, you find yourself holding your breath. In labor, this reaction is definitely a disadvantage, but it sometimes occurs with unprepared women. Instead of holding your breath, you will learn new behavior—breathing patterns to use along with conscious relaxation—to help you cope with the contractions of your uterus. Through practice, the breathing patterns will become automatic, so that during labor you will respond to the stimulus from the contracting uterus by using one of the patterned breathing techniques. Correct breathing not only increases your pain threshold and allows you to handle your contractions more effectively but also allows the uterus to function more efficiently.

Breathing patterns are important for the following reasons:

1. Muscles need oxygen to contract efficiently, and the uterus is no exception. If the uterus cannot contract efficiently because of lack of oxygen, labor may be prolonged. Controlled breathing during each contraction assures the availability of oxygen to the uterine muscle.

2. If the uterine muscle does not receive adequate oxygen it becomes more sensitive, and consequently, causes more pain for the mother.

3. If the mother becomes tense and holds her breath during contractions, she reduces the oxygen level in her blood; she is not only depriving her uterus of oxygen but her baby as well.

4. Because breathing patterns act as a focus of attention, the stimulus from the uterus is not perceived so completely.

5. Chest breathing, rather than abdominal breathing, is the basis of the Lamaze breathing patterns. By chest breathing, you are less likely to disturb the contracting uterus with the abdominal muscles. As the contractions increase in intensity, the breathing patterns become more

Controlled Breathing Patterns for Labor

shallow, reducing the downward movement of the diaphragm on the contracting uterus.

Breathing patterns can be practiced and used as follows:

1. The breathing patterns are used during contractions only. Between contractions, resume your normal rate of breathing. However, if between contractions you are uncomfortable, you may want to use conscious relaxation and first level breathing.

2. To help determine if you are chest breathing, place your hands on your lower ribs on each side. If your rib cage expands as you inhale, while your abdomen remains relatively quiet, you are breathing correctly. Because your abdominal muscles are attached to your rib cage, you will see some motion in the abdomen, but you should not be actively using your abdominal muscles for the breathing. Keep your shoulder and neck muscles relaxed.

3. To help you concentrate while simulating or actually having a contraction, you will keep your eyes on a focal point.

4. While practicing, your coach will give you the cue to start and stop a breathing pattern by saying, "contraction begins," and "contraction ends."

You can simulate contractions for practice and practice when you have Braxton-Hicks contractions. In labor, you will use the onset of a contraction as your cue to begin the breathing patterns and relaxation.

5. Begin and end each breathing pattern with a *deep, cleansing (or releasing) breath.* Take a deep breath in through your nose and exhale through your mouth.

Think of the cleansing (or releasing) breath as a cue to your body to relax completely. It also signals your coach and nurse that a contraction is beginning or ending.

6. Be sure your breathing is even and rhythmic. Inhale and exhale equal amounts of air so that you don't upset the oxygen and carbon dioxide balance in your system. If you inhale and exhale unequal amounts, you may hyperventilate (see discussion of hyperventilation later in this chapter).

7. Practice the breathing patterns twice daily, at least once with your coach. If you become dizzy or light-headed, decrease the length of the simulated contraction to twenty seconds and then gradually increase it. You may also benefit by practicing the breathing pattern more slowly.

8. Change positions during practice sessions, as you will do in labor.

9. Do not start using your breathing patterns for labor until you need them. Your first tool in labor should be *active relaxation.* When this technique alone is no longer effective, add *first-level breathing.* Do not switch to a more difficult breathing pattern until the one you are using is no longer effective in helping you maintain control. The easier the breathing pattern, the less energy it requires.

THE COACH'S ROLE

1. During practice, time the mother's contractions. Tell her when the contraction begins:

"You're going to have a contraction. Get ready. Contraction begins. Take a cleansing breath."

If helpful to the mother, tell her how she is progressing through the contraction; for example,

"Twenty seconds—you're getting toward the peak. Half over. Contraction's nearly over now."

Remind her to take a cleansing breath at the end of the contraction.

"Contraction's over. Take a cleansing breath."

2. During practice and labor, check her for relaxation and help her relax by giving her verbal and tactile cues.
3. Make sure her breathing is rhythmical. It may help to count or gently tap to the appropriate rhythm. If necessary, breathe with her.
4. Keep her breathing as quiet, relaxed, and slow as possible.
5. You may simulate a contraction's pressure during practice sessions by applying firm, even pressure on the muscle area above her knee or elbow. Don't pinch. Gradually increase the pressure, maintain it, and then decrease it as a contraction would accelerate, peak, and then ease off.

FIRST-LEVEL BREATHING: SLOW AND DEEP

The contractions are of mild intensity, and the mother is able to maintain the same slow, even breathing throughout the contraction. The apex is moderately harder than the rest of the contraction.

1. This breathing is slow, even, chest breathing.
2. Breathe in through your nose and out through your nose or mouth. As you inhale, allow your rib cage to expand.
3. Take between six and nine breaths per 60-second contraction.
4. Initially, it is helpful for the coach to count out the contraction, and later, for the mother to count the pattern to herself. The counting will help keep her mind occupied and the breathing even.
5. If you were going to take six breaths per minute, you would be slowly inhaling for five seconds and exhaling for five seconds. You could count like this, with one count every second:

> In two three four five
> Out two three four five . . .
> and so on throughout the contraction.

6. If this count seems too slow, merely decrease the number to which you count, and you will be breathing faster.

The pattern looks like the following:

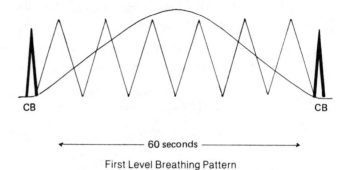

CB   CB

←————————— 60 seconds —————————→

First Level Breathing Pattern

SECOND-LEVEL BREATHING: ACCELERATED-DECELERATED

The need for second-level breathing arises because the contraction's apex is now too strong for the mother to comfortably control with first-level breathing. She feels the need to breathe faster at the peak of the contraction.

1. The breathing pattern is accelerated (more shallow and rapid) as the intensity of the contraction increases, is fairly rapid at the peak, and decelerates (slows and gets deeper) as the contraction decreases in intensity.
2. Breathe in through your nose and out through your mouth.
3. Remember that as your breathing accelerates, it *must* become more *shallow*. It may help you to place your hand at your throat as a reminder.
4. Initially it is helpful to use a set pattern of counting. You would count in the following way, keeping in mind that each count is approximately one second:

> In   two   three   four
> Out   two   three   four
> In   two   three
> Out   two   three
> In   two
> Out   two

This count takes approximately 20 seconds, or the time in which the contraction is increasing in intensity.

At the apex of the contraction (approximately 20 seconds) breathe

In   out
In   out . . . and so on.

At the end of the apex, as the contraction begins to decrease in intensity, count

In   two
Out   two
In   two   three
Out   two   three
In   two   three   four
Out   two   three   four

The pattern looks like the following:

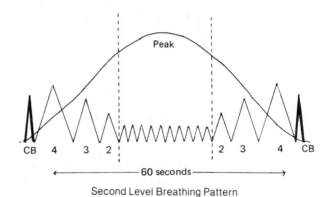

Second Level Breathing Pattern

5. Once you have learned this pattern, you will need to learn how to vary the breathing to fit your individual contractions. Some women's contractions will peak faster, last longer than 60 seconds, or have a longer peak.

For instance, if you find the peak of your contraction lasting longer, stay with the shallow in-out pattern until you feel the contraction easing. The pattern would look like the following:

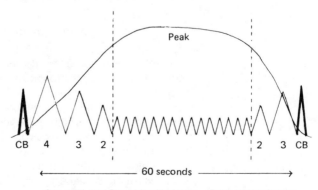

Second Level Breathing Variation—Peak lasting longer

If your contractions suddenly peak sooner than 20 seconds, you may be caught off guard. Remember that you can switch to peak breathing regardless of where you are in the counting. Adapt your breathing pattern for the next contractions by shortening the buildup counting. The pattern might look like the following:

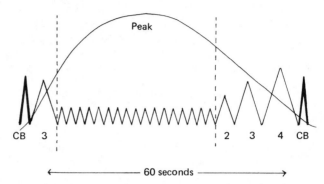

CB   3   2   3   4   CB

←———————————— 60 seconds ————————————→

Second Level Breathing Variation—Contraction which peaks suddenly

You need to accommodate this breathing pattern by remembering:

You breathe as slowly as you can as long as you can.
When you have to, you breathe faster and shallower.
As soon as you can, you slow the breathing down.

Trust your body's sensations and adapt the breathing pattern to them. This pattern will be more effective if you are not too rigid about the counting during labor.

THIRD-LEVEL BREATHING: TRANSITION

By transition, the woman's contractions are consistently long and intense. They may seem to be all peak or to have multiple peaks. The woman breathes a rapid pattern throughout the contraction.

1. This breathing is more rapid and *must be shallow.*
2. You will need to breathe through your mouth.
3. The pattern consists of three "Hees" and a "Hoo."
4. Keep your mouth in a semismiling position during the Hee-Hee-Hee portion of the pattern. Slightly purse your lips during the Hoo portion. If this breathing pattern makes your mouth dry, place your tongue against the roof of your mouth.
5. These contractions get hard very quickly, so you need to start the pattern with a rapid cleansing breath. Then breathe in through your mouth (the "ah" sound) and exhale by making a *quiet* "Hee" sound.

Do this three times. After you inhale the fourth time, exhale by making a *quiet* ''Hoo'' sound. Repeat this pattern through the contraction, and end with a few cleansing breaths.

6. This pattern is not counted, as were the two previous ones. It looks like the following:

> (ah) Hee
> (ah) Hee
> (ah) Hee
> (ah) Hoo . . . and so on.

7. Do not exaggerate the Hoo sound nor pause on it before beginning the next series. Keep the breathing at the same rate all the way through, just as if you were breathing to the rhythm of a metronome. Try not to speed up as the contraction gets harder.

The pattern looks like the following:

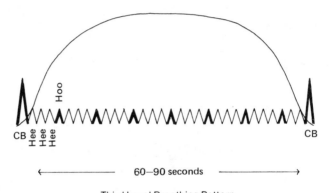

60—90 seconds

Third Level Breathing Pattern

8. For some people this breathing pattern is too naturally easy and rhythmic. To make it more difficult, involving more concentration, you can vary the number of Hees and Hoos. For instance:

4 Hees and 1 Hoo (or)
5 Hees and 1 Hoo (or)
2 Hees and 1 Hoo for strongest part of contraction (or)
The pattern: 2 Hees and 1 Hoo, 4 Hees and 1 Hoo, and 6 Hees and 1 Hoo.
Reverse the order or repeat.

BREATHING FOR A PREMATURE URGE TO PUSH

During a transition contraction, you may feel an urge to push or bear down. It is very important not to push until you have been told that your cervix is completely dilated. If you were to push too soon, you might cause swelling or laceration of the cervix. Controlling the urge to push before you are dilated can be very difficult, but this breathing can help.

1. If you have the urge to push, breathe in and blow out gently through your mouth, keeping your cheeks and lips floppy and relaxed. Do not blow hard, pursing your lips, as if you were trying to blow out all the candles on a birthday cake. Blowing hard may cause you to hyperventilate or to bear down with your abdominal muscles.
2. When and if the urge to push subsides, return to the Hee–Hee–Hee–Hoo pattern until the contraction is over.
3. The urge to push can come and go more than once during a contraction. Use the blowing each time you feel it.

The transition pattern, with the breathing for the urge to push, now looks like the following:

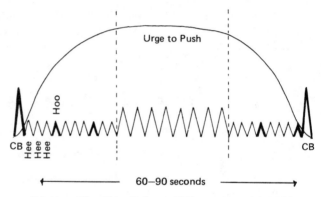

Third Level Breathing Pattern—With urge to push breathing

HYPERVENTILATION

Sometimes women *hyperventilate* when they use the controlled breathing techniques, either in practice or in labor. Technically, hyperventilation results from an imbalance of carbon dioxide and oxygen in the body; specifically, exhaling too much carbon dioxide. The result is too much oxygen in the body.

You may hyperventilate if you

● Lose control or lose the rhythm of the breathing patterns.
● Breathe in and out unequal amounts of air, i.e., exhale more air than you inhale.

- Are unable to relax, especially your shoulder and neck muscles.
- Become panicky.

If you hyperventilate, you may have the following sensations:

- Tingling and/or numbness in your fingers, toes, upper lip, and tip of your nose.
- Dizziness, feeling light-headed, or faint.
- Spots in front of your eyes.
- Muscle cramps.
- Spasms in one or both hands.

If you hyperventilate, you and/or your coach should do the following:

1. At the *first* signs of hyperventilation, rebreathe your carbon dioxide

Breathing Pattern	Possible Problem	Possible Cure
Level 1 Slow and Deep	Breathing too fast Breathing too deeply	Slow down or switch to accelerated— decelerated (Level 2)
Level 2 Accelerated- Decelerated	Inhaling and exhaling unequal amounts of air, especially exhaling too much Breathing too deeply over the accelerated peak	Count the inhale and exhale in an effort to make breathing more rhythmic Breathe more shallowly and rhythmically
Level 3 Transition	Breathing too deeply Emphasizing the exhale in the Hee-Hee-Hee-Hoo pattern Speeding up breathing pattern or allowing it to become irregular	Breathe more shallowly Do not emphasize; breathe quietly Regain slower, more regular pattern

by breathing into a surgical mask, paper bag, or cupped hands covering your mouth and nose both during and between contractions until your symptoms disappear. You may continue to use the breathing patterns during contractions.

2. Your coach should encourage relaxation, especially in your shoulders and neck, by light massage and verbal cues. The coach may need to breathe with you, counting or tapping out the rhythm of the pattern during difficult contractions.

3. Hold your breath a few seconds at the end of the contractions until all your symptoms are gone.

4. If hyperventilation is severe or your symptoms do not disappear with these suggestions, stop the breathing pattern and breathe normally into a mask or bag. Resume the breathing pattern when you feel better.

5. It is important for you to be alert for symptoms and take measures to cure them right away. Left untreated, hyperventilation can be potentially serious to you and your baby and can affect your ability to stay in control of your contractions. Tell your nurse or doctor if you are hyperventilating.

6. Practice will help you master the breathing patterns and make it less likely that you will hyperventilate during labor.

10

This chapter deals with some of the variations that can occur in labor. Included are back labor, breech presentation, induction, fetal monitoring, and multiple birth.

BACK PAIN DURING LABOR

Continuous back pain during labor is referred to as *back labor.* The pain has been described as everything from a dull ache to a sharp knife-like pain. It can be present during contractions or both during and between contractions. The pain can be localized in one spot or radiate over the entire low back and even into the thighs. You may not be aware of contractions in your abdomen.

There are many theories concerning the actual cause of the back pain, but the general consensus is that the hard, bony part of the back of the baby's head presses on the mother's muscles, bones, and ligaments, resulting in pain. This situation occurs when the baby is in a posterior position, either head first or breech. The more usual anterior position means that the softer front parts of the baby's face are resting against the mother's back, and therefore not causing as much discomfort in the back.

The symptoms of a possible posterior presentation, which may result in back labor, are as follows:

1. More backache in the last few weeks of pregnancy.
2. Irregular labor contractions, especially during the active phase; the length, interval, and intensity vary. The pattern is often one longer, stronger contraction followed by one or two shorter, milder contractions.[1]

[1] Joy Clausen *et al., Maternity Nursing Today* (New York: McGraw-Hill Book Company, 1973), p. 473.

Variations in Childbirth

3. Physical and emotional fatigue due to slow, prolonged labor.
4. Restlessness and difficulty in relaxing.
5. Longer pushing stage if the baby fails to rotate. Your doctor may use forceps or manually rotate the baby so that he is born in a face-down (anterior) position.

To relieve pain from back labor:

1. Use only those positions that keep the baby's head from resting directly on your spine:
    a. Sit up in the bed or chair and lean forward against the bedside table.
    b. Lie on the side opposite the baby's back.
    c. Get on your hands and knees.
2. Change your position frequently.
3. If possible, try pelvic tilting on all fours; this movement may also facilitate fetal rotation.
4. A change in temperature may help: hot water bottle, heating pad, or cold compress.
5. *Very firm sacral pressure in the lower back* by the labor coach is often helpful. The coach uses the heel and palm of his hand to apply firm, steady pressure to the base of the mother's spine. He should be careful to apply steady pressure and not jar the mother during a contraction. It may be helpful to apply powder or lotion to her back first. You will be able to use this remedy more effectively during labor if you have practiced beforehand.
6. The coach should provide much needed emotional support and relate information to the mother regarding her progress.
7. Use relaxation and breathing techniques. Breathing at a slower rate and concentrating on counting out the pattern seem to help keep the mind occupied. Striving for relaxation is very important.
8. Although it is discouraged, if you must lie on your back, lie on a rolled towel, bath blanket, or sheet, which will provide counter-pressure to the painful area of your back. During a contraction, the coach should put his hands between your back and the bed and push up against your back. You can also rest against two clean tennis balls placed on either side of your spine to provide counterpressure where you feel the most pain.

BREECH PRESENTATION

Breech presentation refers to the buttocks, feet, or knees preceding the head through the birth canal. The incidence of breech is 3 to 4 percent[2] with a term baby but higher with prematurity. A vaginal breech delivery

[2]Harry Oxorn and William R. Foote, *Human Labor and Birth,* 3rd ed. (New York: Appleton-Century-Crofts, 1975), p. 193.

may be possible when the baby is a complete or frank breech, depending upon the position of his legs and the maternal pelvic measurements.

Since the part of the baby helping to dilate the cervix is soft and smaller than the head, it may take more time for the cervix to reach complete dilatation. Also, because of the smaller size of the presenting part, it could move through the cervix before complete dilatation, causing a premature urge to push. During labor, the baby's head under your ribs may be uncomfortable, and raising the backrest of the bed should help. Statistically, breech labors and deliveries are not significantly longer.[3]

Sometimes a breech presentation requires a Cesarean birth because the doctor believes that it would be safer for both mother and infant to avoid the stress of labor or that the baby's head would not fit through the pelvis (see Chapter Twelve). The incidence of Cesarean birth increases with a premature breech baby because the head is larger than the chest. The chest of a term baby is about equal to the head size, so it helps to dilate the cervix for the head. The doctor wants to avoid a situation in which the premature baby's body slips through the cervix without dilating it sufficiently for the head.

Because of decreased maneuverability of the presenting part, some breech deliveries are a little harder. Also more common is prolapse of the umbilical cord, in which the cord comes through the cervix before the baby's body and is compressed between the mother's bony pelvis and the presenting part. If the cord is compressed, the baby's oxygen supply would be decreased.

The passing of meconium during labor is not unusual in a breech delivery. The contractions cause pressure on the lower part of the baby's body, pressing it against the mother's pelvis.

When a breech is going to be delivered vaginally, the mother may be x-rayed during labor to make sure that her pelvic measurements are adequate for the baby's head measurements. She may be given a trial labor before the method of delivery is determined. Also, the doctor will probably request that minimal anesthesia, if any, be used, enabling the mother to feel completely the expulsion contractions and to push more effectively. Vaginal breech deliveries are often accomplished through the pushing efforts of the mother and use of forceps to deliver the head. An episiotomy is usually necessary to enlarge the vaginal outlet for the head and forceps.

Breech babies are sometimes born with swollen or bruised buttocks and genitals, much like molding in vertex deliveries. This condition will soon disappear.

The mother and coach can cooperate in a breech delivery as follows:

1. Relaxation and breathing techniques can help the mother maintain control.

[3]*Ibid.*, p. 194.

2. The urge to push before complete dilatation is usual, so it is important for the coach to assist the mother in breathing for a premature urge to push.
3. Coaching is of utmost importance, since anesthesia may not be permitted. Praise for the mother's efforts is important.
4. Since a vaginal breech delivery is more uncommon than a vertex one, it is important that the mother receive information and assurance that nothing is wrong.

INDUCTION

An induction is a labor that is started artificially. It is one means of protecting the life of the mother and the infant when it is determined that a baby must be born and labor has not begun on its own.

Inductions are performed for the following reasons:

1. For the mother's health and well-being, as in the case of severe maternal toxemia or a history of previous *precipitous* (extremely rapid) labors.
2. For the infant's health and well-being, as in the case of maternal diabetes or documented (dates are certain) postmaturity. Diabetes can sometimes cause problems for the baby toward the end of pregnancy. With postmaturity, the placenta does not always function adequately, endangering the baby's life.
3. For the health and well-being of both mother and baby; if a mother's membranes are ruptured for over 24 hours without spontaneous labor, there is a danger of intrauterine infection, jeopardizing both mother and baby.
4. For elective reasons; inductions for reasons of convenience or when not medically necessary are generally discouraged. There are more risks to induction than to a spontaneous labor.

The doctor evaluates the baby's condition and readiness to be born as follows:

1. The *Oxytocin Challenge Test* (OCT) may be given. A small amount of *Pitocin* (synthetic oxytocin) is administered through an IV, and the mother is given a trial labor. The baby's heart rate is monitored and evaluated to see how he responds to three labor contractions in a ten-minute period. During a contraction, blood flow through the placenta is decreased, and the baby's heart rate drops. If the heart rate recovers before the end of the contraction it is a good indication. From this test the doctor can determine whether the baby would be under stress if an induction were performed.

2. The doctor can also evaluate a series of *estriol levels*. The baby's adrenal gland produces a substance that is converted to estriol by the placenta. The level of estriol in the baby's system can be measured in

maternal blood or urine samples. The doctor expects to see the estriol level rise after 28 weeks of gestation and continue this trend until term. A significant drop in estriol levels over a period of time may indicate that the baby is at risk and should be delivered.[4]

For a urinary estriol test, the mother collects all urine for a 24-hour period. For a blood estriol, a blood sample is taken from the mother. The latter method is considerably faster and less vulnerable to error.

3. The *nonstress test* is a noninvasive method of determining fetal well-being. The mother is monitored externally for ten minutes to obtain a baseline reading of the fetal heart rate.

The rate is again observed during a twenty-minute period which includes at least two fetal movements. The doctor hopes to see the heart rate accelerate with the fetal movements. This is a good indication that the baby is functioning adequately in his uterine environment.

4. The *fetal movement test* is another noninvasive method of determining fetal well-being. The mother counts the number of fetal movements she feels in a certain period of time. Generally, she would feel about ten movements in a two-hour period after 36 weeks of gestation.

The doctor can use a measure known as the Bishop Score to evaluate the mother's readiness for induction. This measure takes into account the following conditions:

1. *Dilatation of the cervix:* Is there any dilatation prior to labor or is the cervix still closed?
2. *Effacement of the cervix:* Is there any effacement prior to labor?
3. *The baby's station:* Is the head engaged in the pelvis or even lower (+ station), or is the head still free-floating (− station)?
4. *The consistency of the cervix:* Is it firm or is it ripe (soft) in preparation for labor?
5. *The position of the cervix:* Is it still posterior or has it moved forward in preparation for labor?

The doctor evaluates these conditions and makes a decision about the probable success of induction.

Two procedures can act as inducers if the mother's cervix is favorable: *enema* and *rupture of the membranes*. Labor is usually started, however, by synthetic oxytocics. *Pitocin* (sometimes called "pit") is commonly used. It is an artificial substitute for the natural hormone secreted by the pituitary gland, and it causes the uterus to contract.

Pitocin is most safely administered through an intravenous infusion (IV) into the mother's arm. The amount is carefully monitored. Continuous assessment of the baby's response to the Pitocin-induced contractions—his heart rate—is made. The mother's response—strength of

[4]Dyanne Affonso and Ann Clark, *Childbearing: A Nursing Perspective* (Philadelphia: Davis and Company, 1976), p. 313.

uterine contractions—is also monitored. Usually a fetal monitor will be used for these assessments (see discussion of fetal monitors later in this chapter). The number of Pitocin drops per minute is varied to arrive at a safe rate for both mother and baby, usually producing 60-second contractions every two to three minutes.

Your labor will be different if an induction is performed. An induction means that the latent phase is probably eliminated. The mother does not go through a slow, progressive buildup of contractions, that is, 30-second contractions every 20 minutes, gradually increasing over a period of hours to 60-second contractions every 5 minutes. Once Pitocin is administered and takes effect, you will have contractions of good strength, length, and frequency, and you will miss the opportunity to accustom yourself gradually to the contractions of active labor. Thus, labor may seem harder to control. Also, these strong contractions may not produce a change in the cervix right away, which can be quite discouraging to the mother and coach. On the plus side, if the cervix is ready, inductions generally result in labors shorter than spontaneous ones.

If you are to have an induction,

1. Be sure you have thoroughly discussed it with your doctor and know exactly what to expect. If you have questions, *ask*; don't worry. Pain is intensified by fear.

2. Be sure to sleep the night before the induction; pain is intensified by fatigue. If you think you won't be able to sleep because of excitment or anticipation, ask your doctor for some safe medication to help you sleep. It will be easier for you to work with your labor if you're well rested.

3. Be prepared for extra medical equipment and personnel. An induction generally means an IV; an external, or sometimes an internal, fetal monitor; and a machine to count drops of Pitocin. It also requires the continual presence of a nurse or other medical personnel. An induction is not the private affair between father and mother that a spontaneous labor sometimes is.

If labor is not progressing at a good rate or if it stops, Pitocin can be used to *augment* labor. An IV, a fetal monitor, and a nurse are present, as in the case of a regular induction. You can expect that the length, intensity, and frequency of the contractions will increase once the Pitocin is administered.

FETAL MONITORING

By means of electronic devices, it is possible to monitor continuously your baby's heart rate and to measure the frequency, length, and strength of your uterine contractions during labor. The monitor produces a printout which enables the nurse and physician to observe the baby's heart rate in response to the mother's contractions. An external or an internal monitor may be used.

By observing the quality of contractions, the doctor can assess how well the mother's uterus is functioning in labor. By observing the baby's heart *rate, variability,* and *periodic changes* in response to the uterine contractions, the doctor can determine how well the baby is responding to the stress of labor. The normal heart rate for the fetus is 120 to 160 beats per minute, and it will be changing within this range in response to the contractions. Certain patterns, depending on when they occur in the contraction, indicate fetal distress.

If a pattern of irregularity or slowing in the baby's heart rate occurs, the medical staff can take steps, such as altering the mother's position, giving her oxygen, or increasing her IV fluids, in order to restore normal circulation to the baby. The staff may also take a sample of the baby's blood from the scalp to confirm fetal distress.

The fetal monitor is not the only way to measure contractions and fetal heart tones. When a monitoring device is not used, the mother's contractions are evaluated by her labor–delivery nurse. She determines the strength, length, and frequency of contractions by resting her fingertips on the fundus of the mother's uterus and timing and evaluating the contraction. The baby's heart tones can be evaluated through a stethoscope, fetoscope, or dopler (an electronic listening device.)

Because electronic monitors provide continuously available information about contractions and fetal heart tones, rather than intermittent readings, some doctors favor their use, especially when the mother is at risk, medication has been used, or the labor has been augmented with Pitocin. However, studies have upheld the belief of some physicians that a well-trained and observant labor–delivery nurse can successfully monitor a laboring woman and pick up signs of fetal distress.

Two small sensing devices are placed against the mother's abdomen by means of a belt fastened around her hips. One device measures the pressure exerted by the contraction. This rise and fall of pressure is reproduced on a moving paper graph, and it is accurate for the duration and frequency, but not the intensity, of the contraction.

At the same time, another small device (usually ultrasound) measures the baby's heart rate and is plotted alongside the pattern of the contraction. The doctor can see that at the beginning of the contraction, the baby's heart rate was x beats per minute, and that it dropped to y beats per minute at the apex of the contraction, and so on. External monitors are not "beat-to-beat" accurate; that is, for every beat of the baby's heart, the machine does not necessarily register a beat. Instead, the machine averages the beats.

Internal Monitors

Internal monitors produce the same information, but it is obtained by sensing devices inserted through the vagina into the uterus.

The contraction is monitored by a small fluid-filled catheter which

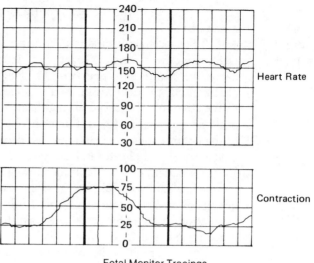

Fetal Monitor Tracings

registers pressure change in millimeters of mercury. This figure is reproduced as a wave on the paper graph. The baby's EKG (electrocardiogram) is monitored by a tiny electrode inserted under his scalp.

Internal Versus External Monitors

External monitors are not as accurate as internal ones. Printouts can be affected when the mother changes position, coughs, and so on. Internal monitoring is considerably more accurate. It requires that the membranes be ruptured and that a certain amount of dilatation be completed already. A patient is usually monitored externally unless a problem arises or a more accurate reading of fetal heart tones is necessary.

Nonmedical Advantage

After the equipment has been explained to him, the father benefits by being able to see the contraction pattern. He can tell his mate when a contraction is beginning, when she is through the apex, and so on. It is a way for the father to be more involved, *as long as the monitor does not become the center of attention.*

Disadvantages

External monitors can be a disadvantage if they limit the mother's movements, although often the nurse is able to reposition the sensing device when the mother moves. Sometimes monitors work well only when the woman is on her back, a most undesirable position in which to labor. Often a situation can be worked out in which occasionally the mother is on her back for a contraction or two to monitor the fetal heart rate, and then she is allowed to resume a more comfortable position. At other times the monitor can be positioned with the mother on her side. Monitors restrict a woman's ability to move about at will.

Internal monitors do not require these restrictions; however, they do require that the membranes be ruptured, which can alter the quality of the mother's contractions, and they do carry a small risk of infection.

No matter which monitor is used, it should be remembered that the mother, not the printout, is the center of attention. The father should not sit with his back to the mother, just to be able to observe the monitor, nor should the hospital personnel.

Research is continuing to verify the safety of fetal monitors.

MULTIPLE BIRTH: TWINS

Twins can be identical or fraternal. Identical twins are the result of one sperm fertilizing one egg, which then divides into two fertilized eggs. Since they have identical genes, these twins are always of the same sex and appearance. Fraternal twins occur because two eggs are fertilized by two sperm. The babies can be the same or different sexes and will look no more alike than any other siblings.

Twins occur once in every 99 conceptions.[5] About three-fourths are fraternal, one-fourth identical. There seems to be a familial tendency for fraternal twins, and the chance of having twins increases with multiparas and the maternal age at conception.

The authorities seem to agree that it can be difficult to diagnose twins, and sometimes the doctor and parents do not know until birth. Some indicating factors include history of twins, especially in the maternal family; abdominal and uterine growth too large for the number of weeks of pregnancy; unexplained excessive weight gain; palpatation of two babies or hearing two heartbeats. Ultrasound or x-ray can usually verify the presence of twins.

Pregnancy

The main difference in carrying twins is that your uterus becomes larger earlier and the discomforts of the third trimester arrive sooner. An increase in backache is common and your cervix may efface and dilate earlier. Some doctors restrict intercourse in the last trimester since premature labor is more common with twins. Mothers are encouraged to get extra rest. If twins are diagnosed during pregnancy, parents can some-

[5]Margaret Duncan Jensen, Ralph C. Benson, and Irene M. Bobak, *Maternity Care: The Nurse and the Family* (St. Louis, Mo.: C. V. Mosby Company, 1977), p. 380.

times identify specific characteristics in each baby; for instance, one may be more active and sleep less. Check with your doctor about your diet and weight gain; you may need extra calories for two babies and need to eat smaller, more frequent meals.

Labor and Delivery

Twins are usually smaller at birth, and the second twin born is usually smaller than the first. The most common presentations are (1) both babies vertex, or (2) the first vertex and the second breech. Medications are usually limited for labor, especially if the babies are small and early. After the first twin is born, the second baby's membranes are ruptured to allow a leak while he is helped into a longitudinal presentation, if necessary, and then delivered. If the second baby does not assume a favorable presentation, a Cesarean delivery would be necessary. Both placentas are then delivered. Because the uterine wall is so stretched and contractions can be less effective, the mother should be sure she is very good at the pushing techniques learned in class.

Postpartum Recovery

The physical recovery is basically the same, but the emotional adjustment of the parents to two babies may deserve some extra attention, especially if the twins were not diagnosed before birth. Caring for two infants can be exhausting. It is probably a good idea to seek some help at home for a while, either from friends or relatives. The increased cost of two babies can be a burden for many parents. If the babies are premature and require continued hospitalization, the parents will have to deal with the anxiety of separation, even though most hospitals welcome parents in their special-care nurseries.

Many women are concerned about being able to breast feed twins. The technique is the same (see Chapter Two), but the babies will usually nurse on only one breast each. Some women choose to nurse both babies at the same time; others prefer one at a time. Most mothers of twins prefer to coax the babies into a similar schedule to avoid the feeling of always feeding a baby. Another approach to breast feeding is to nurse one baby on both sides at a feeding, giving the other baby a supplement; the babies switch sources for the next feeding. Refer to Nutrition in Chapter One and plan your diet to provide extra calories for a milk supply adequate for two babies. Whatever your approach, find a supportive person to call on for assistance, for example, LaLeche League or another mother of twins, and reread your resource book on breast feeding.

Raising twins can be both challenging and rewarding. The twins usually develop a unique and close relationship. After the initial year or so, when the babies are a little more independent, parents usually have more time to relax and enjoy their special family.

National Organization of Mothers of Twins Clubs, Inc.
Executive Offices: 5402 Amberwood Lane
Rockville, Maryland 20853

This organization encourages research and education about twins and tries to make information including a bibliography available to the public.

11

Timing is usually an important concern with later children. Perhaps the children are close enough in age so that they can be companions for one another—which frequently results in a period of time when parents are caring for two babies. The mother's plans for resuming her education or career may contribute to close spacing, or her age may be a factor if she has waited to have her children. Other times, parents have preferred to space their children so that the older child is fairly independent and self-reliant before another baby is born. Sometimes an unexpected pregnancy or infertility determines the spacing of children. No matter what is decided, there are joys and difficulties with any age span.

Another factor that enters into planning for a later baby is your physical well-being. A doctor's medical advice should be sought before another pregnancy to assure that your body has recovered from the previous one before undergoing the strain of another.

Once the spacing is established, parents usually spend time during pregnancy planning how they will deal emotionally with the spacing.

The sex of the child often becomes more important when a family is expecting their second baby. Usually parents would like one of each, but sometimes they prefer two of a kind.

Sometimes parents worry about whether they will have enough love for a second child. Will the love be divided between two children or grow to be enough for two? How can you be mother or father enough for two children? How can you financially support another child?

Having enough time for two (or more) children is another real concern, especially if the older child is still quite young and in need of a lot of time and care. Parents become concerned with meshing the schedules of two children. Often you worry if the older child will suffer because the baby demands so much attention.

When you have one child, it's hard to imagine how a second child could be different from the first. If you are pleased with the older child, you may worry about whether the second child can be as wonderful. If you are upset about the behavior of the first child, you may hope for a better relationship with the second. After having two children who are

Later Births

very different, you become curious about what new and different personality will blossom in the new infant.

Most women have a different experience with each pregnancy. If your first pregnancy was a good one, you will hope for the same again. If the first experience was difficult, you may dread some of the physical and emotional changes that upset you the first time. Remember that each pregnancy can be different.

When you were pregnant the first time, you had no past experience to help you know what to expect each trimester. The second or third time, you know how much your body and emotions are likely to change. You know more about the progress of pregnancy and how it affects you.

If this is to be your last pregnancy, you may feel some nostalgia about the loss of this special state of being, no matter how uncomfortable you may be.

These feelings can apply to childbirth, too. If your first experience was good, you may worry if this delivery can be as smooth and uncomplicated as the first. If your first experience was not all that you hoped for, you may wonder if this birth will be better.

During a woman's second or later pregnancy both mother and father have an added confidence about caring for the baby. Having already cared for a newborn, they are usually not greatly concerned this time, although they might wonder if the knowledge will all come back.

If your first baby was easy to care for, you certainly hope for this good fortune again. If the first baby was difficult to care for, you probably hope that this one will be easier. Having been through postpartum once, you will know basically what to expect; and will probably be more tolerant and relaxed, knowing that the newborn state is temporary.

PREGNANCY, LABOR, AND DELIVERY

What is different about pregnancy, labor, and delivery with subsequent babies?

Before going into labor:

1. The uterus may appear to be round, rather than ovoid, because of weak abdominal muscles.
2. Because of weaker abdominal muscles, lightening (or the "dropping" of the baby) does not usually occur before labor. When the pubic arch widens late in pregnancy, the pelvic floor relaxes, and the lower segment of the uterus softens, engagement will occur and the baby's head will drop further into the pelvis *if* there are firm abdominal muscles. In their absence, the uterus sags further forward and engagement does not usually occur until labor begins.
3. *Multiparas* generally deliver at forty weeks or earlier rather than going beyond their due date, as is common with primiparas.

4. Multiparas generally have weaker pelvic floor muscles, which contribute to greater pressure and more discomfort on the pelvic floor. The pelvic tilt helps tip the uterus out of the pelvis and relieves pressure. Devote extra time to practicing the exercises for the pelvic floor (see Chapter Three).
5. A multipara will probably have more Braxton-Hicks contractions and more false labor than a primipara. Braxton-Hicks contractions often become increasingly uncomfortable with succeeding pregnancies.

During labor:

1. Unlike a primipara, whose cervix may efface before it begins to dilate, a multipara may efface and dilate simultaneously.

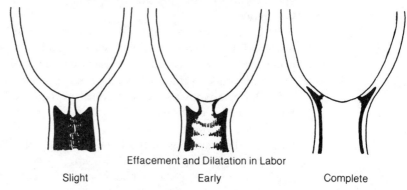

Effacement and Dilatation in Labor

Slight   Early   Complete

2. The *average* length of time spent in labor and delivery is shorter than for a primipara. Friedman has compiled figures showing the *average* duration of labor for a multipara. The following is an adapted graph.[1]

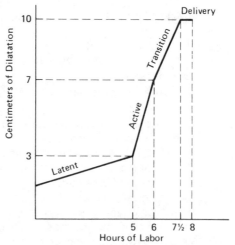

Friedman's Labor Curve for a Multipara

[1]From Emmanuel Friedman, M.D., *Labor: Clinical Evaluation and Management*, 2nd ed., p. 33. Copyright © 1978 by Appleton-Century-Crofts. Used courtesy of Appleton-Century-Crofts and the author.

Early (latent) labor dilatation to 3 cm	5 ¼ hours
Active labor dilatation from 3 to 7 cm	1 hour
Transition dilatation from 7 to 10 cm	1 ½ hours
Delivery	¼ hour
	8 hours

During the active and transition phases of labor, the doctor likes to see a minimum of 1½ cm of dilatation per hour. You may want to compare this graph to the average primipara labor.

During delivery:

1. The average delivery time is eighteen minutes. The maximum time is two hours. Generally, once the cervix has completely dilated, the baby drops immediately to the perineum. The long time needed for the descent of the primipara's baby is eliminated since the walls of the birth canal are not as resistant.
2. An episiotomy may still be performed. Some doctors feel it *might* be avoided or that it will be smaller than before. Be sure to discuss your options with your doctor.
3. Forceps are used less frequently.

After delivery:

Multiparas usually complain of afterpains more frequently than primaparas. In the primipara, the uterus generally stays contracted, but in a multipara, the uterine muscles relax and contract repeatedly. These wave-like contractions may last up to seven days but usually subside after the third. They are intensified by breast feeding since the hormone oxytocin is released when the baby nurses, causing uterine contractions.

To relieve afterpains, it may help to empty your bladder, lie with your abdomen resting on top of a pillow, and use transition breathing. If these suggestions don't help and you're really uncomfortable, ask for an analgesic. If you're nursing, be sure to ask if it's safe.

SIBLING RIVALRY

When a new baby is expected, parents want to know how the older child will react. You may have heard about sibling rivalry and wonder whether it will occur in your family.

Sibling rivalry is a child's behavioral response to the change that results in a family when a new baby arrives. Just as parents feel the changes that a newborn causes—the disrupted schedules, new demands, and altered family relationships—so do children.

Rivalry is a normal phenomenon that occurs between siblings. The two most common behaviors that can appear when a child is seeking attention are temporary regression to an earlier stage of development and acting-out. Your child might give up his potty training, start to hit, or bite his fingernails. He might just be generally crabby.

To a certain extent, the amount of regressive or hostile behavior that occurs when a new baby is born depends on how much attention the older child was receiving as compared to what he's now receiving. If he's eighteen months old, then he's still quite dependent and likely to miss his parent's undivided attention. If he's five years old, he has established some independence from his parents and is less likely to react as strongly to the attention the new baby is receiving. You will probably notice more verbal complaints about the baby and jealousy at this age.

Parents tend to worry about sibling rivalry and look for ways to prevent it, but it's a normal phenomenon. It will probably occur at some point—soon after you bring your new baby home or not until the baby is older and is getting into your first child's toys and possessions. It is unrealistic to expect that your older child won't notice the changes in the family's life style. Your child will be called upon to make some adjustments; his mother may be tired and short-tempered, his lunchtime may be postponed, and his storytime may be interrupted by the baby's demands. At times, parents resent these changes in their life style, and so do kids.

You can prepare for sibling rivalry in the following ways:

1. Prepare your child for the new baby. When you talk about what it will be like when the new brother or sister comes home, don't just talk about the good things. Let the child know that the baby won't be a new playmate right away. Expose your child to a friend's baby. Tell your child that sometimes he may feel angry about the new baby, and when he does, he should tell you.

2. There are some books you can read together that discuss new brothers and sisters at a child's level of understanding. See the Suggested Readings for this chapter at the end of the book.

3. Make every effort to introduce your older child to the new baby while you are still in the hospital. Some hospitals permit siblings to view the baby through the nursery window. Other hospitals are adopting the new, progressive policy of allowing the older child to wash, put on a gown, and hold the new baby in the mother's room. It might help if you are not holding the baby when your child first comes to see you. Children are often fearful during their separation from you, and your warm, loving, uninterrupted greeting can be reassuring.

There are many ideas and opinions about taking the baby home.

1. Go home at night after your child is asleep. Then you can all be together in the morning.
2. Have your child come to take you and the baby home. Let the father carry the baby when possible so you can give attention to the older child.
3. When you get home, have a birthday party for the new baby where everyone gets gifts.
4. Older children enjoy helping to dress the baby for the trip home and having the baby in the car seat in back with them on the drive home.

Once the baby is home:

1. Involve your older child in the care of the new baby. Even very little children can get a diaper and hold or help burp the baby with supervision. Your child might enjoy his own doll to care for, mimicking his mother's and father's actions. This is a good way to begin learning the art of parenting. If you have a son, he might enjoy the story, *William's Doll* by C. Zolotow.
2. Try to avoid comments like "Don't touch the baby," and so on.
3. Spend time alone each day with your older child. Remember, though, if it's twenty minutes or two hours, your child may still feel he hasn't had enough of your attention.
4. You may see your child shift some allegiance from his mother to his father in the postpartum period. This reaction can be quite helpful in reinforcing the father–child relationship.
5. Don't become upset or embarrassed by your child's behavior. If he wets his bed, becomes physically aggressive, or throws toys, acknowledge his behavior—discuss it with an older child and respond appropriately without belittling the child for these regressive behaviors—there is an underlying reason. One effective form of discipline is "time out." Your child is asking for attention in an inappropriate way when he misbehaves, so calmly remove him from your attention by putting him in his room for five or ten minutes. Love and hug him afterwards. If he's old enough to understand, talk to him about the incident.
6. Temporary distraction for the older child from the overwhelming presence of the baby and from seeing his mother caring for the baby can be helpful.
   During the early postpartum period have some outings planned for your older child. Your friends and neighbors can take him to the park or have him over to play for a morning.
7. Some parents find it helpful to buy a small gift and have the new baby bring it home to the older child. Most people are quite con-

siderate and do not bring a gift for the new baby without remembering the older child.

8.   You may want to buy an assortment of small, special treats to give your older child at times of crisis. Depending on his age, these might include a coloring book, matchbox car, paintbrush, clay, eraser, whistle, jumprope, shovel for the sandbox, new game you can play together, or book you can read to him while you're nursing the baby.

9.   Avoid confusing, untruthful statements, such as "This is your baby." "Here is your new playmate," "The stork brought her." The falseness in these statements will eventually become obvious to your child.

12

It is sometimes frightening for couples attending childbirth preparation classes to contemplate the possibility of a Cesarean birth. They have come to class to prepare for a vaginal delivery with the father present. They want to see their baby's birth, to hear the baby's cry, to hold the baby immediately. They want to *participate*. However, for a number of couples who practice childbirth techniques in anticipation of a vaginal delivery, there is the reality of a Cesarean birth. It is important for these couples to know that great strides have been made recently to humanize the Cesarean section so that it is more family-centered—a birth, not just a surgery. The Cesarean birthrate nationally is 10 to 15 percent, although the rate may approach 20 to 25 percent in hospitals with a large high-risk population. An often-heard complaint from couples who have had a Cesarean birth is that they were just not prepared for it: "If only we had known something beforehand."

No one chooses to have a Cesarean birth, but at times it is the safest course for both mother and baby. You can make it a rewarding experience by your attitude. A very important thing for parents to remember is that it is their baby's birthday, not just a surgical procedure. Learning ways to apply your breathing and relaxation techniques during and after a Cesarean birth can make it an easier, more relaxed experience.

A Cesarean section is an operation in which the baby is delivered through incisions made in the mother's abdominal wall and uterus.

A Cesarean birth is necessary when a vaginal delivery is either impossible or difficult and would endanger the well-being of the mother and/or the baby. When deciding whether Cesarean birth is indicated, the physician takes into consideration the safety of a Cesarean delivery in relation to the risk of a vaginal delivery. When the Cesarean birthrate rose, there was a decrease in the number of vaginally delivered babies who were sick or injured because of the birth process.

Sometimes your doctor suspects or knows ahead of time that a Cesarean birth will be necessary. She may tell you that it is a possibility so that you can mentally prepare yourself. Other times your doctor may choose to let you go into labor (trial labor) before deciding on the Cesarean. Sometimes the need for a Cesarean birth arises unexpectedly during labor.

Cesarean Birth

REASONS FOR CESAREAN BIRTH

There are both maternal and fetal reasons for Cesarean birth, none of which can be prevented by the mother.

1. *Cephalopelvic disproportion:* A disproportion exists between the mother's pelvis and the baby's size. The mother's pelvis is too small or contracted, or the baby's head is too large.
2. *Uterine dysfunction:* The mother is having a prolonged labor or one in which the contractions are not causing the cervix to dilate. The active phase of labor (3 to 10 cm) lasts longer than 8 to 10 hours, or the pushing stage lasts longer than 2 hours.
3. *Malposition and malpresentation:* Because of its unusual position or presentation, it would be traumatic or impossible for the baby to be delivered vaginally. Common examples might be some breech babies, transverse lies, and face or brow presentations.
4. *Placenta previa:* The placenta is implanted very low in the uterus and either partially or completely covers the cervix. As the cervix begins to efface and dilate, premature separation of the placenta from the wall of the uterus would occur, with resultant maternal bleeding and oxygen deprivation to the baby.
5. *Abruptio placenta:* The placenta has implanted in a normal place but for some reason is separating from the uterine wall before delivery. There is danger of maternal hemorrhage and oxygen deprivation to the baby.
6. *Fetal distress:* If the baby shows signs of fetal distress, such as severe bradycardia (lowering of the heart rate) or irregular heart tones, and the fetal heart tones cannot be improved, a Cesarean may be performed.
7. *Prolapse of umbilical cord:* When the membranes rupture spontaneously and the presenting part is not well engaged in the pelvis, there is danger that the cord will prolapse into the vagina. If it happens, the baby's oxygen supply is endangered. If the cervix is completely dilated, the baby *may* be delivered vaginally. In the case of incomplete dilatation, a Cesarean birth is necessary.
8. *Previous Cesarean section:* Some doctors feel that "once a section, always a section," because of the danger of uterine rupture at the site of the previous incision. Other doctors (in the minority right now) feel that if the previous Cesarean was for a nonrepeating reason, and if the uterine incision was a lower segment transverse, the woman could be allowed a trial labor.
9. *Vaginal infections:* If a vaginal infection, such as herpes simplex, is present at the end of the mother's pregnancy, delivery through the birth canal can endanger the baby.
10. *Failed induction or failed forceps:* When an induction has been attempted and has failed, or when a doctor feels that forceps are necessary but risky, a Cesarean may be performed.

TESTS OF FETAL MATURITY

Many couples prefer to go into labor before they have a Cesarean birth to help insure that their baby is mature. If this method is what you want, discuss it with your doctor. In the absence of precise due dates your doctor may order one or more of these tests to determine your baby's maturity:

1. *Ultrasound:* Very high-frequency sound waves are used to give a picture of your baby and placenta. Echoes bounce back and are seen as bright lights on an oscilloscope. A photograph of your baby is taken, and measurements are made of his head and chest. These methods give an accurate measure of the baby's size, which can then be used to compute his age, plus or minus two weeks. The procedure is painless, although you may find it uncomfortable to keep your bladder full throughout the test. The test is usually done on an outpatient basis. Often, two or more tests are done over a period of weeks so that measurements can be compared. You may be able to arrange ahead of time for a copy of the photograph that is made of your baby *in utero.*
   Research is continuous in an effort to verify the safety of ultrasound for the fetus and mother.

2. *X-ray pelvimetry:* Late in your pregnancy, or while you are in labor, the size of your pelvis and position of your baby may be checked by x-ray. This test is used with discretion to avoid unnecessarily exposing your baby to radiation.

3. *Estriols:* The amount of estriol in the mother's urine or blood indicates how well the placenta is functioning (see Chapter Ten).

4. *Amniocentesis:* Evaluation of the amniotic fluid surrounding your baby can determine the condition and maturity of the infant. This test can be done in the hospital on an outpatient basis. The mother lies on her back; her abdomen is covered with sterile drapes, and may be shaved and is cleansed with an antiseptic. Usually ultrasound is used to locate the baby and placenta. A local anesthetic is usually injected, a needle is inserted into the abdomen and uterus, and less than an ounce of fluid is withdrawn.
   This fluid is then studied for one or more of the following:
   a. *L/S ratio* (proportion of *lecithin* to *sphingomyelin*): can be used to determine maturity of fetal lungs. When the ratio is greater than two to one, the lungs are mature. This is the most commonly used maturity test of amniotic fluid.
   b. *Absence of bilirubin:* indicates maturity of at least 36 weeks.
   c. *Creatinine:* levels increase with fetal maturity.
   d. *Fat cells:* percentage in fluid can be used to determine weeks of gestation and fetal weight.

PROCEDURES BEFORE THE BIRTH

If your Cesarean birth is planned, you will be asked to check into the hospital either the afternoon before or the morning of your baby's birth.

The night before the birth can be a hard time for the mother. Admitting procedures do not occupy much time, and then you are left to wait. Visitors can be helpful. Bring something to do—a magazine or needlework —or watch television. Your doctor may order some sleeping medication if you would like it. You can also use active relaxation and deep chest breathing to help you relax before going to sleep.

For fathers: Before leaving for the night, you can help your mate relax with massage. Then you get a good night's sleep and eat a good breakfast before returning to the hospital the next morning.

Since most couples in childbirth preparation classes don't have planned, or *elective*, Cesarean births, you will have been admitted to the hospital when you were in labor. Regardless of whether you planned your Cesarean birth or not, the following procedures are followed:

1. Admission and surgery consent forms are signed.
2. Blood and urine samples are obtained.
3. Weight and vital signs are taken. Fetal heart tones are monitored.
4. A brief physical is performed, and your medical history is taken.
5. You and your anesthesiologist will discuss the type and effects of the anesthesia you will have. If you have a preference, be sure to ask if it is suitable to your situation. *Ask any questions you have.*
6. You may be given an enema to clear your bowels.
7. Your abdomen will be prepped or shaved and cleansed with an antiseptic.
8. You *may* be given some preoperative medication.
9. You will be moved from your room to the delivery–operating room. The temperature there is usually kept quite cool because of the amount of surgical clothing the staff must wear. To stabilize the temperature of the newborn, the room temperature may be raised during the time the infant is in the room.

For fathers: This is a time when you and your mate may feel tense and anxious. Being together can be most reassuring. Remind her that she knows what's going to happen and that all will turn out well. It might be helpful to have her do some deep chest breathing to help her relax. Active relaxation and massage may also be reassuring. Waiting can be hard, and you both may have a variety of emotions—joy that the baby is finally almost here and anxiety over the surgery.

Father Not Present at Birth

If hospital policy still does not permit the father to be present during the Cesarean birth, or the father does not choose to be present, the nurse will tell him where to wait. Depending on the type of anesthesia and incision, his total wait will be about 60 to 90 minutes. Once the baby is born, he will probably be taken directly to the nursery. Make sure the nurses know where you are waiting so you can see your new baby. In some hospitals you may accompany the baby to the nursery. When you are able to see your mate will depend on her recovery and hospital procedures. Often you can be with her in the recovery room. Be sure to ask if the three of you can be together.

Father Present at Birth

Some hospitals are now permitting the father to be present during the Cesarean birth of his child. This is a wonderful opportunity because you are able to share the birth and offer support and reassurance to your mate. Usually, couples who are together for the Cesarean birth report very positive feelings regarding the experience.

It is normal for a father to have some concerns about being present during the surgery. However, you will be seated beside the mother's head, and because of the ether screen at her shoulders, you will not see the surgery. Some fathers want to stand up and actually see their baby being delivered, and you should discuss this step beforehand with your doctor.

You will dress in regular delivery room clothes: scrub pants and shirt, hat, mask, and shoe covers. You will be seated in a nonsterile part of the room, so you do not need to scrub or wear gloves.

Some restrictions that *may* be placed on the father include the following:

1. The mother must be awake for the surgery, that is, having spinal or epidural anesthesia. More hospitals are recognizing the importance of the father's presence during the Cesarean birth of his child and are not denying his presence if the mother is asleep.
2. The father does not enter the delivery–operating room until the anesthesia has been administered. Some doctors now recognize that the father's presence can have a calming effect on the mother during this waiting period.
3. Usually, the father must agree that if any member of the medical staff asks him to leave at any point, he will do so. Also the father agrees to remain seated at the mother's head and to avoid touching any sterile drapes or entering the sterile part of the room.

Immediately Preceding Birth

1. *Catheter:* A thin tube is inserted through the urethra into the bladder to continuously drain urine and keep the bladder out of the way of surgery. Insertion of the catheter is usually not painful, although it may be uncomfortable. Relax, use your focal point and first-level breathing.
2. *IV:* An IV containing salt and dextrose will be started in your arm. An armboard is fastened to the operating table for your arm to rest

upon. The IV is used to administer medications, fluids, and blood if necessary.

3. Your other arm will be secured at your side by a sheet, which makes it very difficult to have it released so you can touch the baby. Ask ahead of time if one of your arms could be released after the baby is born. Perhaps both of your arms could be on armboards.

4. A blood pressure cuff will be placed around your arm. Two disks will be placed on your chest to record your heart rate.

5. Your abdomen will be draped with sterile sheets. An ether screen will be placed at your shoulders to prevent you from contaminating the sterile field and seeing the surgery.

6. Your abdomen will be cleansed and painted with an iodine solution.

7. The operating table may be tilted slightly to the left for improved circulation in the blood vessels behind your uterus.

The delivery-operating room will be full of people, all very involved with their equipment and supplies. You may find it confusing and feel left out. If your mate can be with you, his presence is *most* comforting.

Those present may include your obstetrician and his assistant, your anesthesiologist and her assistant, a pediatrician and his assistant, and three or more nurses. All together there will be nine to eleven people in the room, not including the mother and father.

TYPE OF ANESTHESIA

The type of anesthesia you are given depends on whether the Cesarean is an emergency, the preference of the mother and doctors, and the condition of the baby. Either a general or regional anesthetic can be used.

General

With general anesthesia, the mother is asleep during the birth. Once you are prepared for surgery and everyone is ready, *Pentothal* is added to your IV. This drug puts you to sleep within fifteen to twenty seconds. The anesthesiologist may chat with you or ask you to count. Hearing is the last sense you lose, so you may have the feeling that you are asleep but can still hear. Then a muscle relaxant is given when you are asleep, and a tube is placed down your throat and into your lungs. Nitrous oxide (laughing gas) and oxygen are administered as necessary to keep you in a relaxed, comfortable sleep. When the anesthesiologist gives the signal, your doctor will begin the surgery. The baby will be born within minutes. As the doctor is completing the surgery, your anesthesiologist will begin to reduce your medication, so that you are waking up as you are taken to the recovery room.

Spinal and epidural blocks are regional anesthetics used for Cesarean births. A regional anesthetic allows you to remain awake but eliminates pain from your abdomen to your toes. You may feel some tugging or pressure but no pain from the incision.

Spinal. A spinal block is the most frequently used regional anesthetic. To receive a spinal, you may be on your side or sitting upright. The lower back is cleansed and anesthetized and then the injection is administered. The spinal takes effect immediately but may require five to ten minutes to reach a satisfactory level for surgery. A possible side effect of a spinal is headaches caused by leaking spinal fluid at the site of the injection.

Epidural. Occasionally an epidural will be used for a Cesarean, especially if one is already in place from labor. A continuous epidural is administered while you are on your side, curled into a ball. It takes about five minutes to administer an epidural, which can be a difficult time if you are still having labor contractions. The anesthesiologist cleanses your back and applies a local anesthetic. A tiny catheter is threaded through a needle inserted in your back. The anesthetic begins to work fairly soon but may take 20 to 45 minutes to reach a satisfactory level for surgery. Additional anesthesia is given through the catheter. Your blood pressure will be checked frequently, and you will be tilted slightly to your left to improve circulation. You should be aware that occasionally an epidural is administered, but does not numb the mother sufficiently to perform a Cesarean birth, so a general anesthetic must be used. Because epidurals require special expertise, they may not be available everywhere.

PROCEDURES DURING THE OPERATION

The doctor makes the abdominal incision, cutting through the layers of the abdomen. The bladder is moved out of the way, and then an incision is made in the uterus.

The abdominal incisions are either vertical or low and transverse. The latter is called a "Bikini" or Pfannenstiel incision. When the pubic hair grows back, this incision is not very noticeable. The type of abdominal and uterine incision is a medical decision depending on the urgency of the procedure, size and position of the baby, condition of the mother's uterus, and location of the placenta.

The uterine incision can be one of three types.

When retracted or pulled open, the incision in the uterus is about 10 cm, or the size of the completely dilated cervix. After the uterine incision, the doctor will puncture the amniotic sac, suction the amniotic

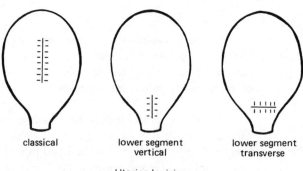

classical | lower segment vertical | lower segment transverse

Uterine Incisions

fluid, and deliver the baby. Then the placenta will be removed. Because of the number of layers of tissue to be stitched, the repair of incisions takes approximately 30 to 60 minutes—much longer than the actual birth. An oxytocic drug will be added to your IV to help contract your uterus following the surgery.

If awake, women may feel more uncomfortable during the repair of the incisions than during the birth. Part of the reason may be that during the birth you were distracted by the anticipation of birth and your mate, if he was with you. Once the baby and mate have gone to the nursery, your attention may focus on the repair. Now you should concentrate on a focal point and one of the breathing patterns. If this technique is not enough, you can safely request more medication since the baby has already been born. You are usually given a tranquilizer to put you in a light sleep, but a general anesthetic may be given. Remember that these extra medications will make you drowsy during the recovery period and may affect your early interaction with the baby.

For fathers: If you have the option to stay with your mate during the repair, you can be her focus of attention and offer emotional support. You and your mate will have to decide whether she or the baby needs you more at this time. If you are allowed to accompany the baby to the nursery, you can spend time cuddling and holding him, beginning the attachment process.

AFTER THE BIRTH

The Baby

The Cesarean baby born without complications receives the same care as the vaginally delivered baby—that is, warmth, clear air passage, and quick physical exam—except that he requires more suctioning of mucous since he did not go through any squeezing from the birth canal. This squeezing helps to bring up excess fluid and mucous. Apgar scores of 7 to 9 are usual for Cesarean babies. Physicians have different opinions about whether the Cesarean baby should be placed in the intensive care nursery for the first 12 to 24 hours of life. Generally, though, by the second day, he is receiving the same care as the vaginally delivered baby. If you are awake for the birth, ask to see and touch the baby right away or to have the baby's bed brought where you can see him.

For fathers: For many mothers it is distressing to be separated from the baby during the incision repair. This separation can be caused by the baby's need for extra care, best given in the nursery, or the cold temperature in the delivery–operating room. It can be reassuring to the mother to know that you are with the baby in the nursery. If it is not possible for the father, mother, and baby to be together immediately, every effort should be made for the parents to be with the baby during his initial alert period in the recovery room.

The Recovery Room

Your care in the recovery room is basically the same as for a vaginally delivered mother except for the effects of anesthesia. If you had a general, you will be waking up when you get to recovery. If you had an epidural, the effects should wear off in one to three hours. If you had a spinal, the effects will wear off in about two to five hours, and you may be asked to remain flat for six to twelve hours to avoid headaches. You will be given medication for pain if you need it when the anesthesia begins to wear off.

Mucous collects in the lungs following anesthesia and must be cleared to avoid infection. Thus, you will be asked to turn, cough, and breathe deeply. Some exercises that will also help are the following:

1. *Abdominal breathing:* When asked to breathe deeply, breathe in through your nose, allowing your abdomen to rise. Flatten your abdomen by pulling in your abdominal muscles while exhaling through your mouth.

2. *Huffing:* When asked to cough, open your mouth, pull in your abdominal muscles, and breathe out quickly, making the sound "huh huh huh huh." Support your incision with your hands or a pillow. Spit out any mucous you bring up. This technique is less painful than coughing.[1]

For fathers: Your presence in the recovery room can comfort your mate, even if she is groggy from the anesthesia. Perhaps you can be the one to show her the baby, help her hold the baby, and tell her the baby's weight and length. You can meet her needs by talking with her about the delivery and the baby.

[1]Elizabeth Noble, *Essential Exercises for the Childbearing Year* (Boston: Houghton Mifflin Company, 1976), pp. 156-57.

The Hospital Recovery

The first 24 hours are usually the most uncomfortable. If you have medication for pain, it will not eliminate your discomfort but make it more tolerable, and it will probably have a sedative effect. During your recovery, remember your breathing and relaxation techniques and use them any time you feel tense or uncomfortable. The usual postpartum stay is five to seven days.

The following procedures will be performed frequently:

- Vital signs will be checked.
- Lochia (vaginal bleeding) will be checked.
- Fluid intake and urine output will be measured.
- Uterine tone or contraction will be checked, and if necessary, uterine massage will be performed. If you find this procedure uncomfortable, relax, find a focal point, and use a breathing pattern.

These exercises will help bridge the gap between being in bed for several hours after your delivery and getting up to walk. Do them before you get up the first time and in between walks for the first few days.

1. *Leg exercises:* As soon as feeling begins to return to your legs, lie in bed with your legs straight or resting on a pillow and do sand-digging exercises (see Chapter 3).
2. *Pelvic tilt:* Lie on your back. Repeatedly tilt your pelvis by pressing the small of your back into the bed and pulling in your abdominal muscles.

You will be helped out of bed the evening or morning after surgery. You probably won't feel like getting up, but the sooner you do, the sooner you'll regain your strength. To get out of bed:

1. Raise the head of the electrically operated bed.
2. Move yourself to the edge by using the side rails. Let your arms move your weight, not your abdominal muscles.
3. Hold your hands or a pillow over your incision if you feel insecure about the stitches.
4. To help avoid faintness, sit at the edge of the bed with your legs dangling for a few minutes before standing.
5. Stand up straight; your tendency will be to lean forward.

Don't get out of bed the first few days without your nurse or mate standing by you. Once you can get around by yourself or with help, do so frequently. Walk the halls.

IV and Catheter. Your IV and catheter remain in place for 24 to 48 hours after surgery. If you should notice any puffiness, inflammation, or itching around your IV, notify the nurse. Your diet will first be fluids through your IV and then clear liquids by mouth, progressing to a soft diet. You may have a loss of appetite and nausea because of medications or as a response to pain. The IV will be removed once you get enough nourishment by eating.

Bowel Function. After abdominal surgery, it is common for bowel functions to be altered, and gas pains are a frequent complaint. Gas can be caused by anesthesia, exposure of your intestines to air during surgery, and immobility after surgery. The problem may be helped by the following:

1. Follow dietary restrictions; no cheating.
2. Drink plenty of fluids.
3. Avoid iced water and carbonated drinks.
4. Walk.
5. Do mild exercises, such as:
   a. *Abdominal tightening:* Begin within the first hour after surgery, and repeat four to five times each waking hour of your hospital stay. Place both hands over your incision for support. Take a deep breath and hold it for a slow count of five. Slowly blow out the air as you pull in your abdominal muscles. Take another deep breath.[2]
   b. *Pelvic tilt:* Lying on your back, repeatedly tilt your pelvis, contracting your abdominal muscles.
   c. *Movement:* Move around in bed, frequently changing your position.

Once you are eating solid foods again, your bowels will become more active. If your first bowel movement is difficult, consult your doctor or nurse. She may increase your fluid intake or give you a rectal tube, laxative, or enema.

Fever and Infection. Low-grade fever following surgery is common. You should drink plenty of fluids to help reduce it.

Watch for signs of uterine infection (for example, change in lochia flow or odor) and report it to the nurse.

Afterpains. You may have afterpains, or abdominal cramping, especially while breast feeding, because the uterus continues to contract down in size.

Incision. Your dressing will be changed several times by your nurse. This procedure is not particularly uncomfortable unless you have an *Elastoplast* dressing, a woven, stretchy fabric, like an Ace bandage, applied to your abdomen with adhesive. It has the advantage of offering

[2]Bonnie Donovan, *The Cesarean Birth Experience* (Boston: Beacon Press, 1977), pp. 134-35.

support to the incision, but it is annoying to have removed. Baby oil will help soften the edges before removal.

Your stitches or clamps will probably be removed before you go home, and many women wonder if the incision is strong enough by then. Your incision is almost at full strength by five days, but you are usually advised not to lift anything heavier than your baby for a while. Be sure to ask any questions you have about the healing process before you go home. Your scar will probably itch, and you should ask your doctor for suggestions to help this problem.

Lochia. You will have lochia, and self-adhesive napkins (or tampons, if your doctor permits) will be more comfortable than a sanitary belt.

You and Your Baby. Depending on your baby's condition, you may ask to see and hold him as soon as you feel able. Early and frequent contact can help begin the attachment process and alleviate any feelings of separation because of the Cesarean. Initially you may feel sleepy, but it may be comforting to have the baby near you in the isolette or held by your mate.

If you plan to breast feed, you will want to begin as soon as you feel able. Remember that early and frequent nursings are conducive to establishing a good milk supply, and your baby will benefit from the colostrum. The most comfortable positions will probably be lying on your side, or lying on your back with the head of the bed elevated, resting the baby on top of a pillow on your abdomen. Relax and ask for help. Also, reread the section in this book on breast feeding and refer to the breast feeding book you brought to the hospital. You may get a slower start because of your own initial discomfort, but don't worry about it, and enjoy your baby.

Once you can get around by yourself and the IV is removed, you can usually begin rooming-in. It keeps your mind off yourself, lets you learn to care for your baby, and helps you get a good start on breast feeding.

For fathers: If you can be at the hospital, you may be able to have rooming-in sooner since you will be there to help care for the baby. The three of you can begin to feel like a family.

THE FOURTH TRIMESTER

Your fourth trimester will not be much different from that of a woman delivered vaginally, except it will take you longer to regain your strength. You may be surprised at how easily you tire. You will probably be able to care for your baby, but try to get help with the house and meals for a few weeks. Ask your doctor when you should begin postpartum exercises.

For fathers: Try to take paternity leave or some of your vacation time to be with your mate the first week, especially if you have other children. Encourage your mate to *take it easy.* Discourage visitors in the hospital and during her first days at home.

As parents you should be aware of the normal range of feelings you may have. It is common to feel disappointment, anger, and guilt about a Cesarean birth if you had planned to share in a vaginal delivery. These feelings will probably be easier to handle if you were able to be together during the Cesarean birth. Try to be open about your feelings, and remember that fatigue makes it more difficult for both parents to cope emotionally. Keep in mind that a positive attitude about a Cesarean birth can do a lot to make it a positive experience. Although your start at parenting might be a little more challenging because you are physically uncomfortable, this condition is temporary, and you will soon be feeling better and enjoying your new baby (see Chapter 13).

13

The fourth trimester is the first three months following the birth of your baby. During this period, major adjustments occur in family relationships. The baby becomes a member of the family, and parents formulate a new life style. The adjustments of the fourth trimester are both physical and emotional. The mother's body recovers from the strain of pregnancy and delivery. She may have concerns about body image, resumption of intercourse, or adjustment to breast feeding. She must become comfortable with her new role as mother. The father must make adjustments also. His relationship with his mate has altered because of the new baby and he may be feeling financial responsibility if he is the sole support of the family. He too must come to terms with his new role. Adjustment requires a different amount of time for each parent and for each couple.

The presence of a baby in the house can be delightful. Parents often become more sensitive to everyday events, experiencing them more fully because they enjoy sharing with the baby. Having a baby to nurture and love and knowing the love will soon be returned are very fulfilling. A baby can bring satisfaction, joy, fun, and pride to his parents, even if there are initial adjustments to be made.

COMMON FEELINGS OF NEW PARENTS

Inadequacy

Going through pregnancy and childbirth doesn't make you feel like a mother or father. Neither does reading everything in the library, although it can help you prepare. All of us learn to be parents through experience, and experience is acquired slowly and with great effort. As you gain experience you feel more confident. A good thing to remember is that babies are really durable and survive despite our well-meaning, but sometimes bumbling, efforts and errors. Their greatest need is *love* from their parents.

All of us worry about whether we're doing the right thing or whether the baby is doing the right things. This isn't a phenomenon of the new-

Fourth Trimester

born period but recurs every time the child enters a new stage of development, and you're faced with decisions regarding appropriate behavior and care.

The worst thing about feelings of inadequacy is that you may be afraid to admit them to anybody, maybe even yourself. It's important to get these feelings out in the open, talk with your mate, a close friend, or another new parent. Feelings of inadequacy are normal. Don't be ashamed of your feelings. You will find that inadequacy is slowly being replaced by confidence as you and your baby become better acquainted.

Don't let your sense of inadequacy as a new mother expand to all other areas of your life. Don't expect the house to be as immaculate as it was previously nor the meals to be their usual gourmet quality nor yourself to be as well put together. Your return to normal functioning will slowly happen. Chaos will not always reign, but sometimes it seems to in the first months, and you can't expect it to be otherwise. Previously, you did not have the responsibility of an infant twenty four hours a day.

Sometimes we feel inadequate because of the messages we're getting from others. Don't take on the role expectations of your mother, sister, or best friend. Your aunt's recollection of how effortlessly she raised two sets of twins without help, baked her own bread, and worked part-time has been blurred by years, and she was probably just as frustrated as you feel at times.

If someone comes to help you, two things are important. It should be someone whom you like, and it should be someone who is willing to *help*. This requirement may seem like a foregone conclusion, but it's not. Help means to clean, cook, shop, do the laundry, answer the phone, and perhaps baby-sit so that you can get out for an hour or so. You will gain confidence in caring for your baby and getting to know him only if you do most of the caring, not your mother or helper. Often, helpers have the notion that *they* will care for the baby. This idea should be strongly discouraged. The baby is your responsibility.

You can acquire some experience in baby care if you elect to have rooming-in at the hospital. For two or three days you can try out mothering skills gradually and call on the nursery for help whenever you need it. Further, you have the luxury of returning the baby to the nursery if you want to nap or bathe. Fathers can also use rooming-in to get used to changing diapers, holding the baby, observing him, and beginning to feel like a father.

Be sure to take advantage of any baby care classes, films, or discussion groups that may be offered by the hospital.

Ambivalence, and Even Some Resentment

Some of us feel immediate love for our babies; others need a little time. How you feel about your labor and delivery can affect your reactions. You may have had high expectations for childbirth that were not met completely, or it may have far exceeded your expectations and left you feeling satisfied and fulfilled. Another factor that can influence your early relationship with the baby is lengthy separation caused by illness of the baby or mother.

At times, all of us have ambivalent feelings about this new role we have undertaken. You may be nostalgic for the life style of earlier days, the once slim waistline, the restful nights, the previous sexual relationship. Or at times you may be angry and resentful.

The nostalgia, the anger, the resentment can all lead to feelings of guilt. The mass media tell us that mothers and fathers *don't* feel this way. However, mothers and fathers *can* feel this way, as all parents can tell you. These feelings can be harmful if they are allowed to continue, and it is much more helpful to work on some of the reasons for them.

One cause of ambivalence for the mother is loss of adult contact, especially for the woman who was working outside the home until delivery. Being home with a nonverbal baby all day, no matter how desired the baby, is a change in roles and a new experience for most women. Any change can result in some tensions. The father comes home from work and needs time to unwind; the mother has been home all day and is dying for some adult conversation. The result can be some 6:00 P.M. tensions.

The mother should consider how she can see adults during the day. Little babies are very mobile and can easily accompany you to a meeting or to a friend's home. Do not plan to depend solely on your mate for adult stimulation.

The father's ambivalence can be stirred by the increased financial burden, especially if the mother is no longer earning a salary. Other causes can be loss of attention from your mate and fatigue from the new responsibilities of fathering or helping at home.

Sometimes we have a hard time imagining life with a baby. We may imagine ourselves in the yard playing ball with a four-year-old. Instead we are confronted with a tiny infant who does relatively little to which we can relate.

As things become more routine and the baby's schedule improves, the ambivalence usually fades. As the baby starts to respond, we begin to feel differently about him. It will help if your relationship with your mate receives some attention, too. This may take some effort, as babies do require a great deal of time.

Another major cause of resentment comes from fatigue. Your baby, although less than ten pounds, places an overwhelming, continual responsibility on you. It constitutes one of the major role changes a man or woman can have in life. This process of changing from the old life style to a new one can leave you extremely tired, and once tired, you can easily become depressed and resentful. *Fatigue is the enemy of all new parents, and you should take vigorous steps to prevent it.*

Recognize and try to accept the fact that there will be some changes in your life style. You can't expect to function as you did previously when you're getting up to feed the baby twice a night. On the other hand, the baby is not always going to be waking up for a night feeding; this is a temporary phase. Try to remember that the baby joined you, you didn't join the baby. Sometimes it's the baby who needs to adapt, and part of your role as a parent is to help your egocentric little baby adapt to his external environment.

In the beginning, remember that you should rest or do something for yourself while the baby naps. In general, you won't feel as relaxed and comfortable when the baby wakes from her nap if you ran around trying to clean the house or do the laundry. Learn to take the phone off the hook when you're napping, and place adhesive tape over the doorbell. Your rest is important to your ability to function. Share the workload with your mate, and cut down on nonessentials. Use paper plates; take advantage of carry-out restaurants; put away any clothes that need ironing. If you have friends that offer to help, let them. Ask them to bring you a casserole or to baby-sit for an hour so you can get out of the house. Also, locate competent baby-sitters.

Postpartum Blues

Learning to be a parent and coping with the newborn can be trying at times. Add fatigue and hormonal changes, and you've got fertile ground for the postpartum blues. Most new mothers feel some degree of depression during the early weeks with the baby.

One very common symptom of the blues is mood swings: one minute you're fine, the next minute you're crying. You might be short-tempered, feeling isolated in your responsibilities and frustration. You may let the common feelings of inadequacy, resentment, and ambivalence depress you.

All these feelings and behaviors are normal and common reactions to the postpartum period. As you begin to gain confidence, get some rest, relax, and enjoy your baby, the symptoms usually disappear.

If you find that tense feelings and periods of depression are becoming worse and are interfering with your ability to function, you should seek some professional assistance to help you adjust to parenthood. There are many qualified professionals—obstetricians, social workers, nurses, psychologists, or psychiatrists—trained to help you resolve these difficulties.

Women have postpartum blues in varying degrees, depending on the stability of home life, the temperament of the baby, and so on. You should remember that they are common during the fourth trimester, and unless they are severe, are normal.

ALL BABIES ARE DIFFERENT

Some babies are easy to take care of; they take nice lengthy naps, seldom spit up, fuss only occasionally, and are just generally content with the world. They love to be held and cuddled. Other babies have a harder time adjusting to life outside the womb. For them, night and day might be reversed, they may have colic, causing persistent crying spells, or they may just seem discontent. This problem isn't your fault; it's just the way some newborns act. Nor does it mean that these behavior patterns will persist throughout their lives.

If you have one of the unhappy babies, don't take it personally—the baby isn't unhappy with you. This stage will pass, and the baby will become more manageable and content. Consequently, don't think that you're the only one who should listen to the crying. Someone else, for example, a baby-sitter, can do it occasionally. Getting away for short periods of time will help you deal with the baby while you're home. Also, make sure you can communicate with your pediatrician about your baby's behavior. He can do a lot to reassure you that this is a normal, temporary phase. Soon your confidence as parents will emerge, your baby will become more content with his new environment, and you will experience the joys of being a family.

PHYSICAL CHANGES IN THE POSTPARTUM PERIOD

The six-week recovery period following childbirth is called the *puerperium,* during which the following changes occur:

Uterus: The uterus involutes or diminishes in size. Immediately after delivery it weighs about two pounds and is the size of a grapefruit. By two weeks post-delivery it weighs only twelve ounces. It remains slightly larger than the prepregnant uterus. *Afterpains,* the contractions of the uterus following delivery, are usually more uncomfortable for multiparas. Generally, afterpains are only bothersome for two to three days.

Lochia: The discharge from the uterus remains bright red for two to three days and contains clots and tissue. It then changes to a pinkish flow and finally is colorless. It smells like menstrual flow. Lochia lasts anywhere from two to six weeks. If it reverts to bright red, you are being too active. If it remains bright red or has a bad odor, call your doctor.

Cervix: Following delivery, the cervix is soft, bruised, and may have small lacerations, but it heals in about a week. The internal portion of the cervix closes completely, but the external portion doesn't. Following delivery it has a jagged, slit appearance.

Vagina and Perineum: The vagina and perineum are swollen following delivery. Gradually this swelling disappears. The episiotomy site may be bothersome for a few days. Ice applied immediately after delivery reduces swelling, and later the frequent application of moist heat will help the healing process. The sutures dissolve by themselves. There is decreased vaginal mucous until ovulation resumes.

Abdominal and Pelvic Floor Muscles: These muscles regain tone in approximately six weeks. Stretch marks remain, and there may be separation of the abdominal muscles (see Chapter Three). Diet, good posture, and resumption of exercise are important.

Breasts: A sense of fullness in the breasts (venous engorgement) occurs due to increased blood circulation following delivery. In breast feeding mothers, sucking stimulates maternal hormonal changes, which begin the production of milk. The breasts initially produce colostrum. The milk comes in twenty-four to seventy-two hours later and milk duct engorgement may occur due to inelastic milk ducts (see Chapter Two).

Ovaries: Ovulation may not occur in the breast-feeding mother until weaning. In the nonbreast-feeding and in some breast-feeding mothers, it will resume by the third month. The first period is generally heavier and longer than normal. Periods may be irregular initially.

GETTING BACK INTO SHAPE

You may be surprised to discover that your body does not resume its prepregnant state immediately after the birth of the baby. According to Dr. Alan Guttmacher, the average patient still weighs about 13½ pounds extra one hour after delivery. In the next 12 days she will lose an additional 3½ pounds. Any weight still left on after 12 weeks is fat, or if she is nursing, breast tissue.[1]

1. Regardless of how much you exercise during pregnancy, your muscles lose some tone. This lack of tone or strength is most evi-

[1]Alan F. Guttmacher, M.D., *Pregnancy, Birth and Family Planning* (New York: Viking Press, Inc., 1973), p. 269.

dent in the stomach muscles. You will need to exercise to get them tight and firm again.

2. Because of the swayed posture you may have assumed during pregnancy, the muscles in your lower back become tight or shorten. You will need to stretch these muscles.

3. These preliminary exercises can be invigorating in an otherwise fatiguing time.

4. Exercises will physically and psychologically make you feel you are doing something for yourself at a time when almost everything else you do is for your family.

You should begin exercising as follows:

1. If you had a normal, uncomplicated vaginal delivery, the exercises may be started 24 to 48 hours after delivery.

2. Do only the exercises listed in this book for the first six weeks, or follow your doctor's recommendations.

3. If you had tearing of the cervix, extensive blood loss, or any other complications, consult your doctor before exercising.

4. Do not exercise if you had a tubal ligation until you have your doctor's permission.

5. Do not do these exercises if you had a Cesarean birth (see Chapter 12).

The following are signals that exercising should be discontinued:

1. If your lochia increases significantly, you're doing too much.

2. If afterpains occur while exercising, discontinue the exercises for as long as you have the afterpains.

3. If any exercise is uncomfortable, temporarily discontinue that particular exercise.

When you exercise:

1. Wear comfortable, loose clothing or a leotard.

2. Do the exercises in bed until you are comfortable on the floor.

3. Do each exercise slowly. Relax briefly between each repetition and for a little longer before starting a new exercise.

4. Inhale during the first part of the exercise and exhale during the last part.

5. Start by doing each exercise four to six times twice daily, and gradually increase the number of repetitions to ten.

Postpartum Exercises

● *Stretching*
  Purpose:
    To stretch the muscles in your body and strengthen those in the abdomen and buttocks.

Position:

Lie on your stomach with a pillow under your hips and with arms above your head.

Exercise:

Stretch from head to toe, making yourself as long as possible. Squeeze your buttocks together and pull in your abdomen. Relax. Repeat.

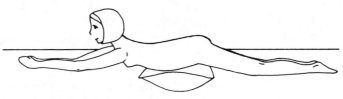

Stretching Exercise

- *Abdominal Breathing*

  Purpose:

  To strengthen abdominal muscles.

  Position:

  Sit or lie on your back.

  Exercise:

  Inhale and let your abdomen enlarge. Exhale slowly through pursed lips and pull in your stomach muscles. Pretend that you are trying to touch your abdominal muscles to your spine.

- *Knee Roll*

  Purpose:

  To trim your waist.

  Position:

  Lie on your back with your knees bent, feet flat on the bed, and arms out to the sides at shoulder level.

  Exercise:

  Roll your knees to the right, keeping your shoulders flat. Return to the starting position and roll your knees to the left. Repeat.

- *Chest Stretch*

  Purpose:

  To prevent rounded shoulders.

  Position:

  Sit or stand with both hands behind your head.

  Exercise:

  Bring your elbows out to the sides and back as far as you can, stretching the muscles under your breasts.

- *Alternate Knee to Chest*

  Purpose:

  To stretch the muscles in your lower back.

  Position:

  Lie on your back with both knees bent, feet on the bed, and pelvis tilted backward (see Chapter Three).

Exercise:
Raise one knee up toward your chest as far as possible. Bring it back to starting position, and repeat with the other knee.

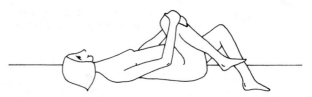

Alternate Knee-to-Chest Exercise

Variation:
If your perineum is not sore from the episiotomy, pull your knee up to your chest as above. Grab your knee with both hands and pull your head and shoulders up. Try to touch your forehead to your knee.

Many of the prenatal exercises can and should be continued after childbirth:

- *For your back:*
  Correct posture.
  Pelvic tilt, Version 1.
- *For your abdominal muscles:*
  Pelvic tilt, Version 2.
  Straight leg raises.
  Partial sit-up. (*Note:* Check for a gap or separation of the abdominal muscles when you raise your head and shoulders. If a gap is present do only Version 1 of the partial sit-ups.)
- *For your chest:*
  Shoulder circles.
  Forearm press.

The Pelvic Floor

The pelvic floor muscles become stretched by the weight of the uterus during pregnancy and by passage of the baby's head at birth. Stretching, in conjunction with an episiotomy, results in loss of tone. If this condition persists you may have any or all of the following problems:

1. Inability to control your bladder, particularly when you cough, sneeze, or laugh.
2. Inability of the pelvic floor muscles to support the uterus, rectum, and/or bladder.
3. Decreased pleasure during intercourse because the pelvic floor muscles lack the ability to tighten the vagina.

You should continue the pelvic floor exercises you did during pregnancy. They will increase the perineal blood circulation to heal your episiotomy and decrease perineal swelling. Don't be surprised if you find it difficult to contract the pelvic floor muscles right after delivery. The muscles have been overstretched and are weak, but you need to start exercising them right away.

SOME POSTPARTUM ADVICE

1. Avoid excessive climbing of stairs during the first couple of weeks. If you live in a two-story home, fix a sleeping and diaper-changing area somewhere downstairs, so you aren't continually running up and down stairs.
2. Avoid heavy lifting, such as grocery bags, furniture, heavy diaper pails, and other children. Have your older children climb into your lap instead of your picking them up.
3. Don't overtire yourself by doing a lot of housework, cooking, and laundry. Most of these jobs can be done minimally for now, and some can be postponed or done by someone else. Aim for two naps a day, but at least make sure you lie down periodically during the day. Develop the habit of lying down when you feed the baby.
4. Avoid too many visitors the first few weeks. If you feel guilty about this stipulation, ask your mate to tell them to visit later; or go visit your friends and relatives. Then you can stay a short while, let them see the baby and entertain you, and then you can leave. When visitors come to your house, you'll feel you need to entertain them. They may not realize how tired you are and stay too long.
5. The first week home, wear your gown and robe, which will help remind you to take it easy.
6. Sometimes pediatricians discourage visitors and outings for a newborn for a few weeks to avoid exposing the baby to infections, viruses, and so on. You can conveniently use this excuse to avoid too many visitors the first few weeks.
7. Try to get some help for the first week or so.
8. Do not overexert yourself by vigorous exercising. Your uterus, cervix, birth canal, and perineum are still healing. Consult your doctor before resuming more vigorous sports, such as bicycling or tennis. Short walks are healthy and invigorating, as long as your lochia does not increase. Long hikes are not recommended during the early postpartum period.
9. Relax and enjoy your baby. They grow up much too fast, so spend lots of time loving and cuddling him and observing his development.
10. If you have questions about the baby, breast feeding, or yourself, be sure to seek answers from doctors, friends, or your Lamaze instructor.

> ### WARNING SIGNS DURING POSTPARTUM
>
> Consult your doctor if *any* of the following occur:
>
> 1. Lochia becomes excessive, returns to bright red, or smells bad.
> 2. Burning sensation when you urinate or a frequent urge to urinate, but little urine is passed; indication of urinary tract infection.
> 3. Spiking fever or sudden elevation in temperature.
> 4. Persistent or prolonged postpartum blues; when the depression begins to interfere with your ability to function.
> 5. Soreness and redness in legs; indication of phlebitis.
> 6. Soreness or redness in breasts; indication of mastitis.

SEXUALITY

The expression of, need for, and interest in sexual and intimate relations after the birth of the baby are as varied as the people involved. Some couples want to resume a sexually active relationship right away. Even before they resume intercourse, they enjoy mutual lovemaking through closeness, touching, hugging, kissing, and fondling, and they resume intercourse as soon as they can. Other couples may have a decrease in sexual desire. Perhaps they are fatigued or engrossed with the baby and prefer to wait for the postpartum medical checkup to resume intercourse. Of course, there are many degrees of interest between these two levels. The important thing is not how active a couple's sex life is but that it meets the needs of each person involved.

Let's look more closely at the physical and emotional reactions new mothers may have. The immediate postpartum period is one of hormonal change. Estrogen levels are low until ovulation returns. These hormonal changes, plus the birth process itself, can cause some temporary physiological changes.

1. There may be decreased vaginal lubrication.
2. There may be discomfort at the site of the episiotomy, in the cervix, or within the vagina.
3. The uterine contractions caused by orgasm may be more uncomfortable than usual.
4. A breast feeding mother's milk may let down when her breasts are stimulated. Some couples don't mind, but others do.
5. Decreased estrogen may make her sexual response slower and less intense. Fatigue can have the same effect.

New mothers display varying emotional responses, which *can* include a decrease in sexual desire. The physical and emotional closeness to the baby, fear of discomfort during intercourse, and tension or anxiety about new responsibilities can make it difficult to become totally involved with lovemaking. The mother's sexual desire can return at varying times.

Fathers also have varying postpartum sexual desires and needs. Sometimes new fathers find the birth and their mate very stimulating and are anxious for closeness and lovemaking right away. Others may fear hurting the mother and prefer to wait to resume intercourse. Some need to adjust to the parenting experience and to seeing their mate in her new role.

Most couples want to know when it is safe to resume intercourse after the baby's birth. Talk to your doctor; ask for specific reasons for the interval of time he suggests you wait and what to expect physically. Your doctor knows your specific case and can best judge your healing time.

Tension in your relationship may develop if the two of you are not ready to resume intercourse at the same time. Be sure you talk about it together and work out ways to meet each other's needs. Be patient; postpartum is temporary.

Some practical measures may include the following:

1. Use a water-soluble jelly such as K-Y to lubricate the vagina.
2. Try to be rested. Relax with a hot shower first.
3. Realize that intercourse may be physically uncomfortable for the woman at first so proceed slowly with tenderness and understanding. If problems persist, talk to your doctor.
4. Communicate your needs to one another; neither of you can read each other's mind. Remember that showing your love for one another can include intimacies other than intercourse.
5. Plan ahead or take advantage of a time when you are fairly sure the baby will sleep and not interrupt you. Put the baby in a different room when you make love.

The adjustments that sometimes accompany life with a new baby— new responsibilities and changing roles—can lead to family tension. It is important for both of you emotionally to nurture your relationship as a couple; the baby cannot meet all your needs. Changes in routines and the adaptation to a new life are easier for both parents if accompanied by the love and security expressed during lovemaking.

CONTRACEPTION

Life with a new baby can be difficult, but life with *two* babies ten to twelve months apart can really be a challenge.

It may not seem possible to you, but you *can* get pregnant even though you just delivered a baby. Ovulation can occur before you again start to menstruate. Ovulation is an unpredictable event.

Therefore, you must consider contraception as soon as you plan to resume intercourse. If you resume before your six-week checkup (as many couples do), the most effective means of contraception is two applications of spermicidal foam and a condom. Foam and a condom used together are considered as effective as the pill.

In any case, discuss contraception with your doctor before you go home from the hospital.

Available Methods

1. *Birth-control pills:* These are synthetic hormone pills which inhibit ovulation. If you are breast feeding, these pills can affect your milk supply if it is not well established. If you are not breast feeding and pills are considered medically safe for you, these are the most effective means of birth control.

2. *IUD* (intrauterine device): IUD's are metal or plastic devices which are inserted into the uterus by your physician. They have threads that extend into the vagina, so you can check the placement of the IUD monthly. How they work to prevent pregnancy is still uncertain. If you are breast feeding, IUD's will not affect your milk supply. They can be inserted once the internal organs have returned to normal size. They are the second most effective means of birth control.

3. *Diaphragm:* If properly and consistently used, the diaphragm is considered the third most effective means of birth control. It is a soft rubber cup which is inserted through the vagina and covers the cervix during intercourse to prevent sperm from entering the uterus. It is used with a contraceptive jelly which provides a chemical barrier to the sperm. A physician must fit you with a diaphragm and teach you to insert it properly. Have your physician check to be sure that *you* can insert it correctly.
   Caution: If you used a diaphragm before this pregnancy, it will no longer fit. Do not use it as a means of birth control; you must be refitted.

4. *Condom:* This is a rubber or synthetic sheath put on the penis before intercourse. It is often used in conjunction with foam or some other spermicidal agent used by the female. The accidental pregnancy rate is about 3 percent,[2] being almost as effective as the diaphragm. It requires no prescription.

5. *Foam:* These are preparations containing spermicidal chemicals to immobilize the sperm and deter their entry into the uterus. Insertion of the foam should occur less than one hour before intercourse and be repeated for subsequent relations. Some physicians

[2]Joy Clausen *et al.*, *Maternity Nursing Today* (New York: McGraw-Hill Book Company, 1973), p. 285.

recommend double applications and use with a condom. Foam is judged to be less effective than condoms.

6. *Rhythm method:* In this method, the couple abstains from intercourse during the fertile period of the woman's menstrual cycle. Irregularities in the menstrual cycle, as well as difficulties in determining the exact fertile period, often make this an unreliable method.

WORKSHEET FOR POSTPARTUM

Considering the stresses of new parenthood, plan together now for the postpartum period.

1. List 5 ways you will bcome informed about the realities of parenthood.

MOTHER	FATHER
1.	1.
2.	2.
3.	3.
4.	4.
5.	5.

2. Make friends with or become better acquainted with couples who have children.
   1.
   2.

3. What household responsibilities can you *both* agree to temporarily eliminate? How can you share chores? Specifically, who will shop for groceries? Who will do laundry? Run the vacuum? Cook dinner? What are the unnecessary jobs? How can you do the necessary ones in the most efficient way?

4. Who could watch the baby for you while you go out?
   1.
   2.
   3.

5. Name two people you can trust and call on for advice or help.

   1.

   2.

6. Name three things you will do for yourselves in the first 6 weeks.

   MOTHER   FATHER

   1.   1.

   2.   2.

   3.   3.

7. Don't give up all your outside activities, but what responsibilities can you temporarily eliminate?

   MOTHER   FATHER

   1.   1.

   2.   2.

   3.   3.

8. Plan 3 enjoyable things you will do together as a couple during the first 6 weeks.

Afterbirth. Placenta and membranes; expelled after the birth of the baby.

Afterpains. Uterine cramps caused by contractions of the uterus after the baby's birth.

Albumin. Protein substance which if found in the pregnant woman's urine may be an indication of toxemia.

Alveoli. Air cells or tiny sacs in the lungs through which oxygen and carbon dioxide are exchanged.

Amniocentesis. Withdrawal of amniotic fluid for the purpose of evaluating the fetus.

Amniotic fluid. The clear, colorless fluid surrounding the baby in the uterus.

Amniotic sac. Bag of waters, or membranes, containing amniotic fluid.

Amniotomy. Artificial rupture of the amniotic membranes.

Analgesic. Drug that relieves pain.

Anesthesiologist. Doctor trained to administer anesthesia.

Anesthetic. Drug that causes loss of sensation.

Anesthetist. A nurse who is trained to monitor a patient once anesthesia has been administered.

Apgar score. Method used to evaluate the condition of the baby one and five minutes after birth.

Bilirubin. Yellowish pigment which is the waste product of broken-down red blood cells; in newborns may cause jaundice 36 to 48 hours after birth.

Birth canal. Vagina.

Bladder. Membranous sac in the pelvic cavity which temporarily holds urine.

Bloody show. Slight bit of blood-tinged mucous (the mucous plug) released from the cervix prior to or during early labor.

Bradycardia. Slow heart rate.

Glossary

Braxton-Hicks contractions. Contractions of the uterus during pregnancy that help prepare it for labor.

Breech. The presenting part of the baby is the buttocks, knees, or feet.

Calorie. Unit of heat used to measure energy produced by a particular food.

Catheter. Thin tube used to drain or inject fluid.

Centimeter (cm). 2/5 of an inch; 2.5 cm is 1 inch.

Cephalopelvic disproportion (CPD): The mother's pelvis will not accommodate the baby's head.

Cervix. The lower, bottleneck portion of the uterus which opens into the vaginal canal.

Cesarean birth. Birth of the baby through incisions in the abdominal and uterine walls.

Colic. Spasms in the stomach or intestines, accompanied by pain.

Colostrum. Fluid high in protein and antibodies, secreted by the mother's breasts before her milk comes in.

Contraction. A shortening or tensing of uterine muscle fibers, followed by a lengthening or relaxation of the fibers.

Creatinine. Normal alkaline constituent of blood and urine; excreted by the kidneys.

Crowning. Appearance of the baby's head at the vaginal outlet.

Descent. Downward movement of the baby into the pelvic cavity.

Diaphragm. Muscle between the abdominal and chest cavities; used in respiration.

Dilatation. Opening of the cervix during the first stage of labor; measured in centimeters.

Dissassociation. Concentrating on a nonpainful characteristic of a painful stimulus.

Dopler. Instrument used for listening to fetal heart tones.

Dystocia. Failure of the cervix to dilate; a difficult labor.

EDC (Estimated date of confinement). Refers to the calculated due date of the baby.

Edema. Swelling caused by an excess of fluid in the tissues.

Effacement. Thinning of the cervix prior to or during labor.

EKG (Electrocardiogram). A recording on a graph of variations in the action of the heart muscle.

Engagement. Descent of the presenting part into the pelvis to zero station, or level, of the ischial spines.

Epidural anesthesia. A type of regional anesthesia which blocks sensory impulses at the nerve roots where they enter the spinal cord; administered in the epidural space outside the spinal cord.

Episiotomy. An incision made in the perineum during delivery to enlarge the vaginal outlet.

Estriol level. Amount of the hormone, estriol, found in the mother's blood or urine; helps determine how well the placenta is functioning.

Explusion. Movement of the baby down the birth canal as a result of uterine contractions and the mother's pushing efforts.

False labor. Irregular uterine contractions which do not result in progressive cervical dilatation.

Fetal distress. Drastic changes in the fetal heart tones, indicating the baby is under too much physical stress.

Fetal heart tones (FHT). The baby's heart rate, which varies between 120 and 160 beats per minute.

Fetal monitor. A machine used to record fetal heart tones and uterine contractions.

Fetus. Refers to the baby in the uterus from three months gestation until its birth.

Fontanels. The soft spots on the baby's head where the skull bones have not united.

Forceps. An instrument that can be used to help deliver the baby.

Fourth trimester. First three months following the birth of the baby.

Fundus. Top portion of the uterus.

Gestational age. Number of weeks of fetal development.

Gravida. A pregnant woman or the number of times a woman has been pregnant.

Hemoglobin. Portion of red blood cells that carries oxygen.

Hemorrhoids. Distention of the blood vessels around the anus.

Hypertension. Increased blood pressure.

Hyperventilation. Imbalance of carbon dioxide and oxygen in the body.

Hypotension. A drop in blood pressure.

Induction. Artificially starting labor, usually by rupturing the membranes or administering Pitocin.

Intravenous infusion (IV). Administration of fluids and medication through the vein.

Involution. Return of the uterus to its near prepregnant state.

Jaundice. Yellow color of skin and whites of the baby's eyes caused by an excess of bilirubin in the blood.

Labor. Uterine contractions causing effacement and dilatation of the cervix leading to delivery.

Lactation. Secretion of milk by the breasts.

Lecithin. A fatty substance found in cell tissue, especially in the brain, blood, and nerves.

Lightening.   Descent of the baby into the pelvis.

LMP.   Last menstrual period.

Lochia.   Vaginal discharge following delivery.

Mastitis.   Infection of the breasts; can be caused by incomplete drainage of a milk duct.

Meconium.   Dark green material in the intestines of a fetus and the first stools of a newborn infant.

Molding.   Overlapping of the newborn's skull bones during labor, resulting in a temporarily misshapen head.

Mucous plug.   A plug of mucous in the cervix which keeps bacteria in the vagina from entering the pregnant uterus.

Multipara.   A mother who has had two or more pregnancies.

Nitrazine paper.   Laboratory test paper which turns a deep blue color (alkaline reaction) to indicate the amniotic membranes have ruptured.

Occiput.   Back of the head.

Ovulation.   Release of an egg or ovum from the ovary. Usually occurs between the 10th and 14th day of a menstrual cycle.

Oxytocin.   Hormone produced by the pituitary gland that causes uterine contractions.

Pelvic exam.   Vaginal examination made to determine the depth of the baby in the pelvis and the amount of effacement and dilatation of the cervix.

Pelvic floor.   Layers of muscle that form a sling across the base of the bony pelvis and support the bladder, uterus, and rectum.

Pelvis.   The bony structure formed by the sacrum, coccyx (tailbone), and two hip bones.

Pentothal.   A barbiturate which produces a prompt hypnotic effect when administered intravenously. Frequently used before gaseous anesthesia.

Perineum.   The pelvic floor muscles between the vaginal outlet and anus.

Pitocin.   A synthetic hormone used to cause uterine contractions before, during, or after childbirth.

Placenta.   The vascular organ through which the baby is nourished and waste products excreted; the afterbirth.

Position.   The relationship between the presenting part of the fetus and the mother's pelvis.

Postmature.   A baby who has remained in the uterus 42 weeks or longer.

Postpartum.   After childbirth.

Precipitous labor.   Extremely rapid labor and delivery—one that is less than three hours.

Pre-eclampsia.   Mild toxemia.

Premature.   An infant born before the 37th or 38th week of gestation.

Presentation.   That part of the baby that is closest to the cervical opening.

Primipara.   A woman having her first baby.

Prolapsed cord.   Protrusion of the umbilical cord ahead of the presenting part.

Puerperium.   Recovery period of six weeks following childbirth.

Psychoanalgesia.   Reduction of pain through the use of mental strategies.

Quickening.   The first movements of the fetus felt by the mother, usually between the 16th and 20th week of gestation.

Relaxin.   A hormone secreted during late pregnancy which relaxes joints and ligaments of the pelvis and the muscles of the pelvic floor in preparation for delivery.

Ripening.   Softening of the cervix.

Rooting reflex.   The baby will turn his head toward the cheek or side of the mouth that is stroked.

Rupture of membranes.   If spontaneous, the amniotic membranes rupture or tear automatically before or during labor. If artificial, the amniotic membranes are ruptured by the doctor or birth attendant.

Spinal anesthesia.   Anesthetic that blocks sensory impulses carried by the spinal cord. The anesthetic is administered into the fluid-filled canal surrounding the spinal cord.

Station.   Measurement of the baby's descent into the bony pelvis.

Term.   38 to 42 weeks gestation.

Third trimester.   The last three months of pregnancy.

Trimester.   A period of three months.

True labor.   Labor consisting of uterine contractions that efface and dilate the cervix.

Ultrasound.   Use of high-frequency sound waves to locate the placenta and the baby within the uterus to obtain measurements of the baby's head and chest which are used to determine gestational age.

Umbilical cord.   Contains two arteries and one vein carrying oxygen, nutrients, and waste products between the placenta and the baby.

Umbilicus.   Belly button; scar where umbilical cord was attached to the uterus.

Uterine inertia.   Ineffective uterine contractions which prolong labor.

Uterus.   The thick-walled, muscular organ which holds the fetus during pregnancy.

Vagina.   Birth canal.

Varicose veins.   Swollen, distended veins; usually in the legs.

Vertex (or cephalic).   The presenting part of the baby is the head.

Vital signs.   Respiration, pulse, and temperature.

Voluntary muscles. Any muscle in the body that can be tightened and relaxed at will.

Wharton's jelly. Soft, jelly-like substance of the umbilical cord.

X-ray pelvimetry. X-rays to determine the size of the pelvis and baby.

Many of the books listed in this section can be ordered through ICEA (International Childbirth Education Association) Book Center. Write to them and ask for "Bookmarks," their book catalogue.

ICEA BOOK CENTER
P.O. Box 70258
Seattle, Washington 98107
(206) 789-4444

ON PREGNANCY

Arms, Suzanne. **A Season To Be Born.** 1973. Photographic essay of a first pregnancy and birth; captures many of the common emotions felt by the pregnant woman. Written by the mother; photographed by the father.

Betts, Donni. **A Shared Journey.** 1977. Diary of a pregnancy, Cesarean birth, and postpartum period. Very good on feelings and photographs.

Bing, Elisabeth, and Libby Colman. **Making Love During Pregnancy.** 1977. The authors address themselves to the interplay of sexuality and pregnancy. Book is enhanced by quotes from men and women and sensitive drawings. Recommended.

Colman, Libby, and Arthur Colman. **Pregnancy: The Psychological Experience.** 1971. Feelings of the mother through three trimesters of pregnancy, culminating in expectations for labor and delivery. Includes information on postpartum and feelings of the father during pregnancy. Worthwhile for parents who are interested in the psychological aspects.

Flanagan, Geraldine L. **The First Nine Months of Life.** 1962. A discussion of the growth processes that occur during the prenatal period—hour by hour, day by day, month by month. Accompanied by photographs of babies at various stages of development. Highly recommended.

Suggested Readings

Furuhjelm, Mirjam, Lennart Nilsson, Axel Ingelman-Sundberg, and Claes Wirsen. **A Child is Born.** 1977. An overview of pregnancy, labor, and delivery. Photographs of fetal development are excellent. This revised edition is more current in its discussions.

ON NUTRITION

Brewer, Faith, and Tom Brewer. **What Every Pregnant Woman Should Know: The Truth About Diets and Drugs in Pregnancy.** 1977. Alerts the reader to the importance of good nutrition during pregnancy, both to the mother and fetus. Includes such topics as toxemia and a basic nutritional program.

Goldbeck, Nikki, and David Goldbeck. **The Supermarket Handbook.** 1973. How to be a good shopper; how to choose nutritious foods; what's really in food. Recommended.

Lappé, Frances Moore. **Diet for a Small Planet.** 1975. Cookbook on protein. How to use vegetable protein and how to combine protein so it has all the essential amino acids. Includes recipes.

Maternal Nutrition and the Course of Pregnancy, Summary Report, National Academy of Sciences, Washington, D.C. 1970. Report of the Commission on Maternal Nutrition, by Food and Nutrition Board, National Research Council. Available at Government Printing Office.

Rombauer, Irma S., and Marion Rombauer Becker. **The Joy of Cooking.** The "bible" of cookbooks. A good investment for its how-to sections.

Williams, Phyllis. **Nourishing Your Unborn Child.** 1974. Basic nutrition and why. Discusses some food hazards, and includes a section on how to buy different kinds of foods. Has an extensive menu and recipe section.

ON INFANT-FEEDING PRACTICES

Castle, Sue. **The Complete Guide to Preparing Baby Foods at Home.** 1973. Probably the best baby-food cookbook available. Includes recipes, label information, and a systematic way of introducing solids. Non-dogmatic attitude.

Citizens Committee on Infant Nutrition. *White Paper on Infant Feeding Practices.* Center for Science in the Public Interest. 1974. Cultural influences on infant feeding: breast versus bottle and early introduction of solids. Should be read by all new parents before they begin feeding their children.

Coffin, Lewis A. **The Grandmother Conspiracy Exposed.** 1974. This book is rapid reading about nutrition. The author, a pediatrician, is especially concerned with high-energy meals and snacks and *low or no sugar* intake for your children. Sound nutritional and dental advice to establish good eating habits.

Lansky, Vicki. **The Taming of the C.A.N.D.Y. Monster (Continuously Advertised Nutritionally Deficient Yummies). 1977.** A practical guide to decreasing your child's consumption of junk foods. Includes a discussion of nutrition (additives, sugar, salt, and so on) and suggestions for packing lunches, snacks, low-sugar desserts, meals for when the baby-sitter comes, travel food, milk-free diets, and shopping. For parents of preschool and elementary school-aged children.

ON CHILDBIRTH

Bing, Elisabeth. **Six Practical Lessons for an Easier Childbirth.** 1977. Well-known childbirth educator presents a guide to labor and delivery and Lamaze techniques in a series of six lessons. Complimentary reading to a class in Lamaze.

Boston's Health Book Collective. **Our Bodies, Ourselves.** 1976. Excellent content on childbirth. This book focuses on women's feelings. Accurate and concise information. A worthwhile reference.

Bradley, Robert A. **Husband Coached Childbirth.** 1974. Another method of prepared childbirth, developed by a Denver obstetrician. Revised edition includes a chapter on "It's not nice to fool mother nature," discussing effects of medical intervention on the normal childbirth process.

Chabon, Irwin. **Awake and Aware.** 1966. A physician discusses the Lamaze method of childbirth, including benefits to parents, baby, and physician. Review of techniques and a section written by parents using the method. Worthwhile reading.

Ewy, Donna, and Rodger Ewy. **Preparation for Childbirth.** 1976. Well-written guide to Lamaze. Worthwhile supplementary reading.

Karmel, Marjorie. **Thank you, Dr. Lamaze.** 1959. Childbirth without pain, as described by an American whose first child was delivered in Paris by Dr. Lamaze. She contrasts this delivery with her second, less satisfying experience in New York. Interesting reading.

Kitzinger, Sheila. **The Experience of Childbirth.** 1972. Well-known British childbirth educator presents her techniques of childbirth. Covers pregnancy through family adjustment. Very strong on relaxation techniques, known as Kitzinger touch relaxation.

Lamaze, Fernand. **Painless Childbirth.** France, 1956; United States, 1970. Discusses psychoprophylactic method (Lamaze) and its philosophy, scientific basis, and class content as it originated in France. Technical reading.

Walton, Vicki E. **Have It Your Way.** 1976. The consumer's guide to pregnancy and childbirth. Enumerates options available in a hospital delivery.

ON BREAST FEEDING

Ewy, Donna, and Rodger Ewy. **Preparation for Breast Feeding.** 1975. Written by the authors of *Preparation for Childbirth*, this book is primarily to help new mothers during the important first weeks. The Ewys feel that knowledge, support, and preparation can lead to a good experience, and they discuss these factors in a practical, concise way.

Pryor, Karen. **Nursing Your Baby.** 1973. A practical book on breast feeding, recommended by La Leche League. It discusses how the breasts function, the quality of milk, doctors who are helpful (or otherwise), the hospital routine, and so on. Has some historical perspectives. Practical information for the nursing mother is included.

ON EXERCISE

Noble, Elizabeth. **Essential Exercises for the Childbearing Year.** 1976. An excellent exercise book; includes prenatal exercises, a discussion of proper posture and body mechanics during pregnancy, and postpartum and post-Cesarean exercises.

ON NEWBORNS

Brazelton, T. Berry. **Infants and Mothers—Differences in Development.** 1969. Dr. Brazelton presents a comparison of three babies with distinctly different personalities, energy levels, and needs. Emphasizes range of differences in both mothers and babies within the so-called "normal." Beneficial and enjoyable reading about the month-by-month development in the first year.

Caplan, Frank. **The First Twelve Months of Life.** 1973. Discusses your baby's growth month-by-month. This is a good gift for an expectant mother to give to the father. Reading about the growth of your child during the coming month can give you a feel for changes, what to look for, and problems common to the age group. Begins with the first week through the twelfth month. Full of photographs. Worth the price.

Child Care. Sutherland Learning Associates, Inc. 1973. A basic, down-to-earth manual concerning child care. Includes information on differences in developmental rates.

Klaus, Marshall H., and John H. Kennell. **Maternal-Infant Bonding.** 1976. Discusses the impact of early infant-parent interaction on family relationships. Includes details of maternal-infant bonding, maternal and paternal behavior toward the baby, and special needs of parents of sick or premature infants. Written for professionals but may be interesting to some parents.

ON SIBLINGS

Barber, Virginia, and Merril Maguire Skaggs. "There's Another Baby in the House," in **The Mother Person.** 1975.

Brazelton, T. Berry. **Toddlers and Parents. A Declaration of Independence.** 1974. A sensitive look at the toddler years and a discussion of the development that takes place in both toddlers and parents. Told through case histories with explanations of behavior. Has section on siblings.

Caplan, Frank, and Theresa Caplan. **The Second Twelve Months of Life.** 1977. Month-by-month development during the second twelve months of life. Enhanced by photographs. Recommended reading.

FOR CHILDREN

Andry, Andrew C., and Steven Schepp. **How Babies Are Made.** Time-Life, 1968. Discusses fertilization of flowers, reproduction in animals, lovemaking by humans, development of the baby, birth process, and breast feeding. Illustrated with paper sculptures. Published in collaboration with SIECUS (Sex Information and Education Council of U.S.).

Gruenberg, Sidonie. **The Wonderful Story of How You Were Born.** 1970. For young children. Beautiful illustrations.

Keats, Ezra Jack. **Peter's Chair.** For preschoolers. Sensitive story of a child's adjustment to a new baby who uses "his" old furniture.

Mayle, Peter. **Where Did I Come From?** 1973. Cartoon illustrations by Arthur Robins. Forthright and explicit, yet humorous. Dedicated to "red-faced parents" everywhere, this book discusses anatomy, making love, reproduction, fetal growth, and birth.

Rogers, Fred. **Mister Rogers Talks About.** 1974. A chapter on "When a New Baby Comes to Your House." Beautiful, large color photographs and clear verbalization of children's thoughts. For the preschooler.

Scott, Ann. **On Mother's Lap.** 1972. Preschool story about adjusting to the new baby.

Sheffield, Margaret. **Where Do Babies Come From?** 1973. Adapted from the award-winning BBC program, this book is explicit yet sensitive. Well illustrated.

Zolotow, Charlotte. **William's Doll.** 1972. Sensitive portrayal of a boy's desire to play with dolls as a way to "role play" being a father.

ON CESAREAN BIRTH

Betts, Donni. **A Shared Journey.** 1976. Diary of the author's pregnancy and birth of her daughter. Cesarean birth incorporated as a positive event.

Breastfeeding After a Cesarean Section. La Leche League International. Reprint #80. Order from La Leche League International, Inc., 9619 Minneapolis Avenue, Franklin Park, Illinois 60131.

Cesarean Birth Support Groups: Many childbirth education organizations now have support groups for parents having Cesarean births. Ask your instructor, postpartum nurse, or doctor to supply current names, addresses, and phone numbers of a group in your area.

C/SEC, Inc. (Cesareans/Support, Education and Concern) is a nonprofit organization founded out of concern for the lack of resources available to couples who anticipate or have had a Cesarean delivery. The group's main objective is to make the delivery a positive and meaningful experience for each couple. Their work is concentrated on three main areas: personal support, education, and policy change. For more information write to C/SEC, Inc., 132 Adams Street, Room 6, Newton, Massachusetts 02158.

Donovan, Bonnie. **The Cesarean Birth Experience: A Practical, Comprehensive and Reassuring Guide for Parents and Professionals.** 1977. The aim of this book is to provide information on all aspects of Cesareans—pregnancy, birth, and postpartum. Included are exercise, breast feeding, anesthesia, presence of father at the birth, vaginal delivery following Cesarean, and much more.

Guttmacher, Alan. **Pregnancy, Birth and Family Planning.** 1973. Includes information about Cesarean birth.

Hausknecht, Richard, and Joan Rattner Heilman. **Having a Cesarean Baby.** 1978. Includes information about Cesarean birth for parents. Discusses such topics as anesthesia, birth and recovery procedures, emotional and physical adjustments, and vaginal delivery for later births.

Noble, Elizabeth. **Essential Exercises for the Childbearing Year.** 1976. Has a unique section for women who have had Cesarean births, including exercises for the hospital and home.

Rozdilsky, Mary Lou, and Barbara Banet. **What Now? A Handbook for New Parents.** Revised 1975. New edition includes a chapter on postpartum for the Cesarean birth parents.

ON THE POSTPARTUM PERIOD

Bing, Elisabeth, and Libby Colman. **Making Love During Pregnancy.** 1977. See Suggested Readings on pregnancy.

McBride, Angela Barron. **The Growth and Development of Mothers.** 1973. When your child is a bit older, you might want to read this book, which looks at some of the reasons women have babies, other than "they love children." She discusses the emotional ups and downs of life with children, concluding with a chapter on coming to terms with yourself.

Rozdilsky, Mary Lou, and Barbara Banet. **What Now? A Handbook for New Parents Postpartum.** Revised 1975. Written by two mothers, this book covers physical problems after the birth, responsibility for an infant, depression, sex, contraception, and so on. Highly recommended.

Salk, Lee. **Preparing for Parenthood.** 1974. Both feelings and practical matters are discussed in this strongly recommended book for new parents. Dr. Salk begins by discussing the mixed feelings that surround parenthood. Both physical and psychological aspects of postpartum are discussed. Practical matters include organizing the home for the baby, breast versus bottle, the hospital stay, and preparing an older child for the new baby. Especially important is the section on mother-father-baby contact immediately after delivery to allow bonding to occur. Also very good is the chapter on "Handling Advice from Others."

Urbanowski, Ferris, with Balaram. **Yoga for New Parents—The Experience and the Practice.** 1975. Presents pregnancy and parenthood from the perspective of those experiencing it. Offers unique postpartum program in the Hatha Yoga method (fathers included). Has excellent photography and presentations of yoga postures, but is expensive for those not sure they will follow the program.

ON PARENTING

Becker, Wesley C. **Parents Are Teachers.** 1971. A programmed learning text by an educator to help parents learn about behavior and discipline. Supplies clear-cut instructions on how to change objectionable behavior by reinforcing good behavior in the child. Principles can be applied at the toddler stage.

Brazelton, T. Berry. **Infants and Mothers—Differences in Development.**

Caplan, Frank **The First Twelve Months of Life.** See Suggested Readings On Newborns.

Consumer Reports, ed. **The Consumers Union Guide to Buying for Babies.** 1975. Rates baby articles, such as cribs, diapers, carriages, clothing, pacifiers. Information is based on research by Consumers Union. Read before purchasing these items.

Dodson, Fitzhugh. **How to Parent.** 1970. The section on infancy is not extensive but consider buying this book when your child becomes a toddler ("first adolescence"). Especially good is the chapter, "Can You Teach a Dolphin to Type?" which provides nine keys to discipline, learning, and behavior. Also excellent is the large appendix on toys, books, and records and their appropriate age levels. A *must* book.

Fraiberg, Selma. **The Magic Years.** 1959. Well-known authority in child psychoanalysis presents the world from a child's viewpoint. She discusses the problems of different stages of development and conveys the understanding necessary by parents to guide their children through the rough times and to enjoy the good times.

Gregg, Elizabeth. **What to Do When There's Nothing to Do.** 1976. Contains many ideas for activities for children on rainy days, when traveling, or when bored. Divided into interests and activities appropriate to age. Emphasis is on low-cost, simple things. Excellent resource to have on hand for use at home, in play-groups, and so on.

Kelly, Marguerite, and Elia Parsons. **The Mother's Almanac.** 1975. "The most complete book ever written on loving and living with small children." This is a real mothercraft book, full of mainly practical, not theoretical, ideas, always approached from each age level, one through six.

Salk, Lee. **What Every Child Would Like His Parents to Know.** 1972. Discusses a child's feelings about everyday occurences and suggests appropriate adult responses.

Abdominal breathing (see Breathing)
Abdominal muscles, 46, 50, 93, 171
Abruptio placenta, 154
Accelerated-decelerated breathing, 128–30
Active labor, 74, 80–81, 106
Active relaxation, 27, 116–22, 126
Admission procedures, 106
Adrenalin production, 116–17
Afterbirth (see Placenta)
Afterpains, 163, 170
Albumin, 23
Alcohol, 60
Allergies, 18, 29
All-fours position, 43
Alternate knee-to-chest exercise, 173
Alveoli, 108
Ambivalence, 167–69
Amino acids, 13
Amniocentesis, 155
Amniotic fluid, 8, 24, 59, 61
Amniotic sac, 59, 61
Analgesia, 104
Anatomy and physiology of childbirth,
    59–72
  maternal pelvis, 66–72
  mother and baby, 59–62
  uterine function, 62–66
Anemia, 11
Anesthesia, 74, 104, 137, 138, 157–59
Anterior position of baby, 70, 145, 146
Antibiotics, newborns and, 110
Antibodies, 8
Anus, 54
Anxiety, 26–28
Apex of contraction (see Peaks of
    contractions)
Apgar, Virginia, 109
Apgar Scoring Systems, 109, 160–61
Appearance of newborns, 111
Areola, 4
Arm stretching exercise, 53
Arrangements before birth, 36

Babies (see Newborns) listed as Newborns
Baby carriers, 33

Backache, 6, 39, 43, 71, 76, 85, 94
Back-lying exercise, 42–43
Back pain during labor, 135–36
Back pressure exercises, 57–58
Bag of waters, 61
Bearing down, 93, 99
Bikini incision, 159–60
Bilirubin, 155
Biofeedback, 117
Birth canal, 26, 54, 89–90
Birth-control pills, 178
Birth education classes, 22
Birthing centers, 102
Birthmarks, 112
Bishop Score, 139
Bladder, 54, 55
Bleeding, postpartum, 101
Bleeding gums, 6
Blood estriol test, 139
Blood pressure, 42, 105
Blood specimen, 105
Body image, 21–22
Body mechanics, 45
Bonding interactions, 102
Bottle feeding, 32
Bowel function, 163
Bradycardia, 154
Bras, 4, 31, 85
Braxton-Hicks contractions, 62–63, 64, 76,
    126, 148
Breast feeding, 18, 104, 164, 171
  beginning, 30–31
  benefits, 28–29
  breast function, 29–30
  father support during, 32
  nutrition and, 13, 15–17
  obstacles to, 31–32
  preparing the nipples, 30
Breathing, 25–28, 57–58, 75, 90, 94, 120,
    125–34, 136, 137
  during exercise, 47–53
  first-level breathing, 126, 127–28, 133
  hyperventilation, 127, 132–34
  postpartum exercise, 172–75
  premature urge to push, 131–32

Index

Breathing: (con't)
  for pushing, 92–93
  role of coach, 127
  second-level breathing, 128–30, 133
  third-level breathing, 81, 130–31, 133
Breech delivery, 68–69, 136–38
Bridging position, 48
Buying for newborns, 32–35

Calcium, 5, 11, 12
Calf cramps, 5
Calf stretching exercise, 51–52
Calories, 10, 18
Cameras, 85, 95, 107
Carbon dioxide, 60, 132, 133–34
Car delivery, 103
Car seats, 33
Catheters, 141, 157, 162–63
Cephalic delivery, 68, 69
Cephalopelvic disproportion, 154
Cervix, 59, 60, 63, 100, 131–32
  dilatation and effacement of, 26, 61–62,
    64–67, 73–75, 77, 78, 80, 137–40, 148
  in multiparas, 148
  postpartum, 171
Cesarean birth, 69, 104, 137, 153–65
  anesthesia, 158–59
  exercise after, 162
  fathers and, 156–58, 160–61, 164, 165
  fourth trimester, 164–65
  procedures before, 156–58
  procedures during operation, 159–60
  reasons for, 154
  recovery after, 160–64
  tests of fetal maturity, 155
Characteristics of newborns, 109, 111–14
Checks for relaxation, 120–22, 127
Chest breathing (see Breathing)
Chest stretch exercise, 173
Childbirth preparation classes, 28
Chills, 100, 101, 109
Chloasma, 6
Circulation, 46, 51
Cleansing breath, 126, 127, 131
Clothing, 5, 6, 85, 118
Coach (see Labor coach)
Coccygeus muscle, 54
Coccyx, 54, 66
Colostrum, 4, 29, 30, 171
Comfort positions, 40–44
Complete breech delivery, 68–69
Conception, 7
Condoms, 178
Conscious Relaxation—Drill 2, 119–20
Constipation, 4, 78
Contraception, 3, 177–79
Contraction/Relaxation—Drill 1, 119
Contractions (see Breathing; Cesarean birth;
  Delivery; Exercise; Labor; Multiparas;
  Relaxation; Third trimester; Variations
  in childbirth)

Controlled breathing patterns (see
  Breathing)
C position, 90, 91
Cramps, 5, 51, 78, 133
Creatinine, 155
Cribs, 33, 99
Crowning, 90, 91, 93

Dehydration, 101
Delivery, 25, 70–72, 74, 89–103
  birth day procedures, 105–7
  breech, 68–69, 136–38
  cephalic, 68, 69
  emergency, 103
  expulsion, 67, 89, 99
  immediate postpartum, 100–102
  of placenta, 67, 99–100
  pushing stage, 83, 89–95
  room, 90, 95–99
  subsequent births and, 147–49
  things to contemplate, 104
  (see also Cesarean birth; Labor)
Descent, 95, 99
Dextrostix, 110
Diabetes, 138
Diapers, 34
Diaphragm, 178
Diarrhea, 76
Diet (see Nutrition)
Dilatation of cervix, 26, 61–62, 64–67, 73–75,
  77, 78, 80, 137, 138, 139, 140, 148
Dizziness, 24, 39, 126, 133
Doctor, choice of, 37
Dopler, 141
Drugs, 60, 104

Early labor (see Latent labor)
Eating habits (see Nutrition)
Eclampsia, 24
Edema, 5, 23, 24
Effacement of cervix, 26, 61–62, 64–67,
  73–75, 77, 78, 80, 131–32, 137–40, 148
Effleurage, 81, 123–24
Egg, 7, 8, 60
EKG (electrocardiogram), 142
Electronic monitoring, 139, 140–43
Elevating legs position, 43–44
Elevator exercise, 93
Embryo, 7–8
Emergency delivery, 103
Emotions:
  in active labor, 80
  of fathers, 2, 22, 101
  in first and second trimester, 1–2
  in fourth trimester, 166–69
  in latent labor, 78
  postpartum, 101
  in third trimester, 21–22
  in transition phase of labor, 82

Enema, 105, 139
Energy, 76 116
Engagement, 72, 75–76, 78
Engorgement, 30
Epidural anesthesia, 157, 159
Episiotomy, 55, 97–98, 100, 101, 104, 137
Ergotrate, 100
Estimated date of confiment (EDC), 73
Estriols, 73, 138–39, 155
Exercise, 5, 38–58
    body mechanics, 45
    breathing, 47–53
    after Cesarean birth, 162
    comfort positions, 40–44
    pelvic floor, 47–48, 53–58, 93, 98, 171,
        174–75
    postpartum, 171–75
    posture, 38–40
    reasons for, 46–47
Expulsion, 67, 89, 99
    of placenta, 67, 99–100
Extension, 96–97
External monitors, 140–43
External rotation, 97

Faintness, 39, 42
Fallopian tubes, 7
False labor, 76–77
Fat cells, 155
Fathers:
    Cesarean birth and, 156–58, 160–61,
        164, 165
    emotions of, 2, 22, 101
    fetal monitors and, 142
    postpartum sexuality and, 177
    support during feeding, 32
Fatigue, 3, 5, 51, 82, 94, 168
Fears, 3, 21, 26–28, 140
Fear-tension-pain cycle, 26, 116
Fertilization, 7
Fetal blood, 60
Fetal growth and development, 7–8, 11
Fetal heart rate, 61, 105, 109, 138–43
Fetal maturity tests, 155
Fetal monitoring, 105, 139, 140–43
Fetal movements, 3, 8, 23, 61, 136, 139
Fetoscope, 141
Fever, 24, 163
Fingerprints, 109
First and second trimester, 1–20
    emotions, 1–2
    fetal growth and development, 7–8, 11
    nutrition, 4, 5, 6, 8–20
    physical changes during, 3–7
    sexual relations during, 2–3
First-level breathing, 126, 127–28, 133
Flexion, 95
Fluid intake, 30–31, 32
Fluid retention, 5, 24
Focal point, 118, 122, 126
Folic acid, 11, 16
Fontanels, 111

Footling breech delivery, 69
Footprints, 109
Forceps, 98–99, 137, 154
Forearm pressing exercise, 53
Fourth trimester, 164–81
    contraception, 177–79
    emotions, 166–69
    exercises, 171–75
    sexual relations, 176–77
    (see also Postpartum)
Frank breech delivery, 69
Fraternal twins, 143–45
Fruits, 12, 16, 17
Fundus, 59, 60, 63, 101, 141

Gag reflex, 114
Gamma globulin, 8
General anesthesia, 158
Genes, 7
Gestation, 73, 112
Gifts, 115, 151–52
Glucose, 110
Grain products, 14–15
Grasp reflex, 114
Gums, 11

Hands-and-knees exercise, 91
Headaches, 5, 24
Heartburn, 4
Heart rate, fetal, 61, 105, 109, 138–43
Heel stick, 110
Hemoglobin, 11
Hemorrhage, 100
Hemorrhoids, 4, 54
Highchairs, 33
Holding newborns, 94, 95, 101, 104, 114,
    115
Home delivery, 103
Hormonal changes, 3, 4, 6, 46, 176
Hospital:
    admission procedure, 106
    articles needed for, 85
    fees, 87–88
Hot water bottles, 85, 136
Hypertension, 23
Hyperventilation, 81, 85, 126, 132–34
Hypoglycemia, 110
Hypothyroidism, 110

Identical twins, 143–45
Identification bracelets, 109
Immediate postpartum (see Postpartum)
Immunities, 29, 30, 60
Implantation, 60
Incision, Cesarean, 163–64
Incontinence, 55
Induction, 138–40, 154

Infection, 23, 138, 163
Infertility, 3
Intensive-care nurseries, 114
Intercourse (see Sexual relations)
Internal monitors, 140–43
Internal rotation, 96
Intra-abdominal pressure, 89
Intrauterine infection, 138
Involution, 60
Iodine, 158
Iron, 11, 16
Ischial spines, 71–72
IUD (intrauterine device), 178
IV, 138, 140, 141, 157–58, 162–63

Jaundice, 113–14

Kneading, 81, 124
Knee-chest position, 43
Kneeling breech delivery, 69
Kneeling position, 91
Knee roll exercise, 173

Labor, 25, 61, 62–66, 70, 73–84, 104
    active stage of, 74, 80–81, 106
    back pain during, 135–36
    breathing (see Breathing)
    false, 76–77
    going into, 73–74
    induction, 138–40, 154
    latent stage of, 74, 78–79, 106, 140
    length of, 74–75
    multiple births, 144
    prelude phase of, 75–77
    subsequent births and, 147–49
    transition stage of, 67, 74, 82–84,
        90, 107, 130–33
    true, 76–77
    (see also Cesarean birth; Delivery)
Labor coach, 26–28, 74, 82, 84, 116–24,
    127
    back labor and, 136
    birth day procedures, 106–7
    breathing, 126, 127
    breech presentation and, 137–38
    during active labor, 81
    during delivery, 94–95
    during latent labor, 79
    pushing technique, 92, 93
    relaxation, 116–24
    in transition phase, 84
Lactation, 10–12
LaLeche League, 31, 144
Lamaze, Fernand, 25
Lamaze Dissassociation—Drill 3, 121–22
Lamaze techniques, 25–27, 116–26

Last menstrual period (LMP), 73
Latent labor, 74, 78–79, 106, 140
Later births, 24, 76, 146–52
LeBoyer techniques, 99, 104
Left occiput anterior position, 70–71
LGA (large for gestational age), 112
Ligaments, 62
Linea nigra, 6
Liquids, 12–13
List making, 33
Lithotomy position, 91–92
Lochia, 162–64, 170, 176
L/S ratio (proportion of lecithin to
    sphingomyelin), 155

Malposition, 154
Malpresentation, 154
Massage, 28, 57, 76, 81, 116–24
Mastitis, 31
Maternal blood, 60
Maternal love, 1, 2
Meconium, 113, 137
Media, 25
Medication, 60, 104
Mediolateral episiotomy, 97
Membranes, 61, 76, 78, 80, 105, 106, 139
    143
Menstruation, 7, 73
Mental retardation, 110
Methergine, 100
Midline episiotomy, 97
Milia, 112
Milk ducts, 30
Milk products, 12, 14–15
Mirrors, during delivery, 94, 95
Miscarriage, 3
Molding of newborn, 111
Morning sickness, 3–4
Moro reflex, 113–14
Mucous, 97, 103, 109, 161
Mucous plug, 59, 61–62, 76, 78
Multiparas, 24, 76, 146–52
Multiple births, 143–45
Muscle tone, 53–56, 109

Nausea, 3–4, 24, 80
Nesting instinct, 76
Newborns, 108–15
    at birth, 108–10
    characteristics of, 109, 111–14
    clothing, 34–35
    holding, 94, 95, 101, 104, 114, 115
    problems with, 114–15
Nipples, 30, 31
Nonstress test, 139
Numbness, 133
Nursing (see Breast feeding)

Nutrition, 10
  breast feeding and, 28
  in first and second trimester, 4, 5, 6,
    8–20

Obesity, 29
Occiput, 70–71
Orgasm, 3, 22, 23
Ovaries, 7, 171
Ovulation, 176, 178
Ovum, 7, 8, 60
Oxygen, 60, 108, 109, 116, 117, 125, 132,
    141
Oxytocin, 29, 100, 117, 138
Oxytocin Challenge Test (OCT), 138

Pain, 24–27, 125
Partial sit-up exercise, 49–50
Peaks of contractions, 63, 64, 92, 127,
    128–30
Pelvic floor exercises, 47–48, 53–58, 93, 98,
    171, 174–75
Pelvis, 66–72, 95–96
Pentothal, 158
Perineum, 41, 50, 54, 55, 90, 91, 93, 94,
    97–98, 100, 101, 171
Petrissage, 81, 124
Pfannenstiel incision, 159–60
Phenylalanine, 110
Phenylketonuria (PKU), 110
Phosphorus, 5, 11
Photography, 85, 95, 107
Physiology of childbirth (see Anatomy and
    physiology of childbirth)
Pitocin (synthetic oxytocin), 100, 106,
    138–41
Placenta, 7, 8, 59, 60, 99, 103, 154
  delivery of, 67, 99–100
Placenta previa, 154
Posterior position of baby, 71, 135
Postmaturity, 73, 138
Postpartum, 67, 100–102, 109, 114–15
  advice, 175–76
  blues, 169
  exercises, 171–75
  multiple births, 144–45
  physical changes in, 170–71
  rooming-in, 102, 104
  worksheet for, 180–81
Posture, 38–40
Pre-eclampsia, 24
Prelude phase of labor, 75–77
Premature urge to push, 131–32
Prematurity, 136, 137
Prenatal exercises (see Exercise)
Primapara, 65, 74, 75, 76
Problem babies, 114

Progesterone, 4, 5
Prolactin, 29
Prolapse, 55
  of umbilical cord, 137, 154
Protein, 10–11, 13, 14, 23, 30
Proteinuria, 23
Prothrombin, 12
Psychological strategies, 27–28
Pubococcygeus, 53–54
Pushing, premature urges, 131–32
Pushing stage, 83, 89–95

Recovery room, 100–101, 104, 107, 110,
    161
Rectum, 53–54, 94
Reflex irritability characteristic, 109
Regional anesthesia, 159
Relaxation, 26–28, 57–58, 75, 116–24, 136,
    137
  active, 27, 116–22, 126
  checks, 120–22, 127
  Conscious Relaxation—Drill 2, 119–20
  Contraction—Relaxation—Drill 1, 119
  effleurage (stroking), 81, 123–24
  Lamaze Disassociation—Drill 3, 121–22
  petrissage (kneading), 8, 124
Relaxin, 6, 68
Resentment, 167–69
Respiratory effort characteristic, 109
Restitution, 97
Rhythm method, 179
Riboflavin, 12
Right occiput anterior position, 70
Rooming-in, 102, 104
Rooting reflex, 114
Round ligament pain, 6
Runner position, 42
Russian method of childbirth preparation, 25

Sacrum, 66, 67
Salt, 5, 18, 24
Sand-digging exercise, 5, 44, 51
Second babies, 76, 146–52
Second-level breathing, 128–30, 133
Second trimester (see First and second
    trimester)
Self image, 46
Semireclining position, 41, 118
Sexual relations:
  in first and second trimester, 2–3
  in fourth trimester, 176–77
  in third trimester, 22–23
SGA (small for gestational age), 112
Shoulder circling exercise, 52
Sibling rivalry, 149–52
Side-lying position, 41–42, 90–91
Sitting, 39–40

Sitz baths, 98
Skin changes, 6
Sleep, 4, 5, 7
Sodium, 5, 18, 24
Sound recording, 107
Spacing of children, 146
Spasms, 133
Special babies, 114
Sperm, 7
Spermicidal foam, 178–79
Sphincter, 53–54
Spinal anesthesia, 157, 159
Squatting position, 44, 91
Standing exercises, 38–39
Station, 71–72, 139
Stepping reflex, 114
Stethoscope, 141
Stimuli during childbirth, 26–28
Stirrups, 92, 95
Straight leg raising exercise, 49
Stretch marks, 6
Stroking, 81, 123–24
Subsequent births, 24, 76, 146–52
Sugar, 18
Sutures, 111
Swelling, 5, 24
Symphysis pubis, 66

Tactile cues, 119, 121, 127
Tailor position, 41, 50, 118
Teeth, 6, 11, 12
Temperature, 105, 136
Tension, 116–17
Thiamine, 12
Third-level breathing (transition), 81,
    130–31, 133
Third trimester, 21–37
    breast feeding (*see* Breast feeding)
    buying for baby, 32–35
    emotions during, 21–22
    preparation for childbirth, 24–28
    sexual relations during, 22–23
    warning signs during, 24
Toxemia, 5, 23, 24, 138
Toys, 34

Transition stage of labor, 67, 74, 82–84,
    90, 107, 130–33
Transverse lie, 69
True labor, 76–77
Twins, 143–45

Ultrasound, 141, 143, 155
Umbilical cord, 59–61, 99, 100, 103, 108
Urinary estriol, 139
Urination, frequency of, 6, 78
Urine, 24, 76
Uterus, 3, 7, 26, 54, 59, 60, 125, 154,
    159–60, 170

Vagina, 24, 26, 53–55, 59, 62, 76, 78,
    89–90, 100, 154, 171
Variations in childbirth, 135–45
    back pain during labor, 135–36
    breech delivery, 68–69, 136–38
    fetal monitoring, 105, 139, 140–43
    induction, 138–40, 154
    multiple births, 143–45
Varicose veins, 5, 39
Vegetables, 14, 16
Vena cava, 42
Verbal cues, 117, 119, 120, 121, 127, 134
Vernix caseosa, 111
Vertex delivery, 68, 69
Vision, 24
Visitors, 107
Visual imagery, 117
Vitamins, 6, 11–12, 16–17, 110
Vomiting, 3–4, 24, 80

Warning signs, during third trimester, 24
Weight, 8, 10, 24, 76, 105, 111
Wharton's jelly, 61, 108
Witches' milk, 112

X-rays, 68, 143, 155

VILLAGE BOOKS

P.O. BOX 440055, AURORA, COLORADO 80044
(303) 751-5924

—QUALITY BOOKS AT A DISCOUNT—

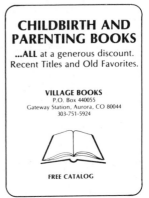
Getting Ready For
CHILDBIRTH ▮ Arlene Fenlon
▮ Ellen Oakes
▮ Lovell Dorchak

OVER 200,000 COPIES SOLD!

Retail price $7.95		
	1 copy	$7.16
	2-14 copies	$6.76 each
	15-29 copies	$5.75 each
	30 or more copies	$5.20 each

You may order books by mail or phone and you will be billed for the
cost of the books, postage, handling, and tax if applicable.
We require full payment within 30 days.

Number of copies ordered_____

SEND TO:

_____
organization if applicable

_____
name

_____
address (street address required by UPS)

_____
city   state   zip

Date_____

BILL TO:

_____
organization if applicable

_____
name

_____
address (street address required by UPS)

_____
city   state   zip

Phone Number (____) _____

VILLAGE BOOKS

P.O. BOX 440055, AURORA, COLORADO 80044
(303) 751-5924

—QUALITY BOOKS AT A DISCOUNT—

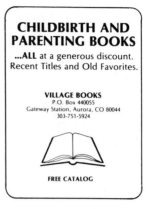

**CHILDBIRTH AND
PARENTING BOOKS**
...ALL at a generous discount.
Recent Titles and Old Favorites.

VILLAGE BOOKS
P.O. Box 440055
Gateway Station, Aurora, CO 80044
303-751-5924

FREE CATALOG

Getting Ready For
CHILDBIRTH ▮ Arlene Fenlon
Ellen Oakes
Lovell Dorchak

OVER 200,000 COPIES SOLD!

Retail price $7.95		
1 copy	$7.16	
2-14 copies	$6.76	each
15-29 copies	$5.75	each
30 or more copies	$5.20	each

You may order books by mail or phone and you will be billed for the
cost of the books, postage, handling, and tax if applicable.
We require full payment within 30 days.

Number of copies ordered_____

SEND TO:

_____
organization if applicable

_____
name

_____
address (street address required by UPS)

_____
city   state   zip

Date_____

BILL TO:

_____
organization if applicable

_____
name

_____
address (street address required by UPS)

_____
city   state   zip

Phone Number (_____)_____

VILLAGE BOOKS

P.O. BOX 440055, AURORA, COLORADO 80044

(303) 751-5924

—QUALITY BOOKS AT A DISCOUNT—

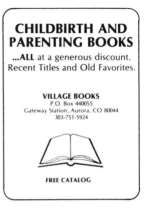
Getting Ready For
CHILDBIRTH ▪ Arlene Fenlon
▪ Ellen Oakes
▪ Lovell Dorchak

OVER 200,000 COPIES SOLD!

Retail price $7.95		
1 copy	$7.16	
2-14 copies	$6.76 each	
15-29 copies	$5.75 each	
30 or more copies	$5.20 each	

You may order books by mail or phone and you will be billed for the cost of the books, postage, handling, and tax if applicable. **We require full payment within 30 days.**

Number of copies ordered_____

SEND TO:

_____
organization if applicable

_____
name

_____
address (street address required by UPS)

_____
city   state   zip

Date_____

BILL TO:

_____
organization if applicable

_____
name

_____
address (street address required by UPS)

_____
city   state   zip

Phone Number (____)_____

IT'S TRUE!

- Foods can be cholesterol-free yet still contain high amounts of fat!
- Smoking, caffeine, refined sugar, and pollution can all raise your cholesterol level!
- An Italian meal may contain as much monosodium glutamate (MSG) as an Oriental meal since both tomatoes and cheese are natural sources of this substance!
- The herb echinacea can protect you from viral and bacterial attack by stimulating your immune system!
- If you work out with weights, complex carbohydrates are as important as meat for muscular maintenance!
- Sweet basil draws poisons out of the skin: use it to relieve bee stings and draw underskin pimples to a head!
- Amino acids arginine and ornithine can help you gain less—even as you eat more!
- Products marked sugarless aren't necessarily low-calorie, and some products using artificial sweeteners contain more calories than if they had natural sugar!
- The herb astragalus fights fatigue and frequent colds!
- If you're under constant stress, a B-vitamin supplement may help you!
- Cancer is more common among people who are obese than people who are at or below their ideal body weight!

It's all here and more in
Earl Mindell's
VITAMIN BIBLE

Also by Earl Mindell

**Earl Mindell's Shaping Up With Vitamins
Unsafe At Any Meal**

Published by
WARNER BOOKS

EARL MINDELL'S

VITAMIN

BIBLE

COMPLETELY REVISED! EXPANDED!

UPDATED FOR THE NINETIES!

WARNER BOOKS

A Time Warner Company

All information regarding brand name products or services was compiled as of January 1991.

WARNER BOOKS EDITION

Cover photo by Don Banks
Cover design by Anne Twomey

Warner Books, Inc.
1271 Avenue of the Americas
New York, N.Y. 10020

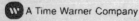 A Time Warner Company

Printed in the United States of America

First printing: November, 1991

10 9 8 7 6

This book is dedicated to
GAIL, ALANNA, EVAN,
our parents and families
and to
the future

The first wealth is health.

RALPH WALDO EMERSON
"The Conduct of Life"

Acknowledgments

I wish to express my deep and lasting appreciation to my friends and associates who have assisted me in the preparation of this book, especially J. Kenney, Ph.D.; Linus Pauling, Ph.D.; Harold Segal, Ph.D.; Bernard Bubman, R.Ph.; Mel Rich, R.Ph.; Sal Messineo, R.Ph.; Arnold Fox, M.D.; Dennis Huddleson, M.D.; Stuart Fisher, M.D.; Robert Mendelson, M.D.; Gershon Lesser, M.D.; David Velkoff, M.D.; Rory Jaffee, M.D.; Vickie Hufnagel, M.D.; Donald Cruden, O.D.; Joel Strom, D.D.S.; Nathan Sperling, D.D.S.; Peter Mallory; Teri Cox; and Hester Mundis.

I would also like to thank the Nutrition Foundation; the International College of Applied Nutrition; the American Medical Association; the New York Blood Center; the American Academy of Pediatrics; the American Dietetic Association; the National Academy of Sciences; the National Dairy Council; the Society for Nutrition Education; the United Fresh Fruit and Vegetable Association; the Albany College of Pharmacy; Edward Leavitt, D.V.M.; Jane Bicks, D.V.M.; Betty Haskins; Stephanie Marco; Susan Towlson; Ronald Borenstein; Laura Borenstein; Glenn Williams; and Richard Curtis, without whom a project of this scope could never have been completed.

Contents

A Note to the Reader   *xix*
Preface   *xxi*

I. Getting into Vitamins   **1**
   (1) Why I did—(2) What vitamins are—(3) What
   vitamins are not—(4) How they work—(5) Should you
   take supplements?—(6) What are nutrients?—(7) The
   difference between micronutrients and macronutrients—
   (8) How nutrients get to work—(9) Understanding your
   digestive system—(10) Name that vitamin—(11) Name
   that mineral—(12) Your body needs togetherness—(13)
   Eye-opening nutrition facts—(14) Any questions about
   chapter I?

II. A Vitamin Pill Is a Vitamin Pill Is a . . .   **16**
   (15) Where vitamins come from—(16) Why vitamins
   come in different forms—(17) Oil v. dry or water
   soluble—(18) Synthetic vs. natural and inorganic vs.
   organic—(19) Chelation, and what it means—(20) Time
   releases—(21) Fillers, binders, or what else am I
   getting?—(22) Storage and staying power—(23) When
   and how to take supplements—(24) What's right for you
   —(25) Any questions about chapter II?

**III. Everything You Always Wanted to Know About
      Vitamins but Had No One to Ask**   **26**
   (26) Vitamin A—(27) Vitamin B1 (thiamine)—(28)
   Vitamin B2 (riboflavin)—(29) Vitamin B6 (pyridoxine)

—(30) Vitamin B12 (cobalamin)—(31) Vitamin B13 (orotic acid)—(32) B15 (pangamic acid)—(33) Vitamin B17 (laetrile)—(34) biotin (coenzyme R or vitamin H) —(35) Vitamin C (ascorbic acid, cevitamin acid)—(36) Calcium pantothenate (pantothenic acid, panthenol, vitamin B5)—(37) Choline—(38) Vitamin D (calciferol, viosterol, ergosterol, "sunshine vitamin")—(39) Vitamin E (tocopherol)—(40) Vitamin F (unsaturated fatty acids—linoleic, linolenic, and arachidonic)—(41) Folic acid (folacin, folate)—(42) Inositol—(43) Vitamin K (menadione)—(44) Niacin (nicotinic acid, niacinamide, nicotinamide)—(45) Vitamin P (C complex, citrus bioflavonoids, rutin, hesperidin)—(46) PABA (para-aminobenzoic acid)—(47) Vitamin T—(48) Vitamin U—(49) Any questions about chapter III?

IV. Your Mineral Essentials   69
(50) Calcium—(51) Chlorine—(52) Chromium—(53) Cobalt—(54) Copper—(55) Fluorine—(56) Iodine (iodide)—(57) Iron—(58) Magnesium—(59) Manganese —(60) Molybdenum—(61) Phosphorus—(62) Potassium —(63) Selenium—(64) Sodium—(65) Sulfur—(66) Vanadium—(67) Zinc—(68) Water—(69) Any questions about chapter IV?

V. Protein—and Those Amazing Amino Acids   100
(70) The protein-amino acid connection—(71) How much protein do you need, really?—(72) Types of protein—what's the difference?—(73) Protein myths— (74) Protein supplements—(75) Amino acid supplements —(76) Let's talk tryptophan—(77) The phenomenal phenylalanine—(78) DL-phenylalanine (DLPA)—(79) Looking at lysine—(80) All about arginine—(81) Growth hormone (G.H.) releasers—(82) Other amazing amino acids—(83) Any questions about chapter V?

VI. Fat and Fat Manipulators   122
(84) Lipotropics—what are they?—(85) Who needs them and why—(86) The cholesterol story—(87)

Leveling about cholesterol levels—(88) Saturated fat vs. unsaturated fat—(89) Foods and nutrients that can lower your cholesterol naturally—(90) Do you know what's raising your cholesterol?—(91) Any questions about chapter VI?

VII. Carbohydrates and Enzymes   131
(92) Why carbohydrates are necessary—(93) The truth about enzymes—(94) The twelve tissue salts and their functions—(95) Any questions about chapter VII?

VIII. Other Wonder Workers   137
(96) Acidophilus—(97) Ginseng—(98) Alfalfa, garlic, chlorophyll, and yucca—(99) Fiber and bran—(100) Kelp—(101)Yeast—(102) Any questions about chapter VIII?

IX. Herbs and Folk Remedies   148
(103) What you should know about natural remedies—(104) Basil—(105) Echinacea—(106) Saw-Palmetto (berries)—(107) Poke weed—(108) Aconite—(109) Aloe vera—(110) Anise (seed)—(111) Astragalus—(112) Blessed thistle—(113) Chamomile—(114) Comfrey—(115) Juniper (berries)—(116) Licorice—(117) Evening primrose oil—(118) Parsley (seeds and leaves)—(119) Pennyroyal—(120) Peppermint (leaves)—(121) Rosemary (leaves)—(122) Thyme—(123) Dangerous herbs—(124) Any questions about chapter IX?

X. How to Find Out What Vitamins You Really Need   161
(125) What is a balanced diet and are you eating it?—(126) How to test for deficiencies—(127) Possible warning signs—(128) Cravings—what they might mean—(129) Getting the most vitamins from your food—(130) Any questions about chapter X?

XI. Read the Label   189
(131) The importance of understanding what's on labels
—(132) How does that measure up?—(133) Breaking
the RDA code—(134) What to look for—(135) Any
questions about chapter XI?

XII. Your Special Vitamin Needs   195
(136) Selecting your regimen—(137) Women—(138)
Men—(139) Infants—(140) Children—(141) Pregnant
women—(142) Nursing mothers—(143) Runners—(144)
Joggers—(145) Executives—(146) Students—(147)
Senior citizens—(148) Athletes—(149) Body builders—
(150) Night workers—(151) Truck drivers—(152)
Dancers—(153) Construction workers—(154) Gamblers
—(155) Salespersons—(156) Actors—stage, screen,
radio and TV performers—(157) Singers—(158)
Doctors and nurses—(159) Handicapped—(160) Golfers
—(161) Tennis players—(162) Racketball players—
(163) Teachers—(164) Smokers—(165) Drinkers—
(166) Excessive TV watchers—(167) Travelers on the
go—(168) Any questions about chapter XII?

XIII. The Right Vitamin at the Right Time   210
(169) Special situation supplements—(170) Acne—(171)
Athlete's foot—(172) Bad breath—(173) Baldness or
falling hair—(174) Bee stings—(175) Bleeding gums—
(176) Broken bones—(177) Bruises—(178) Burns—
(179) Cold feet—(180) Cold sores and herpes simplex—
(181) Constipation—(182) Cuts—(183) Dry skin—(184)
Hangovers—(185) Hay fever—(186) Headaches—(187)
Heartburn—(188) Hemorrhoids—(189) Insomnia—(190)
Itching—(191) Jet lag—(192) Leg pains—(193)
Menopause—(194) Menstruation—(195) Motion
sickness—(196) Muscle soreness—(197) The pill—
(198) Poison ivy—(199) Polyps—(200) Postoperative
healing—(201) Prickly heat—(202) Prostate problems—
(203) Psoriasis—(204) Stopping smoking—(205)
Sunburn—(206) Teeth grinding—(207) Varicose veins

—(208) Vasectomy—(209) Warts—(210) Any questions about chapter XIII?

XIV. Getting Well and Staying That Way   **223**
(211) Why you need supplements during illness—(212) Allergies—(213) Arthritis—(214) Asthma—(215) Blood pressure—high and low—(216) Bronchitis—(217) Candida albicans—(218) Chicken pox—(219) Chronic fatigue syndrome—(220) Colds—(221) Colitis—(222) Diabetes—(223) Eye problems—(224) Heart conditions —(225) Hypoglycemia—(226) Impetigo—(227) Measles —(228) Mononucleosis—(229) Mumps—(230) P.M.S. (premenstrual syndrome)—(231) Shingles—(232) Tonsillitis—(233) Ulcers—(234) Venereal disease— (235) Any questions about chapter XIV?

XV. It's Not All in Your Mind   **238**
(236) How vitamins and minerals affect your moods— (237) Nutrients that combat depression, anxiety and stress—(238) Other drugs can add to your problem— (239) Any questions about chapter XV?

XVI. Drugs and You   **244**
(240) Let's start with caffeine—(241) You're getting more than you think—(242) Caffeine alternatives— (243) What alcohol does to your body—(244) What you drink and when you drink it—(245) Vitamins to decrease your taste for alcohol—(246) The lowdown on marijuana and hashish—(247) Cocaine costs a lot more than you think—in more ways than one—(248) Help for coming down or kicking the cocaine habit—(249) Whether Rx or over-the-counter, there are alternatives to drugs—(250) The great medicine rip-off—(251) Any questions about chapter XVI?

XVII. Losing It—Diets by the Pound   **259**
(252) The Atkins' diet—(253) The Stillman diet—(254) The Scarsdale Diet—(255) Weight Watchers—(256) The drinking man's diet—(257) Liquid protein and

Cambridge diets—(258) Zen macrobiotic diet—(259) Fructose diet—(260) Kelp, lecithin, vinegar, B6 diet—(261) Mindell dieting tips—(262) Mindell vitamin-balanced diet to lose and live by—(263) Supplements for eating more and gaining less—(264) Any questions about chapter XVII?

XVIII. So You Think You Don't Eat Much Sugar
       and Salt   272
(265) Kinds of sugars—(266) Other sweeteners—(267) Dangers of too much sugar—(268) How sweet it is—(269) Dangers of too much salt—(270) High-salt traps—(271) How salty is it?—(272) Any questions about chapter XVIII?

XIX. Staying Beautiful—Staying Handsome   279
(273) Vitamins for healthy skin—(274) Vitamins for healthy hair—(275) Vitamins for hands and feet—(276) Natural cosmetics—what's in them?—(277) Not so pretty drugs—(278) Any questions about chapter XIX?

XX. Staying Young, Energetic, and Sexy   287
(279) Retarding the aging process—(280) Basic keep yourself young program—(281) High-pep energy regimen—(282) High-pep supplements—(283) Vitamins and sex—(284) Food and supplements for better sex—(285) Any questions about chapter XX?

XXI. Pets Need Good Nutrition Too   296
(286) Vitamins for your dog—(287) Arthritis and dysplasia—(288) Vitamins for your cat—(289) Any questions about chapter XXI?

XXII. Vitamins "Yeses" and "Nos"
      You Should Know   301
(290) Cautions—(291) Quick reference cancer defense guide—(292) Any questions about chapter XXII?

XXIII. Locating a Nutritionally-Oriented Doctor   310
(293) How to go about it—(294) Finding specialized
nutrition help—(295) Free calls for fast answers

Afterword   *319*
Glossary   *320*
Bibliography and Recommended Reading   *327*
Index   *335*

A Note to the Reader About This Newly Revised Edition

Since the first publication of *The Vitamin Bible* in 1979, and its revision in 1985, the connection between diet and disease has grown from possibility to probability; actually, it has become irrefutable. Where once preventive medicine was considered speculative and the domaine of an off-beat few, it is now accepted as fact by even the most conservative members of the medical establishment. Nutritional fitness has become the credo of the '90s.

This new edition has been updated and expanded to include not only the National Research Council's revised vitamin and mineral requirements but the latest nutritional discoveries affecting our daily health and lives today. Although the format remains unchanged, there is new information in every chapter. There are also seventeen completely new sections—including a quick-reference cancer defense guide to foods you should (or shouldn't) be eating; everything you need to know about cholesterol; the lowdown on the latest wonder-working herbs and amino acids; natural alternatives to steroids; nutrients that may help alleviate Chronic Fatigue Syndrome; warnings about the water you're drinking; natural remedies for candida albicans; what you're entitled to know about artificial sweeteners, fake fats, and much, much more. It's all here, along with a greatly expanded list of cautions and suggested nutritional regimens.

ONE IMPORTANT REMINDER

The regimens throughout this book are recommendations, not prescriptions, and are not intended as medical advice. Before starting any new program, check with your physician or a nutritionally oriented doctor (see section 293), especially if you have a specific physical problem or are taking any medication.

Preface

This book is written for *you*—the untold legions of men and women who are forever trying to fit yourselves into statistical norms only to find that the charts are designed for some mythical average person who is taller, shorter, fatter, skinnier, less or more active than you'll ever be. It is a guide to healthy living for individuals, not statistics. Wherever feasible I have given personal advice, for this, I believe, is the only way to lead anyone to optimal health, which is the purpose of this book.

In these pages I have combined my knowledge of pharmacy with that of nutrition to best explain the confusing, often dangerous, interrelation of drugs and vitamins. I've attempted to personalize and be specific so as to eliminate much of the confusion about vitamins that has arisen with generalizations.

In using the book you will occasionally find that your vitamin needs fall into several different categories. In this case, let common sense dictate the necessary adjustment. (If you are already taking B6, for example, there's no need to double up on it unless a higher dosage is called for.)

The recommendations I've made are not meant to be prescriptive but can easily be used as flexible programs when working with your doctor. No book can substitute for professional care.

It is my sincere hope that I have provided you with information that will help you attain the longest, happiest, and healthiest of lives.

EARL MINDELL, R.PH., PH.D.

I

Getting into Vitamins

1. Why I Did

My professional education was strictly establishment when it came to vitamins. My courses in pharmacology, biochemistry, organic and inorganic chemistry, and public health hardly dealt with vitamins at all—except in relation to deficiency diseases. Lack of vitamin C? Scurvy. Out of B1? Beriberi. Not enough vitamin D? Rickets. My courses were the standard fare, with the usual references to a balanced diet and eating the "right foods" (all unappetizingly illustrated on semiglossy charts).

There were no references to vitamins being used for disease prevention or as ways to optimum health.

> Both of us were working fifteen hours a day,
> but only *I* looked and felt it.

In 1965 I opened my first pharmacy. Until then I never realized just how many drugs people were taking, not for illness but simply to get through the day. (I had one regular patron who had prescriptions for pills to supplant virtually all his bodily functions—and he wasn't even sick!) My partner at the time was very vitamin-oriented. Both of us were working fifteen hours a day, but only *I* looked and felt it. When I asked him what his secret was, he said it was not secret at

1

all. It was vitamins. I realized what he was talking about had very little to do with scurvy and beriberi and a lot to do with me. I instantly became an eager pupil, and have never since regretted it. He taught me the benefits that could be reaped from nature's own foods in the form of vitamins, how B complex and C could alleviate stress, how vitamin E would increase my endurance and stamina, and how B12 could eliminate fatigue. After embarking on the most elementary vitamin regimens I was not only convinced. I was converted.

Suddenly nutrition became the most important thing in my life. I read every book I could find on the subject, clipped articles and tracked down their sources, dug out my pharmacy school texts and discovered the amazingly close relationship that did indeed exist between biochemistry and nutrition. I attended any health lecture I could. In fact, it was at one such lecture that I learned of the RNA-DNA nucleic complex and its age-reversing properties. (I have been taking RNA-DNA supplements since then, as well as SOD—Super-Oxide Dismutase. Today, because of these, most people guess me to be five to ten years younger than I am.) I was excited about each new discovery in the field, and it showed.

A whole new world had opened up for me and I wanted others to share it. My partner understood completely. We began giving out samples of B complex and B12 tablets to patrons, suggesting they try decreasing their dependency on tranquilizers, pep pills, and sedatives with the vitamins and vitamin-rich foods.

The results were remarkable! People kept coming back to tell us how much better and more energetic they felt. Instead of the negativity and resignation that often accompanies drug therapies, we received overwhelming positiveness. I saw a woman who had spent nearly all her young adult life on Librium, running from doctor to therapist and back again, become a healthy, happy, drug-free human being; a sixty-year-old architect, on the brink of retirement because of ill health, regain his well-being and accept a commission for what is now one of the foremost office buildings in Los Angeles; a middle-aged pill-dependent actor kick his habit and land a sought-after supporting role in a TV series that still nets him handsome residuals.

By 1970 I was totally committed to nutrition and preventive medicine. Seeing the paucity of knowledge in the area, I went into partnership with another pharmacist for the prime purpose of making natural vitamins and accurate nutrition information available to the public.

Today, as a nutritionist, lecturer, and author, I'm still excited about that world that opened up to me over twenty years ago—a world that continues to grow with new discoveries daily—and I'm eager to share it.

2. What Vitamins Are

> We must obtain vitamins from natural foods, or dietary supplements in order to sustain life.

When I mention the word "vitamin," most people think "pill." Thinking "pill" brings to mind confusing images of medicine and drugs. Though vitamins can and certainly often do the work of both medicine and drugs, they are neither.

• Quite simply, vitamins are organic substances necessary for life. Vitamins are essential to the normal functioning of our bodies and, save for a few exceptions, cannot be manufactured or synthesized internally. Necessary for our growth, vitality, and general well-being, they are found in minute quantities in all natural food. We must obtain vitamins from these foods or from dietary supplements.

What you have to keep in mind is that supplements, which are available in tablet, capsule, liquid, powder, and even injection forms, are still just food substances, and, unless synthetic, are also derived from living plants and animals.

• It is impossible to sustain life without *all* the essential vitamins.

3. What Vitamins Are Not

> Vitamins are neither pep pills nor
> substitutes for food.

A lot of people think vitamins can replace food. They cannot. In fact, vitamins cannot be assimilated without ingesting food. There are a lot of erroneous beliefs about vitamins, and I hope this book can clear up most of them.

• Vitamins are not pep pills and have no caloric or energy value of their own.
• Vitamins are not substitutes for protein or for any other nutrients, such as minerals, fats, carbohydrates, water—or even for each other!
• Vitamins themselves are not the components of our body structures.
• You cannot take vitamins, stop eating, and except to be healthy.

4. How They Work

If you think of the body as an automobile's combustion engine and vitamins as spark plugs, you have a fairly good idea of how these amazing minute food substances work for us.

> Vitamins regulate our metabolism through
> enzyme systems. A single deficiency can
> endanger the whole body.

Vitamins are components of our enzyme systems which, acting like spark plugs, energize and regulate our metabolism, keeping us tuned up and functioning at high performance.

Compared with our intake of other nutrients like proteins, fats, and carbohydrates, our vitamin intake (even on some megadose regimens) is minuscule. But a deficiency in even one vitamin can endanger the whole human body.

5. Should You Take Supplements?

> "Everyone who has in the past eaten
> sugar, white flour, or canned food has
> some deficiency disease. . . ."

Since vitamins occur in all organic material, some containing more of one vitamin than another and in greater or lesser amounts, you could say that if you ate the "right" foods in a well-balanced diet, you would get all the vitamins you need. And you would probably be right. The problem is, very few of us are able to arrange this mythical diet. According to Dr. Daniel T. Quigley, author of *The National Malnutrition*, "Everyone who has in the past eaten processed sugar, white flour, or canned food has some deficiency disease, the extent of the disease depending on the percentage of such deficient food in the diet."

> Because most restaurants tend to reheat food or keep it warm under heat lamps, if you frequently eat out you run the risk of vitamin A, B1, and C deficiencies. (And if you're a woman between the ages of 13 and 40, this sort of work-saving dining is likely to cost you invaluable calcium and iron.)

Most of the foods we eat have been processed and depleted in nutrients. Take breads and cereals, for example. Practically all of them you find in today's supermarkets are high in nothing but carbohydrates. "But they are enriched!" you say. It's written right on the label: *Enriched*.

Enriched? Enrichment means replacing nutrients in foods that once contained them but because of heat, storage, and so forth no longer do. Foods, therefore, are "enriched" to the levels found in the natural product before processing. Unfortunately, standards of enrichment leave much to be desired nutritionally. For example, the standards of enrichment for white flour is to replace the twenty-two natural nutrients that are removed with three B vitamins, vitamin D, calcium and iron salts. Now really, for the staff of life, that seems a pretty flimsy stick.

I think you can see why my feeling about taking supplements is clear.

6. What Are Nutrients?

They're more than vitamins, though people often think they are the same thing.

```
                    Six important nutrients
```

Carbohydrates, proteins (which are made up of amino acids*), fats, minerals, vitamins, and water are all nutrients—absorbable components of foods—and necessary for good health. Nutrients are necessary for energy, organ function, food utilization, and cell growth.

7. The Difference Between Micronutrients and Macronutrients

Micronutrients, like vitamins and minerals, do not themselves provide energy. The macronutrients—carbohydrates, fat, and protein—do that, but only when there are sufficient micronutrients to release them.

```
              With nutrients, less is often the
                    same as more.
```

The amount of micronutrients and macronutrients you need for proper health is vastly different—but each is important. (See Section 70 for "The Protein-Amino Acid Connection.")

8. How Nutrients Get To Work

```
              The Body simplifies nutrients in
                    order to utilize them.
```

*See Section 75.

Nutrients basically work through digestion. Digestion is a process of continuous chemical simplification of materials that enter the body through the mouth. Materials are split by enzymatic action into smaller and simpler chemical fragments, which can then be absorbed through walls of the digestive tract—an open-ended muscular tube, more than thirty feet long, which passes through the body—and finally enter the bloodstream.

9. Understanding Your Digestive System

Knowing how your digestive system works will clear up, right at the start, some of the more common confusions about how, when, and where nutrients operate.

Mouth and Esophagus
Digestion begins in the mouth with the grinding of food and a mixture of saliva. An enzyme called ptyalin in the saliva already begins to split starches into simple sugars. The food is then forced to the back of the mouth and into the esophagus, or gullet. Here is where peristalsis begins. This is a kneading "milking" constriction and relaxation of muscles that propels material through the digestive system. To prevent backflow of materials, and to time the release of proper enzymes—since one enzyme cannot do another enzyme's work—the digestive tract is equipped with valves at important junctions.

Stomach
This is the biggest bulge in the digestive trace, as most of us are well aware. But it is located higher than you might think, lying mainly behind the lower ribs, not under the navel, and it does not occupy the belly. It is a flexible bag enclosed by restless muscles, constantly changing form.

• Virtually nothing is absorbed through the stomach walls except alcohol.

> An ordinary meal leaves the stomach
> in three to five hours.

Watery substances, such as soup, leave the stomach quite rapidly. Fats remain considerably longer. An ordinary meal of carbohydrates, proteins, and fats is emptied from the average stomach in *three* to *five* hours. Stomach glands and specialized cells produce mucus, enzymes, hydrochloric acid, and a factor that enables vitamin B12 to be dissolved through intestinal walls into the circulation. A normal stomach is definitely on the acid side, and gastric juice, the stomach's special blend, consists of many substances:

Pepsin   The predominant stomach enzyme, a potent digester of meats and other proteins. It is active only in an acid medium.

Rennin   Curdles milk.

HCL (Hydrochloric acid)   Produced by stomach cells and creates an acidic state.

The stomach is not absolutely indispensable to digestion. Most of the process of digestion occurs beyond it.

Small Intestine

> Virtually all absorption of nutrients
> occurs in the small intestine.

Twenty-two feet long, here is where digestion is completed and virtually all absorption of nutrients occurs. It has an alkaline environment, brought about by highly alkaline bile, pancreatic juice, and secretions of the intestinal walls. The alkaline environment is necessary for the most important work of digestion and absorption. The *duodenum,* which begins at the stomach outlet, is the first part of the small intestine. This joins with the *jejunum* (about ten feet long), which joins with the *ileum* (ten to twelve feet long). When semiliquid contents of the small intestine are moved along by peristaltic action, we often say we hear our stomach "talking." Actually our stomach lies above these rumblings (called borborygmi), but even with the truth known it's doubtful the phrase will change.

Large Intestine (Colon)

> It takes twelve to fourteen hours for
> contents to make the circuit of the large intestine.

Any material leaving the ileum and entering the cecum (where the small and large intestine join) is quite watery. Backflow is prevented at this junction by a muscular valve.

Very little is absorbed from the large intestine except water.

The colon is primarily a storage and dehydrating organ. Substances entering in a liquid state become semisolid as water is absorbed. It takes twelve to fourteen hours for contents to make the circuit of the intestine.

The colon, in contrast to the germ-free stomach, is lavishly populated with bacteria, normal intestinal flora. A large part of the feces is composed of bacteria, along with indigestible material, chiefly cellulose, and substances eliminated from the blood and shed from the intestinal walls.

Liver

> The main storage organ for
> fat-soluble vitamins.

The liver is the largest solid organ of the body and weighs about four pounds. It is an incomparable chemical plant. It can modify almost any chemical structure. It is a powerful detoxifying organ, breaking down a variety of toxic molecules and rendering them harmless. It is also a blood reservoir and a storage organ for vitamins such as A and D and for digested carbohydrate (glycogen), which is released to sustain blood sugar levels. It manufactures enzymes, cholesterol, proteins, vitamin A (from carotene), and blood coagulation factors.

One of the prime functions of the liver is to produce bile. Bile contains salts that promote efficient digestion of fats by detergent action, emulsifying fatty materials.

Gallbladder

> Even the sight of food may empty
> the gallbladder.

This is a saclike storage organ about three inches long. It holds bile, modifies it chemically, and concentrates it tenfold. The taste or sometimes even the sight of food may be sufficient to empty it out. Constituents of gallbladder fluids sometimes crystallize and form gallstones.

Pancreas

> The pancreas provides the body's most
> important enzymes.

This gland is about six inches long and is nestled into the curve of the duodenum. Its cell clusters secrete insulin, which accelerates the burning of sugar in the body. Insulin is secreted into the blood, not the digestive tract. The larger part of the pancreas manufactures and secretes pancreatic juice, which contains some of the body's most important digestive enzymes—*lipases*, which split fats; *proteases*, which split protein; and *amylases*, which split starches.

10. Name That Vitamin

Because at one time no one knew the chemical structure of vitamins and therefore could not give them a proper scientific name, most are designated by a letter of the alphabet. The following vitamins are known today; many more may yet be discovered.

> Known vitamins from A to U

Vitamin A (retinol, carotene); vitamin B-complex group: B1 (thiamine), B2 (riboflavin), B3 (niacin, niacinamide), B4 (adenine), B5 (pantothenic acid), B6 (pyridoxine), B10, B11 (growth factors), B12 (cobalamin, cyanocobalamin), B13 (orotic acid), B15 (pangamic acid), B17 (amygdalin), Bc (folic acid), Bt (carnitine), Bx or PABA (para-aminobenzoic acid); choline; inositol; C (ascorbic acid); D (calciferol, viosterol, ergosterol); E (tocopherol); F (fatty acids); G (riboflavin); H (biotin); K (menadione); L (necessary for lactation); M (folic acid); P (bioflavonoids); Pp (niacinamide); P4 (troxerutin); T (growth-promoting substances); U (extracted from cabbage juice).

11. Name That Mineral

> The top seven minerals are: calcium, iodine,
> iron, magnesium, phosphorus, selenium,
> and zinc.

Although about eighteen known minerals are required for body maintenance and regulatory functions, Recommended Dietary Allowance (RDA) have only been established for seven—calcium, iodine, iron, magnesium, phosphorus, selenium, and zinc.

The active minerals in your body are: calcium, chlorine, chromium, cobalt, copper, fluorine, iodine, iron, magnesium, manganese, molybdenum, phosphorus, potassium, selenium, sodium, sulfur, vanadium, and zinc. Trace minerals such as boron, silicon, nickel and arsenic are also necessary for optimal growth and membrane function.

12. Your Body Needs Togetherness

> Vitamins alone are not enough.

As important as vitamins are, they can do nothing for you without minerals. I like to call minerals the Cinderellas of the nutrition world, because, though very few people are aware of it, vitamins cannot function, cannot be assimilated, without the aid of minerals. And though the body can synthesize some vitamins, it cannot manufacture a *single* mineral.

13. Eye-opening Nutrition Facts

- One cigarette destroys 25–100 mg. of vitamin C!
- Milk with synthetic vitamin D (which means almost all store-bought milk) can rob the body of magnesium!
- People who live in smoggy cities are not getting the vitamin D that their country cousins get because the smog absorbs the sun's ultraviolet rays!
- Daily "happy hours" of more than one cocktail can cause a depletion of vitamins B1, B6, and folic acid!
- Eighty percent of American women are deficient in calcium!
- Ten million American women take oral contraceptives and most of them are unaware that the pills can interfere with the availability of vitamins B6, B12, folic acid, and vitamin C!
- American men rank thirteenth in world health, American women sixth.
- Children need one-and-a-half to two times more protein per pound of body weight than adults—and babies need three times more!
- Cancer researchers at the Massachusetts Institute of Technology have found that vitamins C and E and certain chemicals called indoles, found in cabbage, brussels sprouts, and related vegetables in the crucifer family, are potent and apparently safe inhibitors of certain carcinogens!
- Vitamin B1 can help fight air and seasickness.
- If you're on a high-protein diet your need for B6 *increases*!
- Onions, garlic, radishes, and leeks all contain a natural antibiotic called *allicin*, which can destroy disease germs without sweeping away the friendly bacteria in the process!
- Aspirin can triple the rate of excretion of your vitamin C!
- Eighteen pecan halves can furnish an entire day's supply of vitamin F.
- Frequent consumption of foods containing artificial flavors, colors, MSG, and other additives can diminish the effectiveness of the immune system.

- Raw peanuts contain enzyme inhibitors that make it difficult for your body to digest protein.
- Bran is not a balanced food.
- Pasta packed in clear cellophane, or with large cellophane windows, is subject to nutrient loss.
- Water softeners can unhealthily increase your daily salt intake.
- A main ingredient of margarine—hardened vegetable oil —may be even worse for your health than saturated fat.
- Blueberries, blackberries, and red cabbage are actually better for you if cooked!
- Yellow and red onions, red grapes, and broccoli are rich in quercetin, a newly discovered anticancer agent that the University of California lab studies have shown can suppress malignant cells before they form tumors.
- Olive oil is one of the best heart disease-fighting natural foods available.
- The easiest way to rid your body of excess sodium is to flush it out by drinking 6 to 8 glasses of salt-free water daily.
- There may be a connection between toothpaste (with its crystalline abrasives, foaming agents and other additives) and bowel diseases such as ulcerative colitis, Chrohn's disease and irritable bowel syndrome. It's advisable to always rinse your mouth well after brushing and to try to avoid swallowing any toothpaste.
- There is more to smoking than the average seven-year drop in life expectancy reported by the American Cancer Society. ELEVEN YEARS MORE! New studies show that life expectancy between smokers and non-smokers differs by 18 years!
- The mineral "boron" (found in apples, grapes, grape juice and raisins) may retard bone loss in women after menopause. Also, boron helps women on ERT (estrogen replacement therapy) keep the estrogen in their blood longer.
- Avoiding black coffee may help you avoid cancer of the esophagus. Tannin, found in coffee and tea, is a suspected carcinogen. The protein in milk, though, neutralizes tannin, rendering it non-absorbable by the body.

• Bugs Bunny was right! Carrots may help keep plaque from forming on artery walls and help prevent heart attacks in people with artherosclerosis. Eating one large carrot daily will give you approximately 11,000 IU of vitamin A from beta-carotene!

14. Any Questions About Chapter I?

I've seen quite a few amino acid supplements in health food stores lately. Are these considered nutrients? Are they as important as vitamins?

Emphatically yes, and yes again! Amino acids (see section 70) are the building blocks of one of our most important nutrients—protein.

Every cell in your body contains (and needs) protein. It's used to build new tissue and repair damaged cells, as well as to make hormones and enzymes, keep the acid-alkaline blood content balanced, and eliminate the unwanted garbage, among other things. As protein is digested, it's broken down into smaller compounds called amino acids. When these amino acids reach the cells in your body, they're formed into protein again. It's a wonderful cycle.

The importance of vitamins and amino acids in nutrition is equal, because you'll get no value from one without the proper amount of the other. As for amino acid supplements and their value to you as an individual, I'd suggest looking over sections 70 and 75, which discuss some of the remarkable benefits supplementation has been shown to provide.

I know that vitamins can't work properly without minerals, but do some minerals make them work more effectively than others?

Definitely. Vitamin A, for instance, works best with the minerals calcium, magnesium, phosphorous, selenium, and zinc. The B vitamins are also potentiated by these minerals, along with cobalt, copper, iron, manganese, potassium, and sodium. For vitamin C, the five minerals found to promote the most effectiveness are calcium, cobalt, copper, iron, and sodium; for vitamin D, they are calcium, copper, magnesium, selenium, and sodium; and for vitamin E, they are calcium, iron manganese, phosphorous, potassium, selenium, sodium, and zinc. To find out what minerals—and other vitamins— can increase the effectiveness of individual vitamins, see sections 26–49.

What is this new mineral "boron"?

First of all, it's not new. And it's classified more as a trace element than a mineral. But this does not diminish its newly discovered importance in working with calcium, magnesium and vitamin D to help prevent osteoporosis. As a supplement, the daily recommended dosage is 3 mg.

II

A Vitamin Pill Is a Vitamin Pill Is a . . .

15. Where Vitamins Come From

> Most vitamins are extracted from
> basic natural sources.

Because vitamins are natural substances found in foods, the supplements you take—be they capsules, tablets, powders, or liquids—also come from foods. Though many of the vitamins can be synthesized, most are extracted from basic natural sources.

For example: Vitamin A usually comes from fish liver oil. Vitamin B complex comes from yeast or liver. Vitamin C is best when derived from rose hips, the berries found on the fruit of the rose after the petals have fallen off. And vitamin E is generally extracted from soybeans, wheat germ, or corn.

16. Why Vitamins Come in Different Forms

Everyone's needs are different, and for this reason manufacturers have provided many vitamins in a variety of forms.

> Vitamins come in different forms
> because people do.

Tablets are the most common and convenient form. They're easier to store, carry, and have a longer shelf life than powders or liquids.

Capsules, like tablets, are convenient and easy to store, and are the usual supplement for oil-soluble vitamins such as A, D, and E.

Caplets are capsule-shaped tablets. Sometimes these are "enteric coated" so that they dissolve in the intestine, not in the stomach (which is acid).

Gel-caps are soft gelatin capsules that many people find easier to swallow than regular capsules.

Powders have the advantages of extra potency (1 tsp. of many vitamin-C powders can give you as much as 4,000 mg.) and the added benefit of no fillers, binders, or additives for anyone with allergies.

Liquids are available for easy mixing with beverages and for people unable to swallow capsules or tablets.

Nasal inhalers have recently become a popular form of providing nutrients—particularly B and C vitamins, which are quickly absorbed through the mucous membranes in the nose.

Patches and implants, which can supply continuous, measured amounts of nutrients—in a variety of formulations— will also soon be available.

17. Oil v. Dry or Water Soluble

The oil-soluble vitamins, such as A, D, E, and K, are available and advisable in "dry" or water-soluble form for people who tend to get upset stomachs from oil, for acne sufferers, or anyone with a skin condition where oil ingestion is not advised, and for dieters who have cut most of the fat from their meals. (Fat-soluble vitamins need fat for proper assimilation. If you're on a low-fat diet and taking A, D, E, or K supplements, I suggest you use the dry form.)

18. Synthetic vs. Natural and Inorganic vs. Organic

> Synthetic vitamins might be less likely to
> upset your budget—but not your stomach.

When I'm asked if there's a difference between synthetic and natural vitamins, I usually say only one—and that's to you. Though synthetic vitamins and minerals have produced satisfactory results, the benefits from natural vitamins, on a variety of levels, surpass them. Chemical analysis of both might appear the same, but there's more to natural vitamins because there's more to those substances in nature.

Synthetic vitamin C is just that, ascorbic acid and nothing more. Natural C from rose hips contains bioflavonoids, the entire C complex, which make the C much more effective.

Natural vitamin E, which can include all the tocopherols, not just alpha, is more potent than its synthetic double.

According to Dr. Theron G. Randolph, noted allergist: *A synthetically derived substance may cause a reaction in a chemically susceptible person when the same material of natural origin is tolerated, despite the two substances having identical chemical structures.*

On the other hand, people who are allergic to pollen could experience an undesirable reaction to a natural vitamin C that had possible pollen impurities.

Nonetheless, as many who have tried both can attest, there are less gastrointestinal upsets with natural supplements, and far fewer toxic reactions when taken in higher than recommended dosage.

The difference between inorganic and organic is not the same as the one between synthetic and natural, though that is the common misconception. All vitamins are organic. They are substances containing carbon.

19. Chelation, and What It Means

> Only 2 to 10 percent of inorganic iron taken
> into the body is actually absorbed.

First, pronounce it correctly. *Key' lation*. This is the process by which mineral substances are changed into their digestible form. Common mineral supplements such as bonemeal and dolomite are often not chelated and must first be acted upon in the digestive process to form chelates before they are of use to the body. The natural chelating process is not performed efficiently in many people, and because of this a good deal of the mineral supplements they take is of little use.

When you realize that the body does not use whatever it takes in, that most of us do not digest our foods efficiently, that only 2 to 10 percent of inorganic iron taken into the body is actually absorbed, and, even with this small percentage, 50 percent is then eliminated, you can recognize the importance of taking minerals that have been chelated. Amino acid-bound chelated mineral supplements provide three to ten times greater assimilation than the nonchelated ones, and are well worth the small additional cost.

20. Time Release

A major step forward in vitamin manufacturing has been the introduction of time-release supplements. Time (or sustained) release is a process by which vitamins are enrobed in micro-pellets (tiny time pills) and then combined into a special base for their release in a pattern that assures six- to twelve-hour absorption. Most vitamins are water soluble and cannot be stored in the body. Without time release, they are quickly absorbed into the bloodstream, and, no matter how large the dose, are excreted in the urine within two to three hours.

> A way to twenty-four hour vitamin protection.

Time-release supplements can offer optimum effectiveness, minimal excretory loss, and stable blood levels all during the day and through the night.

21. Fillers, Binders, Or What Else Am I Getting?

There's more to a vitamin supplement than meets the eye—and sometimes more than meets the label. Fillers, binders, lubricants, and the like do not have to be listed and often aren't. But if you'd like to know what you're swallowing, the following list should help.

Diluents or fillers   These are inert materials added to the tablets to increase their bulk, in order to make them a practical size for compression. Dicalcium phosphate, which is an excellent source of calcium and phosphorus, is used in better brands. It is derived from purified mineral rocks. It is a white powder. Sorbitol and cellulose (plant fiber) are used occasionally.

Binders   These substances give cohesive qualities to the powdered materials, otherwise the binders or granulators are the materials that hold the ingredients of the tablet together. Cellulose and ethyl cellulose are used most often. Cellulose is the main constituent of plant fiber. Occasionally, lecithin and sorbitol are used. Other binders that can be used, but that you should be aware of—and look out for—are:

Acacia (gum arabic)—a vegetable gum that has been declared GRAS (Generally Recognized As Safe) by the FDA (Food and Drug Administration) but which can cause mild to severe asthma attacks and rashes in asthmatics, pregnant women, and anyone prone to allergies.

Algin (alginic acid or sodium alginate)—a plant carbohydrate derived from seaweed, but one that's potentially harmful. It is currently being investigated as a possible mutagen, capable of causing reproductive problems and birth defects. I'd suggest that if you're pregnant, trying to conceive, or a nursing mother, you should avoid products containing any alginates.

Lubricants   A slick substance added to a tablet to keep it from sticking to the machines that punch it out. Calcium stearate and silica are commonly used. Calcium stearate is derived from natural vegetable oils. Silica is a natural white powder. Magnesium stearate can also be used.

Disintegrators   Substances such as gum arabic, algin, and alginate are added to the tablet to facilitate its breakup or disintegration after ingestion.

Colors   They make the tablet more aesthetic or elegant in appearance. Colors derived from natural sources, like chlorophyll, are best.

Flavors and sweeteners   Used only in chewable tablets, the sweeteners are usually fructose (fruit sugar), malt dextrins, sorbitol, or maltose. Sucrose (sugar) is rarely used in better brands.

Coating material   These substances are used to protect the tablet from moisture. They also mask unpleasant flavor or odor and make the tablet easier to swallow. Zein is one of the substances. It is natural, derived from corn protein, and a clear film-coating agent. Brazil Wax, which is a natural product derived from palm trees, is also frequently used.

Drying agents   These substances prevent water-absorbing (hydroscopic) materials from picking up moisture during processing. Silica gel is the most common drying agent.

22. Storage and Staying Power

Vitamin and mineral supplements should be stored in a cool dark place away from direct sunlight in a well-closed—preferably opaque—container. They do not have to be stored in the refrigerator unless you live in a desert climate. To guard against excessive moisture, place a few kernels of rice at the bottom of your vitamin bottle. The rice works as a natural absorbent.

> Vitamins can last two to three years
> in a well-sealed container.

If vitamins are kept cool and away from light, and remain well sealed, they should last for two to three years. To insure freshness, though, your best bet is to buy brands that have an expiration date on the label. Once a bottle is opened you can expect a twelve-month shelf life.

Our bodies tend to excrete in urine substances we take in on a four-hour basis, and this is particularly true of water-soluble vitamins such as E and C. On an empty stomach, B and C vitamins can leave the body as quickly as two hours after ingestion.

The oil-soluble vitamins, A, D, E, and K, remain in the body for approximately twenty-four hours, though excess amounts can be stored in the liver for much longer. Dry A and E do not stay in the body as long.

23. When and How To Take Supplements

The human body operates on a twenty-four-hour cycle. Your cells do not go to sleep when you do, not can they exist without continuous oxygen and nutrients. Therefore, for best results, space your supplements as evenly as possible during the day.

> If you take your supplements all
> at once, do so after dinner,
> not breakfast.

The prime time for taking supplements is after meals. Vitamins are organic substances and should be taken with other foods and minerals for best absorption. Because the water-soluble vitamins, especially B complex and C, are excreted fairly rapidly in the urine, a regimen of after breakfast, after lunch, and after dinner will provide you with the highest body level. If after each meal is not convenient, then half the amount should be taken after breakfast and the other half after dinner.

If you must take your vitamins all at once, then do so after the largest meal of the day. In other words, for best results, after dinner, not after breakfast, is the most desirable.

And remember, minerals are essential for proper vitamin absorption, so be sure to take your minerals and vitamins together.

24. What's Right for You

If you're unsure as to whether you'd be better off with a powder, a liquid, or a tablet, regular vitamin E or dry, taking supplements three times a day or time released, my advice to you is to experiment. If the supplement you're taking doesn't agree with you, try it in another form. Vitamin-C powder mixed in a beverage might be much easier to take than several large pills when you're coming down with a cold. If your face breaks out with vitamin E, try the dry form. Check sections 26 through 69 and the cautions in section 290 to make sure you know all you should about your supplement.

25. Any Questions About Chapter II?

When vitamins smell awful, does that mean they're spoiled, and could they be harmful?

Strong odors don't necessarily signify spoilage, but it is possible. If you've been keeping your vitamins in sunlight and warmth (great for you but not for them) it's more than possible, it's probable. But even if your vitamins have spoiled, they won't harm you. The worst that can happen is that they lose their effectiveness.

Every so often I detect a sort of alcohol smell in a bottle of vitamins. Does this indicate some sort of deterioration, and are these vitamins still safe to take?

No, the vitamins are not deteriorating, and yes they are safe to take. Alcohol is often used as a drying agent to prevent any moisture contamination. Occasionally, if the product is packed too quickly, some of the alcohol smell remains. My advice is put a few kernels of rice in the bottle. These will absorb the moisture and the smell.

Sometimes I find that a few of my B vitamin pills are cracked. Are these safe to take?

Yes they are, as are your C's and any others. Poor tablet coating causes the cracks, but the vitamins themselves are still effective and safe.

If binders like acacia gum and alginic acid have been declared GRAS (Generally Recognized As Safe) by the FDA, why aren't they?

Just because an additive has been declared GRAS doesn't mean that it can't harm you. Here's why: when the food additive law requiring scientific testing of all chemicals for safe usage in foods went into effect in 1958, the FDA established the GRAS list to eliminate expensive testing of what were unquestionably assumed to be safe chemicals (sugar, starch, salt, baking soda, etc.). As a result of the FDA's action, all additives in use before that year were deemed GRAS; regrettably, many were later found to be otherwise.

If a vitamin supplement is available in both capsule and tablet form, which one is better?

That's a tough but good question. There are pros and cons for both. On the capsule pro side: many people find them easier to swallow than tablets; they dissolve faster; they appear to have no fillers or binders; and, because many prescription medicines come in capsule form, they seem more potent and effective.

On the con side: capsules are not as effective as tablets in protecting vitamins from oxidation; the slow release effected by capsules is more natural where nutrients are concerned;

capsules are usually more expensive than tablets, and the belief that they have no fillers or binders is untrue. (See section 21.)

What you may find to be a deciding factor—if you're a vegetarian—is that capsules are made with gelatin, an animal product. Tablets, on the other hand, can be totally vegetarian. (Be forwarned, though, that not *all* of them are.)

When in doubt, call the manufacturer—or consult a nutritionally oriented doctor. (See section 293.)

III

Everything You Always Wanted to Know About Vitamins but Had No One to Ask

26. Vitamin A

FACTS:

Vitamin A is fat soluble. It requires fats as well as minerals to be properly absorbed by your digestive trace.

It can be stored in your body and need not be replenished every day.

It occurs in two forms—performed vitamin A, called retinol (found only in foods of animal origin), and provitamin A, known as carotene (provided by foods of both plant and animal origin).

Vitamin A is measured in USP Units (United States Pharmocopea), IU (International Units), and—most recently—RE (Retinol Equivalents). (See section 132.)

1,000 RE (or 5,000 IU) is the recommended daily dosage for adult males to prevent deficiency. For females it's 800 RE (4,000 IU). During pregnancy the new RDAs do not recommend an increase, but for nursing mothers an additional 500 RE is suggested for the first six months and an additional 400 RE for the second six months.

NOTE: Throughout this book, beta-carotene will be the preferred form of vitamin A. I find it preferable because it does not have the same toxicity potential of vitamin A. Moreover, it has been shown to be a preventive for certain types of cancer, helpful in lowering levels of harmful cholesterol (see section 89) and a significant factor in reducing the risk of heart disease.

WHAT IT CAN DO FOR YOU:

Counteract night blindness, weak eyesight, and aid in the treatment of many eye disorders. (It permits formation of visual purple in the eye.)

Build resistance to respiratory infections.

Aid in the proper function of the immune system.

Shorten the duration of diseases.

Keep the outer layers of your tissues and organs healthy.

Help in the removal of age spots.

Promote growth, strong bones, healthy skin, hair, teeth, and gums.

Help treat acne, superficial wrinkles, impetigo, boils, carbuncles, and open ulcers when applied externally.

Aid in the treatment of emphysema and hyperthyroidism.

DEFICIENCY DISEASE:

Xerophthalmia, night blindness. (For deficiency symptoms, see section 127.) Deficiency often occurs as a result of chronic fat malabsorption. It's most commonly found in children under five years, usually because of insufficient dietary intake.

BEST NATURAL SOURCE:

Fish liver oil, liver, carrots, dark green and yellow vegetables, eggs, milk and dairy products, margarine, and yellow fruits. (Note: The color intensity of a fruit or vegetable is not necessarily a reliable indicator of its provitamin A content.)

SUPPLEMENTS:

Usually available in two forms, one derived from natural fish liver oil and the other water dispersible. Water-dispersible supplements are either acetate or palmitate and recommended for anyone intolerant to oil, particularly acne sufferers. 5,000 to 10,000 IU are the most common daily doses.

Vitamin A acid (retin A), which has often been used in the treatment of acne, and is now being marketed as a treatment for eradicating superficial wrinkles, is available only by prescription.

TOXICITY:

More than 50,000 IU daily, if taken for many months, can produce toxic effects in adults.

More than 18,500 IU daily can produce toxic effects in infants.

Toxicity symptoms include hair loss, nausea, vomiting, diarrhea, scaly skin, blurred vision, rashes, bone pain, irregular menses, fatigue, headaches, and liver enlargement. (See section 290, "Cautions.")

ENEMIES:

Polyunsaturated fatty acids with carotene work against vitamin A unless there are antioxidants present. (See section 49 for antioxidants, and section 250 for drugs that deplete vitamins.)

PERSONAL ADVICE:

You need at least 10,000 IU vitamin A if you take more than 400 IU vitamin E daily.

If you are on the pill, your need for A is *decreased*.

If your weekly diet includes ample amounts of liver, carrots, spinach, sweet potatoes, or cantaloupe, it's unlikely you need an A supplement.

Vitamin A should *not* be taken with mineral oil.

Vitamin A works best with B complex, vitamin D, vitamin E, calcium, phosphorus, and zinc. (Zinc is what's needed by the liver to get vitamin A out of its storage deposits.)

Vitamin A also helps vitamin C from oxidizing.

Don't supplement your dog's or cat's diet with vitamin A unless a vet specifically advises it.

If you are on a cholesterol-reducing drug such as Questran (*cholestyramine*), you'll have decreased vitamin A absorption and probably need a supplement.

27. Vitamin B1 (Thiamine)

FACTS:

Water soluble. Like all the B-complex vitamins, any excess is excreted and not stored in the body. It must be replaced daily.

Measured in milligrams (mg.).

Being synergistic, B vitamins are more potent together than when used separately. B1, B2, and B6 should be equally balanced (i.e., 50 mg. of B1, 50 mg. of B2, and 50 mg. of B6) to work effectively.

The official RDA for adults is 1.0 to 1.5 mg. (During pregnancy and lactation 1.5 to 1.6 mg. is suggested.)

Need increases during illness, stress, and surgery.

Known as the "morale vitamin" because of its beneficial effects on the nervous system and mental attitude.

Has a mild diuretic effect.

WHAT IT CAN DO FOR YOU:

Promote growth.

Aid digestion, especially of carbohydrates.

Improve your mental attitude.

Keep nervous system, muscles, and heart functioning normally.

Help fight air or seasickness.

Relieve dental postoperative pain.

Aid in treatment of herpes zoster.

DEFICIENCY DISEASE:

Beriberi. (For deficiency symptoms, see section 127.)

BEST NATURAL SOURCES:

Brewer's yeast, rice husks, unrefined cereal grains, whole

wheat, oatmeal, peanuts, organic meats, lean pork, most vegetables, bran, milk.

Supplements:

Available in low- and high-potency dosages—usually 50 mg., 100 mg., and 500 mg. It is most effective in B-complex formulas, balanced with B2 and B6. It is even more effective when the formula contains antistress pantothenic acid, folic acid, and B12. 100 to 300 mg. are the most common daily doses.

Toxicity:

No known toxicity for this water-soluble vitamin. Any excess is excreted in the urine and not stored to any degree in tissues or organs.

Rare excess symptoms (when doses exceed 5–10 g. daily) include tremors, herpes, edema, nervousness, rapid heartbeat, and allergies.

(See section 290, "Cautions.")

Enemies:

Cooking heat easily destroys this B vitamin. Other enemies of B1 are caffeine, alcohol, food-processing methods, air, water, estrogen, antacids, and sulfa drugs. (See section 250 for drugs that deplete vitamins.)

Personal Advice:

If you are a smoker, drinker, or heavy sugar consumer, you need more vitamin B1.

If you are pregnant, nursing, or on the pill you have a greater need for this vitamin.

If you're in the habit of taking an after-dinner antacid, you're losing the thiamine you might have gotten from the meal.

As with all stress conditions—disease, anxiety, trauma, postsurgery—your B-complex intake, which includes thiamine, should be increased.

28. Vitamin B2 (Riboflavin)

FACTS:

Water soluble. Easily absorbed. The amount excreted depends on bodily needs and may be accompanied by protein loss. Like the other B vitamins it is not stored and must be replaced regularly through whole foods or supplements.

Also known as vitamin G.

Measured in milligrams (mg.).

Unlike thiamine, riboflavin is *not* destroyed by heat, oxidation, or acid.

For normal adults, 1.2 to 1.7 mg. is the RDA. During pregnancy, 1.6 mg. is suggested. For nursing mothers, 1.8 mg. is recommended for the first six months and 1.7 mg. for the second six months.

Increased need in stress situations.

America's most common vitamin deficiency is riboflavin.

WHAT IT CAN DO FOR YOU:

Aid in growth and reproduction.

Promote healthy skin, nails, hair.

Help eliminate sore mouth, lips, and tongue.

Benefit vision, alleviate eye fatigue.

Function with other substances to metabolize carbohydrates, fats, and proteins.

DEFICIENCY DISEASE:

Ariboflavinosis—mouth, lips, skin, genitalia lesions. (For deficiency symptoms, see section 127.)

BEST NATURAL SOURCES:

Milk, liver, kidney, yeast, cheese, leafy green vegetables, fish, eggs.

SUPPLEMENTS:

Available in both low and high potencies—most commonly in 100-mg. doses. Like most of the B-complex vitamins, it is most effective when in a well-balanced formula with the others.

100 to 300 mg. are the most common daily doses.

TOXICITY:

No known toxic effects.

Possible symptoms of minor excess include itching, numbness, sensations of burning or prickling.

(See section 290, "Cautions.")

ENEMIES:

Light—especially ultraviolet light—and alkalies are destructive to riboflavin. (Opaque milk cartons now protect riboflavin that used to be destroyed in clear glass milk bottles.) Other natural enemies are water (B2 dissolves in cooking liquids), sulfa drugs, estrogen, alcohol.

PERSONAL ADVICE:

If you are taking the pill, pregnant, or lactating, you need more vitamin B2.

If you eat little red meat or dairy products you should increase your intake.

There is a strong likelihood of your being deficient in this vitamin if you are on a prolonged restricted diet for ulcers or diabetes. (In all cases where you are under medical treatment for a specific illness, check with your doctor before altering your present food regimen or embarking on a new one.)

All stress conditions require additional B complex.

This vitamin works best with vitamin B6, vitamin C, and niacin.

If you're taking an antineoplastic (anticancer) drug such as *methotrexate*, too much vitamin B2 can cut down the drug's effectiveness.

29. Vitamin B6 (Pyridoxine)

FACTS:

Water soluble. Excreted within eight hours after ingestion and, like the other B vitamins, needs to be replaced by whole foods or supplements.

B6 is actually a group of substances—pyridoxine, pyridoxal, and pyridoxamine—that are closely related and function together.

Measured in milligrams (mg.).

Requirement increased when high-protein diets are consumed.

Must be present for the production of antibodies and red blood cells.

There is some evidence of synthesis by intestinal bacteria, and that a vegetable diet supplemented with cellulose is responsible.

The recommended adult intake is 1.6 to 2.0 mg. daily, with 2.2 mg. doses suggested during pregnancy and 2.1 mg. for lactation.

Required for the proper absorption of vitamin B12.

Necessary for the production of hydrochloric acid and magnesium.

Dairy products are relatively poor sources of B6.

WHAT IT CAN DO FOR YOU:

Properly assimilate protein and fat.

Aid in the conversion of tryptophan, an essential amino acid, to niacin.

Help prevent various nervous and skin disorders.

Alleviate nausea (many morning-sickness preparations that doctors prescribe include vitamin B6).

Promote proper synthesis of antiaging nucleic acids.

Help reduce dry mouth and urination problems caused by tricyclic anti-depressants.

Reduce night muscle spasms, leg cramps, hand numbness, certain forms of neuritis in the extremities.

Work as a natural diuretic.

DEFICIENCY DISEASE:

Anemia, seborrheic dermatitis, glossitis. (For deficiency symptoms, see section 127.)

BEST NATURAL SOURCES:

Brewer's yeast, wheat bran, wheat germ, liver, kidney, soy beans, cantaloupe, cabbage, blackstrap molasses, unmilled rice, eggs, oats, peanuts, walnuts.

SUPPLEMENTS:

Readily available in a wide range of dosages—from 50 to 500 mg.—in individual supplements as well as in B-complex and multivitamin formulas.

To prevent deficiencies in other B vitamins, pyridoxine should be taken in equal amounts with B1 and B2.

Can be purchased in time-disintegrating formulas that provide for gradual release up to ten hours.

TOXICITY:

Daily doses of 2–10 grams can cause neurological disorders.

Possible symptom of an oversupply of B6 is night restlessness and too vivid dream recall.

Doses over 500 mg. are not recommended. (See section 290, "Cautions.")

ENEMIES:

Long storage, canning, roasting or stewing of meat, freezing fruits and vegetables, water, food-processing techniques, alcohol, estrogen. (See section 250.)

PERSONAL ADVICE:

If you are on the pill, you are more than likely to need increased amounts of B6.

Heavy protein consumers need extra amounts of this vitamin.

Vitamin B6 might decrease a diabetic's requirement for insulin, and if the dosage is not adjusted, a low-blood-sugar reaction could result.

Arthritis sufferers being treated with Cuprimine (*penicillamine*) should be taking supplements of this vitamin.

This vitamin works best with vitamin B1, vitamin B2, pantothenic acid, vitamin C, and magnesium.

Supplements for this vitamin should *not* be taken by anyone under *levodopa* treatment for Parkinson's disease! (Ask your doctor about Sinemet, a drug which can bypass this particular adverse vitamin interaction.)

30. Vitamin B12 (Cobalamin)

FACTS:

Water soluble and effective in very small doses.

Commonly known as the "red vitamin," also cyanocobalamin.

Cyanocobalamin is the commercially available form of vitamin B12 used in vitamin pills.

Measured in micrograms (mcg.)

The only vitamin that contains essential mineral elements.

Not well assimilated through the stomach. Needs to be combined with calcium during absorption to properly benefit body.

Recommended adult dose is 2 mcg., with 2.2 mcg. suggested for pregnant women and 2.6 mcg. for nursing mothers.

A diet low in B1 and high in folic acid (such as a vegetarian diet) often hides a vitamin-B12 deficiency.

A properly functioning thyroid gland helps B12 absorption. Symptoms of B12 deficiency may take more than five years to appear after body stores have been depleted.

In the human diet, vitamin B12 is supplied primarily by animal products, since plant foods (with minor exceptions) don't contain it.

WHAT IT CAN DO FOR YOU:

Form and regenerate red blood cells, thereby preventing anemia.

Promote growth and increase appetite in children.
Increase energy.
Maintain a healthy nervous system.
Properly utilize fats, carbohydrates, and protein.
Relieve irritability.
Improve concentration, memory, and balance.

DEFICIENCY DISEASE:

Pernicious anemia, neurological disorders. (For deficiency symptoms, see section 127.)

BEST NATURAL SOURCES:

Liver, beef, pork, eggs, milk, cheese, kidney.

SUPPLEMENTS:

Because B12 is not absorbed well through the stomach, I recommend the sublingual form of the vitamin, or the time-release form—accompanied by sorbitol—so that it can be assimilated in the small intestine.

Supplements are available in a variety of strengths from 50 mcg. to 2,000 mcg.

Doctors routinely give vitamin-B12 injections. If there is a severe indication of deficiency or extreme fatigue, this method might be the supplementation that's called for.

Daily dosages most often used are 5 to 100 mcg.

TOXICITY:

There have been no cases reported of vitamin-B12 toxicity, even on megadose regimens.

(See section 290, "Cautions.")

ENEMIES:

Acids and alkalies, water, sunlight, alcohol, estrogen, sleeping pills. (See section 250.)

PERSONAL ADVICE:

If you are a vegetarian and have excluded eggs and dairy products from your diet, then you need B12 supplementation.

If you keep regular "Happy Hours" and drink a lot, B12 is an important supplement for you.

Combined with folic acid, B12 can be a most effective revitalizer.

Surprisingly, heavy protein consumers may also need extra amounts of this vitamin, which works synergistically with almost all other B vitamins as well as vitamins A, E, and C.

Elderly people frequently have difficulty absorbing vitamin B12 and require supplementation by injection.

Women may find B12 helpful—as part of a B complex— during and just prior to menstruation.

31. Vitamin B13 (Orotic Acid)

FACTS:

Not available in the United States.
Metabolizes folic acid and vitamin B12.
No RDA has been established.

WHAT IT CAN DO FOR YOU:

Possibly prevent certain liver problems and premature aging.

Aid in the treatment of multiple sclerosis.

DEFICIENCY DISEASE:

Deficiency symptoms and diseases related to this vitamin are still uncertain.

BEST NATURAL SOURCES:

Root vegetables, whey, the liquid portion of soured or curdled milk.

SUPPLEMENTS:

Available as calcium orotate in supplemental form outside of the United States.

TOXICITY:

Too little is known about the vitamin at this time to establish guidelines.
(See section 290, "Cautions.")

ENEMIES:

Water and sunlight.

PERSONAL ADVICE:

Not enough research has been done on this vitamin for recommendations to be made.

32. B15 (Pangamic Acid)

FACTS:

Water soluble.
Because its essential requirement for diet has not been proved, it is not a vitamin in the strict sense.
Measured in milligrams (mg.).
Works much like vitamin E in that it is an antioxidant.
Introduced by the Soviets who are thrilled with its results, while the U.S. Food and Drug Administration wants it off the market.
Action is often improved by being taken with vitamins A and E.

WHAT IT CAN DO FOR YOU:*

Extend cell life span.
Neutralize the craving for liquor.

*U.S. research in the case of B15 has been limited. The list of benefits given here is based on my study of Soviet tests.

Speed recovery from fatigue.
Lower blood cholesterol levels.
Protect against pollutants.
Relieve symptoms of angina and asthma.
Protect the liver against cirrhosis.
Ward off hangovers.
Stimulate immunity responses.
Aid in protein synthesis.

DEFICIENCY DISEASE:

Again, research has been limited, but indications point to glandular and nerve disorders, heart disease, and diminished oxygenation of living tissue.

BEST NATURAL SOURCES:

Brewer's yeast, whole brown rice, whole grains, pumpkin seeds, sesame seeds.

SUPPLEMENTS:

Usually available in 50-mg. strengths.
Daily doses most often used are 50 to 150 mgs.

TOXICITY:

There have been no reported cases of toxicity. Some people say they have experienced nausea on beginning a B15 regimen, but this usually disappears after a few days and can be alleviated by taking the B15 supplements after the day's largest meal.
(see section 290, "Cautions.")

ENEMIES:

Water and sunlight.

PERSONAL ADVICE:

Despite the controversy, I have found B15 effective and believe most diets would benefit from supplementation.

If you are an athlete or just want to feel like one, I suggest one 50-mg. tablet in the morning with breakfast and one in the evening with dinner.

An important supplement for residents of big cities and high-density pollution areas.

33. Vitamin B17 (Laetrile)

FACTS:

One of the most controversial "vitamins" of the decade.

Chemically a compound of two sugar molecules (one benzaldehyde and one cyanide) called an amygdalin.

Known as nitrilosides when used in medical doses.

Made from apricot pits.

One B vitamin that is not present in brewer's yeast.

Unaccepted as a cancer treatment in most of the United States at this date. (Legal in twenty-five states.) Rejected by the Food and Drug Administration on the grounds it might be poisonous due to its cyanide content.

WHAT IT CAN DO FOR YOU:

It is purported to have specific cancer-controlling and preventive properties.

DEFICIENCY DISEASE:

May lead to diminished resistance to cancer.

BEST NATURAL SOURCES:

A small amount of laetrile is found in the whole kernels of apricots, apples, cherries, peaches, plums, and nectarines.

SUPPLEMENTS:

Daily doses most often used at 0.25 to 1.0 g.

TOXICITY:

Though no toxicity levels have been established yet, taking

excessive amounts of laetrile could be dangerous. Cumulative amounts of more than 3.0 g. can be ingested safely, but not more than 1.0 g. at any one time.

According to the *Nutrition Almanac*, five to thirty apricot kernels eaten throughout the day, but never all at the same time, can be a sufficient preventive amount.

(See section 290, "Cautions.")

PERSONAL ADVICE:

If you are interested in laetrile as a cancer preventive or treatment, check with a nutrition-oriented physician. See section 293.

There is now extensive literature available on laetrile. I strongly advise personal research and a consultation with a physician before embarking on any regimen involving B17.

34. Biotin (Coenzyme R or Vitamin H)

FACTS:

Water soluble, sulfur containing, and another member of the B-complex family.

Usually measured in micrograms (mcg.).

Synthesis of ascorbic acid requires biotin.

Essential for normal metabolism of fat and protein.

The RDA for adults is 100 to 300 mcg.

Can be synthesized by intestinal bacteria.

Raw eggs prevent absorption by the body.

Synergistic with B2, B6, niacin, A, and in maintaining healthy skin.

WHAT IT CAN DO FOR YOU:

Aid in keeping hair from turning gray.

Help in preventive treatment for baldness.

Ease muscle pains.

Alleviate eczema and dermatitis.

DEFICIENCY DISEASE:

Eczema of face and body, extreme exhaustion, impairment of fat metabolism, anorexia, alopecia, depression. (For deficiency symptoms, see section 127.)

BEST NATURAL SOURCES:

Beef liver, egg yolk, soy flour, brewer's yeast, milk, kidney, and unpolished rice.

SUPPLEMENTS:

Biotin is usually included in most B-complex supplements and multiple-vitamin tablets.

Daily doses must often used are 25 to 300 mcg.

TOXICITY:

There are no known cases of biotin toxicity.
(See section 290, "Cautions.")

ENEMIES:

Raw egg white (which contains avidin, a protein that prevents biotin absorption), water, sulfa drugs, estrogen, food-processing techniques, and alcohol. (See section 250.)

PERSONAL ADVICE:

If you drink a lot of eggnogs made with raw eggs you probably need biotin supplementation.

Be sure you're getting at least 25 mcg. daily if you are on antibiotics or sulfa drugs.

Balding men might find that a biotin supplement may keep their hair there longer.

Keep in mind that biotin works synergistically—and more effectively—with B2, B6, niacin, and A.

Biotin levels fall progressively throughout pregnancy. Although there's been no association with low birth weight, you might want to check with your doctor about a supplement which could help keep your spirits up.

35. Vitamin C (Ascorbic Acid, Cevitamin Acid)

FACTS:

Water soluble.

Most animals synthesize their own vitamin C, but humans, apes, and guinea pigs must rely upon dietary sources.

Plays a primary role in the formation of collagen, which is important for the growth and repair of body tissue cells, gums, blood vessels, bones, and teeth.

Helps in the body's absorption of iron.

Measured in milligrams (mg.).

Used up more rapidly under stress conditions.

The RDA for adults is 60 mg. (higher doses recommended during pregnancy and lactation—70 to 95 mg.).

Smokers and older persons have greater need for vitamin C. (Each cigarette destroys 25–100 mg.)

Recommended as a preventive for crib death or Sudden Infant Death Syndrome (SIDS).

WHAT IT CAN DO FOR YOU:

Heal wounds, burns, and bleeding gums.

Increases effectiveness of drugs used to treat urinary tract infections.

Accelerate healing after surgery.

Help in decreasing blood cholesterol.

Aid in preventing many types of viral and bacterial infections and generally potentiate the immune system.

Offer protection against cancer-producing agents.

Help counteract the formation of nitrosamines (cancer-causing substances).

Act as a natural laxative.

Lower incidence of blood clots in veins.

Aid in treatment and prevention of the common cold.

Extend life by enabling protein cells to hold together.

Increase the absorption of inorganic iron.

Reduce effects of many allergy-producing substances.

Prevent scurvy.

DEFICIENCY DISEASE:

Scurvy. (For deficiency symptoms, see section 127.)

BEST NATURAL SOURCES:

Citrus fruits, berries, green and leafy vegetables, tomatoes, cauliflower, potatoes, and peppers.

SUPPLEMENTS:

Vitamin C is one of the most widely taken supplements. It is available in conventional pills, time-release tablets, syrups, powders, chewable wafers, in just about every form a vitamin can take.

The form that is *pure* vitamin C is derived from corn dextrose (although no corn or dextrose remains).

The difference between "natural" or "organic" vitamin C and ordinary ascorbic acid is primarily in the individual's ability to digest it.

The best vitamin-C supplement is one that contains the complete C complex of bioflavonoids, hesperidin, and rutin. (Sometimes these are labeled citrus salts.)

Tablets and capsules are usually supplied in strengths up to 1,000 mg., and in powder form sometimes 5,000 mg. per tsp.

Daily doses most often used are 500 mg. to 4 g.

Rose hips vitamin C contains bioflavonoids and other enzymes that help C assimilate. They are the richest natural source of vitamin C. (The C is actually manufactured under the bud of the rose—called a hip.)

Acerola C is made with acerola berries.

TOXICITY:

Excessive intake may cause oxalic acid and uric acid stone formation (though taking magnesium, vitamin B6, and a sufficient amount of water daily can rectify this.) Occasionally, very high doses (over 10 g. daily) can cause unpleasant side effects, such as diarrhea, excess urination, and skin rashes. If any of these occur, cut back on your dosage.

Vitamin C should not be used by cancer patients undergoing radiation or chemotherapy.

(See section 290, "Cautions.")

ENEMIES:

Water, cooking, heat, light, oxygen, smoking. (See section 250.)

PERSONAL ADVICE:

Because vitamin C is excreted in two to three hours, depending on the quantity of food in the stomach, and it is important to maintain a constant high level of C in the bloodstream at all times, I recommend a time-release tablet for optimal effectiveness.

Large doses of vitamin C can alter the results of laboratory tests. If you're going to have any blood or urine testing, be sure to inform your doctor that you're taking vitamin C so that no errors will be made in diagnosis. (Vitamin C can mask the presence of blood in stool.)

Diabetics should be aware that testing the urine for sugar could be inaccurate if you're taking a lot of vitamins C. (But there are testing kits available that aren't affected by vitamin C. Ask your pharmacist or physician.)

If you're taking over 750 mg. daily, I suggest a magnesium supplement. This is an effective deterrent against kidney stones.

Carbon monoxide destroys vitamin C, so city dwellers should definitely up their intake.

You need extra C if you are on the pill.

To maximize the effectiveness of vitamin C, remember that it works best in conjunction with bioflavonoids, calcium, and magnesium.

I recommend increasing C doses if you take aspirin, which triples the excretion rate of vitamin C.

If you take ginseng, it's better to take it three hours before or after taking vitamin C or foods that are high in the vitamin.

36. Calcium Pantothenate (Pantothenic Acid, Panthenol, Vitamin B5)

FACTS:

Water soluble, another member of the B-complex family.

Helps in cell building, maintaining normal growth, and development of the central nervous system.

Vital for the proper functioning of the adrenal glands.

Essential for conversion of fat and sugar to energy.

Necessary for synthesis of antibodies, for utilization of PABA and choline.

The RDA (as set by the FDA) is 10 mg. for adults.

Can be synthesized in the body by intestinal bacteria.

WHAT IT CAN DO FOR YOU:

Aid in wound healing.

Fight infection by building antibodies.

Treat postoperative shock.

Prevent fatigue.

Reduce adverse and toxic effects of many antibiotics.

DEFICIENCY DISEASE:

Hypoglycemia, duodenal ulcers, blood and skin disorders. (For deficiency symptoms, see section 127.)

BEST NATURAL SOURCES:

Meat, whole grains, wheat germ, bran, kidney, liver, heart, green vegetables, brewer's yeast, nuts, chicken, crude molasses.

SUPPLEMENTS:

Most commonly found in B-complex formulas in a variety of strengths from 10 to 100 mg.

10 to 300 mg. are the daily doses usually taken.

TOXICITY:

No known toxic effects.
(See section 290, "Cautions.")

ENEMIES:

Heat, food-processing techniques, canning, caffeine, sulfa drugs, sleeping pills, estrogen, alcohol. (See section 250.)

PERSONAL ADVICE:

If you frequently have tingling hands and feet, you might try increasing your pantothenic acid intake—in combination with other B vitamins.

Pantothenic acid can help provide a defense against a stress situation that you foresee or are involved in.

1,000 mg. daily has been found effective in reducing the pain of arthritis, in some cases.

If you suffer from allergies, relief could be just a vitamin B5 and C away. Try taking 1,000 mg. of each—with food —morning and evening.

37. Choline

FACTS:

A member of the B-complex family and a lipotropic (fat emulsifier).

Works with inositol (another B-complex member) to utilize fats and cholesterol.

One of the few substances able to penetrate the so-called blood-brain barrier, which ordinarily protects the brain against variations in the daily diet, and go directly into the brain cells to produce a chemical that aids memory.

The RDA has not yet been established, though it's estimated that the average adult diet contains between 500 and 900 mg. a day.

Seems to emulsify cholesterol so that it doesn't settle on artery walls or in the gall bladder.

WHAT IT CAN DO FOR YOU:

Help control cholesterol buildup.

Aid in the sending of nerve impulses, specifically those in the brain used in the formation of memory.

Assist in conquering the problem of memory loss in later years. (Doses of 1–5 g. a day.)

Help eliminate poisons and drugs from your system by aiding the liver.

Produce a soothing effect.

Aid in the treatment of Alzheimer's disease.

DEFICIENCY DISEASE:

May result in cirrhosis and fatty degeneration of liver, hardening of the arteries, and possibly Alzheimer's disease. (For deficiency symptoms, see section 127.)

BEST NATURAL SOURCES:

Egg yolks, brain, heart, green leafy vegetables, yeast, liver, wheat germ, and, in small amounts, in lecithin.

SUPPLEMENTS:

Six lecithin capsules, made from soybeans, contain 244 mg. each of inositol and choline.

The average B-complex supplement contains approximately 50 mg. of choline and inositol.

Daily doses most often used are 500 to 1,000 mg.

TOXICITY:

None known.
(See section 290, "Cautions.")

ENEMIES:

Water, sulfa drugs, estrogen, food processing, and alcohol. (See section 250.)

PERSONAL ADVICE:

Always take choline with your other B vitamins.

If you are often nervous or "twitchy" it might help to increase your choline.

If you are taking lecithin, you probably need a chelated calcium supplement to keep your phosphorous and calcium in balance, since choline seems to increase the body's phosphorus.

Try getting more choline into your diet as a way to a better memory.

If you're a heavy drinker, make sure you're giving your liver the choline it needs to do the extra work.

38. Vitamin D (Calciferol, Viosterol, Ergosterol, "Sunshine Vitamin")

FACTS:

Fat soluble. Acquired through sunlight or diet. Ultraviolet sunrays act on the oils of the skin to produce the vitamin, which is then absorbed into the body.)

When taken orally, vitamin D is absorbed with fats through the intestinal walls.

Measured in International Units (IU), or micrograms of cholecalciferol mcg.).

The RDA for adults is 200–400 IU, or 5–10 mcg.

Smog reduces the vitamin-D-producing sunshine rays.

After a suntan is established, vitamin-D production through the skin stops.

WHAT IT CAN DO FOR YOU:

Properly utilize calcium and phosphorus necessary for strong bones and teeth.

Taken with vitamins A and C it can aid in preventing colds.

Help in treatment of conjunctivitis.

Aid in assimilating vitamin A.

DEFICIENCY DISEASE:

Rickets, severe tooth decay, osteomalacia, senile osteoporosis. (For deficiency symptoms, see section 127.)

BEST NATURAL SOURCES:

Fish liver oils, sardines, herring, salmon, tuna, milk and dairy products.

SUPPLEMENTS:

Usually supplied in 400 IU capsules, the vitamin itself derived from fish liver oil.
Daily doses most often taken are 400 to 1,000 IU.

TOXICITY:

20,000 IU daily over an extended period of time can produce toxic effects in adults.
Dosages of over 1,800 IU daily may cause hypervitaminosis D in children.
Signs of toxicity are unusual thirst, sore eyes, itching skin, vomiting, diarrhea, urinary urgency, abnormal calcium deposits in blood-vessel walls, liver, lungs, kidney, and stomach.
(See section 290, "Cautions.")

ENEMIES:

Mineral oil, smog. (See section 250.)

PERSONAL ADVICE:

City dwellers, especially those in areas of high smog density, should increase their vitamin-D intake.
Night workers, nuns, and others whose clothing or lifestyle keeps them from sunlight should increase the D in their diet.
If you're taking an anticonvulsant drug, you most probably need to increase your vitamin D intake.
Children who don't drink D-fortified milk should increase their intake of D.

Dark-skinned people living in northern climates usually need an increase in vitamin D.

Do not supplement your dog's or cat's diet with vitamin D unless your vet specifically advises it.

Vitamin D works best with vitamin A, vitamin C, choline, calcium, and phosphorus.

39. Vitamin E (Tocopherol)

FACTS:

Fat soluble and stored in the liver, fatty tissues, heart, muscles, testes, uterus, blood, adrenal and pituitary glands.

Formerly measured by weight, but now generally designated according to its biological activity in International Units (IU). With this vitamin 1 IU is the same as 1 mg.

Composed of compounds called tocopherols. Of the eight tocopherols—alpha, beta, gamma, delta, epsilon, zeta, eta, and theta—alpha-tocopherol is the most effective.

An active antioxidant, prevents oxidation of fat compounds as well as that of vitamin A, selenium, two sulfur amino acids, and some vitamin C.

Enhances activity of vitamin A.

The RDA for adults is 8 IU to 10 IU. (This requirement is based on the National Research Council's latest revised allowances.)

60 to 70 percent of daily doses are excreted in feces. Unlike other fat-soluble vitamins, E is stored in the body for a relatively short time, much like B and C.

Important as a vasodilator and an anticoagulant.

Products with 25 mcg. of selenium for each 200 units of E increases E's potency.

WHAT IT CAN DO FOR YOU:

Keep you looking younger by retarding cellular aging due to oxidation.

Supply oxygen to the body to give you more endurance.

Protect your lungs against air pollution by working with vitamin A.

Prevent and dissolve blood clots.

Alleviate fatigue.

Prevent thick scar formation externally (when applied topically—it can be absorbed through the skin) and internally.

Accelerate healing of burns.

Working as a diuretic, it can lower blood pressure.

Aid in prevention of miscarriages.

Helps alleviate leg cramps and "charley horse."

Lower risk of ischemic heart disease.

DEFICIENCY DISEASE:

Destruction of red blood cells, muscle degeneration, some anemias and reproductive disorders. (For deficiency symptoms, see section 127.)

BEST NATURAL SOURCES:

Wheat germ, soybeans, vegetable oils, nuts, brussels sprouts, leafy greens, spinach, enriched flour, whole wheat, whole-grain cereals, and eggs.

SUPPLEMENTS:

Available in oil-base capsules as well as water-dispersible dry tablets.

Usually supplied in strengths from 100 to 1,500 IU. The dry form is recommended for anyone who cannot tolerate oil or whose skin condition is aggravated by oil. It's also best for people over 40.

Daily doses most often used are 200 to 1,200 IU.

TOXICITY:

Essentially nontoxic.

(See section 290, "Cautions.")

ENEMIES:

Heat, oxygen, freezing temperatures, food processing, iron, chlorine, mineral oil. (See section 250.)

PERSONAL ADVICE:

If you're on a diet high in polyunsaturated oils, you might need additional vitamin E.

Inorganic iron (ferrous sulfate) destroys vitamin E, so the two should not be taken together. If you're using a supplement containing any ferrous sulfate, E should be taken at least eight hours before or after.

Ferrous gluconate, peptonate, citrate, or fumerate (organic iron complexes) do not destroy E.

If you have chlorinated drinking water, you need more vitamin E.

Pregnant or lactating women, as well as those on the pill or taking hormones, need increased vitamin E.

I advise women going through menopause to increase their E intake. (Mixed tocopherols are recommended. 400–1,200 IU daily.)

40. Vitamin F (Unsaturated Fatty Acids— Linoleic, Linolenic, and Arachidonic)

FACTS:

Fat soluble, made up of unsaturated fatty acids obtained from foods.

Measured in milligrams (mg.).

No RDA has been established, but the National Research Council has suggested that at least 1 percent of total calories should include essential unsaturated fatty acids.

Unsaturated fat helps burn saturated fat, with intake balanced two to one.

Twelve teaspoons sunflower seeds or eighteen pecan halves can furnish a day's complete supply.

If there is sufficient linoleic acid, the other two fatty acids can be synthesized.

Heavy carbohydrate consumption increases need.

WHAT IT CAN DO FOR YOU:

Aid in preventing cholesterol deposits in the arteries.
Promote healthy skin and hair.

Give some degree of protection against the harmful effects of X-rays.

Aid in growth and well-being by influencing glandular activity and making calcium available to cells.

Combat heart disease.

Aid in weight reduction by burning saturated fats.

DEFICIENCY DISEASE:

Eczema, acne. (For deficiency symptoms, see section 127.)

BEST NATURAL SOURCES:

Vegetable oils—wheat germ, linseed sunflower, safflower, soybean, and peanut—peanuts, sunflower seeds, walnuts, pecans, almonds, avocados.

SUPPLEMENTS:

Comes in capsules of 100- to 150-mg. strengths.

TOXICITY:

No known toxic effects, but an excess can lead to unwanted pounds.

(See section 290, "Cautions.")

ENEMIES:

Saturated fats, heat, oxygen.

PERSONAL ADVICE:

For best absorption of vitamin F, take vitamin E with it at mealtimes.

If you are a heavy carbohydrate consumer, you need more vitamin F.

Anyone worried about cholesterol buildup should be getting the proper intake of F.

Though most nuts are fine sources of unsaturated fatty acids, Brazil nuts and cashews are *not*!

Watch out for fad diets high in saturated fats.

41. Folic Acid (Folacin, Folate)

FACTS:

Water soluble, another member of the B complex, also known as Bc or vitamin M.

Measured in micrograms (mcg.).

Essential to the formation of red blood cells.

Aid in protein metabolism.

The official Recommended Daily Allowance for adults is 180–200 mcg., twice that amount for pregnant women, and for nursing mothers, 280 mcg. the first six months and 260 mcg. the second six months.

Important for the production of nucleic acids (RNA and DNA).

Essential for division of body cells.

Needed for utilization of sugar and amino acids.

Can be destroyed by being stored, unprotected, at room temperature for extended time periods.

WHAT IT CAN DO FOR OU:

Improve lactation.

Protect against intestinal parasites and food poisoning.

Promote healthier-looking skin.

Act as an analgesic for pain.

May delay hair graying when used in conjunction with pantothenic acid and PABA.

Help prevent birth defects.

Increase appetite, if you are debilitated (run down.)

Act as a preventive for canker sores.

Help ward off anemia.

DEFICIENCY DISEASE:

Nutritional macrocytic anemia. (For deficiency symptoms, see section 127.)

BEST NATURAL SOURCES:

Deep-green leafy vegetables, carrots, tortula yeast, liver,

egg yolk, cantaloupe, apricots, pumpkins, avocados, beans, whole and dark rye flour.

SUPPLEMENTS:

Usually supplied in 400-mcg. strengths. Strengths of 1 mg. (1,000 mcg.) are available by prescription only in the United States.

400 mcg. are sometimes supplied in B-complex formulas, but often only 100 mcg. (Check labels.)

Daily doses most often used are 400 mcg. to 5 mg.

TOXICITY:

No known toxic effects, though a few people experience allergic skin reactions.

(See section 290, "Cautions.")

ENEMIES:

Water, sulfa drugs, sunlight, estrogen, food processing (especially boiling), heat. (See section 250.)

PERSONAL ADVICE:

If you are a heavy drinker, it is advisable to increase your folic-acid intake.

High vitamin-C intake increases excretion of folic acid, and anyone taking more than 2 g. of C should probably up his folic acid.

If you are on Dilantin or take estrogens, sulfonamides, phenobarbital, or aspirin, I suggest increasing folic acid.

I've found that many people taking 1 to 5 mg. daily, for a short period of time, have reversed several types of skin discoloration. If this is a problem to you, it's worth checking out a nutritionally oriented doctor about the possibility.

If you are getting sick, or fighting an illness, make sure your stress supplement has ample folic acid. When folic acid is deficient, so are your antibodies.

Large doses of folic acid may bring on convulsions in epileptics taking the medication phenytoin.

42. Inositol

FACTS:

Water soluble, another member of the B complex, and a lipotropic.

Measured in milligrams (mg.).

Combines with choline to form lecithin.

Metabolizes fats and cholesterol.

Daily dietary allowances have not yet been established, but the average healthy adult gets approximately 1 g. a day.

Like choline, it has been found important in nourishing brain cells.

WHAT IT CAN DO FOR YOU:

Help lower cholesterol levels.

Promote healthy hair—aid in preventing fallout.

Help in preventing eczema.

Aid in redistribution of body fat.

Produce a calming effect.

DEFICIENCY DISEASE:

Eczema. (For deficiency symptoms, see section 127.)

BEST NATURAL SOURCES:

Liver, brewer's yeast, dried lima beans, beef brains and heart, cantaloupe, grapefruit, raisins, wheat germ, unrefined molasses, peanuts, cabbage.

SUPPLEMENTS:

As with choline, six soybean-based lecithin capsules contain approximately 244 mg. each of inositol and choline.

Available in lecithin powders that mix well with liquids. Most B-complex supplements contain approximately 100 mg. of choline and inositol.

Daily doses most often used are 250 to 500 mg.

TOXICITY:

No known toxic effects.
(See section 290, "Cautions.")

ENEMIES:

Water, sulfa drugs, estrogen, food processing, alcohol, and coffee. (See section 250.)

PERSONAL ADVICE:

Take inositol with choline and your other B vitamins.
If you are a heavy coffee drinker, you probably need supplemental inositol.
If you take lecithin, I advise a supplement of chelated calcium to keep your phosphorus and calcium in balance, as both inositol and choline seem to raise phosphorus levels.
A good way to maximize the effectiveness of your vitamin E is to get enough inositol and choline.

43. Vitamin K (Menadione)

FACTS:

Fat soluble.
Usually measured in micrograms (mcg.)
There is a trio of K vitamins. K1 and K2 can be formed by natural bacteria in the intestines. K3 is a synthetic.
The RDA for adults is 65–80 mcg.
Essential in the formation of prothrombin, a blood-clotting chemical.

WHAT IT CAN DO FOR YOU:

Help in preventing internal bleeding and hemorrhages.
Aid in reducing excessive menstrual flow.
Promote proper blood clotting.

DEFICIENCY DISEASE:

Celiac disease, sprue, colitis. (For deficiency symptoms, see section 127.)

BEST NATURAL SOURCES:

Leafy green vegetables, yogurt, alfalfa, egg yolk, safflower oil, soybean oil, fish liver oils, kelp.

SUPPLEMENTS:

Available in 100 mcg. tablets (though the abundance of natural vitamin K generally makes supplementation unnecessary).

It is not included ordinarily in multiple-vitamins.

TOXICITY:

More than 500 mcg. of synthetic vitamin K is not recommended.

(See section 290, "Cautions.")

ENEMIES:

X-rays and radiation, frozen foods, aspirin, air pollution, mineral oil. (See section 250.)

PERSONAL ADVICE:

Excessive diarrhea can be a symptom of vitamin K deficiency, but before self-supplementing, see a doctor.

Green leafy vegetables are your best defense against a vitamin-K deficiency.

If you have nosebleeds often, try increasing your K through natural food sources. Alfalfa tablets might help.

If you are taking an anticoagulant (blood thinner), be aware that this vitamin (even in natural foods) can reverse the drug's effect.

If you are on a chronic broad-spectrum antibiotic regimen, you're high risk for a vitamin K deficiency. Increase the K-rich foods in your diet—and I suggest you check with a nutritionally oriented doctor about a supplement. (See section 293.)

44. Niacin (Nicotinic Acid, Niacinamide, Nicotinamide)

FACTS:

Water soluble and a member of the B-complex family, known as B3.

Usually measured in milligrams (mg.).

Using the amino acid tryptophan, the body can manufacture its own niacin.

A person whose body is deficient in B1, B2, and B6 will not be able to produce niacin from tryptophan.

Lack of niacin can bring about negative personality changes.

The RDA, according to the National Research Council, is 13 to 19 mg. for adults. For nursing mothers the recommendation is 20 mg.

Essential for synthesis of sex hormones (estrogen, progesterone, testosterone), as well as cortisone, throxine, and insulin.

Necessary for healthy nervous system and brain functions.

Niacinamide is more generally used since it minimizes the flushing and itching of the skin that frequently occurs with the nicotinic acid form of niacin. (The flush, by the way, is not serious and usually disappears in about twenty minutes. Drinking a glass of water helps.)

One of the few vitamins that is relatively stable in foods and can withstand cooking and storage with little loss of potency.

WHAT IT CAN DO FOR YOU:

Aid in promoting a healthy digestive system, alleviate gastrointestinal disturbances.

Give you healthier-looking skin.

Help prevent and ease severity of migraine headaches.

Increase circulation and reduce high blood pressure.

Ease some attacks of diarrhea.

Reduce the unpleasant symptoms of vertigo in Meniere's syndrome.

Increase energy through proper utilization of food.
Help eliminate canker sores and, often, bad breath.
Reduce cholesterol and triglycerides.

DEFICIENCY DISEASE:

Pellagra, severe dermatitis. (For deficiency symptoms, see section 127.)

BEST NATURAL SOURCES:

Liver, lean meat, whole wheat products, brewer's yeast, kidney, wheat germ, fish, eggs, roasted peanuts, the white meat of poultry, avocados, dates, figs, prunes.

SUPPLEMENTS:

Available as niacin and niacinamide. (The only difference is that niacin—nicotinic acid—might cause flushing and niacinamide-nicotinamide—will not. If you prefer niacin, you can minimize the flushing by taking your pill on a full stomach or with an equivalent amount of inositol.)

Usually found in 50- to 1,000-mg. doses in pill and powder form.

50 to 100 mg. are ordinarily included in the better B-complex formulas and multivitamin preparations. (Check labels.)

TOXICITY:

Essentially nontoxic, except for side effects resulting from doses above 100 mg.

Some sensitive individuals might evidence burning or itching skin.

Do not give to animals, especially dogs. It can cause flushing and sweating and great discomfort for the animal.

(See section 290, "Cautions.")

ENEMIES:

Water, sulfa drugs, alcohol, sleeping pills, estrogen. (See section 250.)

PERSONAL ADVICE:

If you're taking antibiotics and suddenly find your niacin flushes becoming severe, don't be alarmed. It's quite common. You'll probably be more comfortable if you switch to niacinamide.

If you have a cholesterol problem, increasing your niacin intake can help.

Skin that is particularly sensitive to sunlight is often an early indicator of niacin deficiency.

CAUTION: A recent report in *Post Graduate Medicine* magazine revealed that large amounts of niacin can interfere with the body's ability to dispose of sugar, causing possible deterioration of glucose control in borderline diabetes and percipitating the full-blown disease. Also, it can interfere with the control of uric acid, bringing on attacks of gout in people prone to that disease.

NOTE: Recent research has shown that much smaller amounts of niacin are needed to produce cholesterol-lowering results (without the uncomfortable side effects) if the niacin is taken in combination with chromium. A chromium-niacin complex is now available. Apparently, the synergistic effect of these two nutrients is powerful, because the complex is effective with only 200 mcg. of chromium bound to 2 mg. of niacin.

45. Vitamin P (C Complex, Citrus Bioflavonoids, Rutin, Hesperidin)

FACTS:

Water soluble and composed of citrin, rutin, and hesperidin, as well as flavones and flavonals.

Usually measured in milligrams (mg.).

Necessary for the proper function and absorption of vitamin C.

Flavonoids are the substances that provide that yellow and orange color in citrus foods.

Also called the capillary permeability factor. (P stands for permeability.) The prime function of bioflavonoids is to increase capillary strength and regulate absorption.

Aids vitamin C in keeping connective tissues healthy.

No daily allowances has been established, but most nutritionists agree that for every 500 mg. of vitamin C you should have at least 100 mg. of bioflavonoids.

Works synergistically with vitamin C.

WHAT IT CAN DO FOR YOU:

Prevent vitamin C from being destroyed by oxidation.

Strengthen the walls of capillaries, thereby preventing bruising.

Help build resistance to infection.

Aid in preventing and healing bleeding gums.

Increase the effectiveness of vitamin C.

Help in the treatment of edema and dizziness due to disease of the inner ear.

DEFICIENCY DISEASE:

Capillary fragility. (For deficiency symptoms, see section 127.)

BEST NATURAL SOURCES:

The white skin and segment part of citrus fruit—lemons, oranges, grapefruit. Also in apricots, buckwheat, blackberries, cherries, and rose hips.

SUPPLEMENTS:

Available usually in a C complex or by itself. Most often there are 500 mg. of bioflavonoids to 50 mg. of rutin and hesperidin. (If the ratio of rutin and hesperidin is not equal, it should be twice as much rutin.)

All C supplements work better with bioflavonoids.

Most common doses of rutin and hesperidin are 100 mg. three times a day.

TOXICITY:

No known toxicity.
(See section 290, "Cautions.")

ENEMIES:

Water, cooking, heat, light, oxygen, smoking. (See section 250.)

PERSONAL ADVICE:

Menopausal women can usually find some effective relief from hot flashes with an increase in bioflavonoids taken in conjunction with vitamin D.

If your gums bleed frequently when you brush your teeth, make sure you're getting enough rutin and hesperidin.

Anyone with a tendency to bruise easily will benefit from a C supplement with bioflavonoids, rutin, and hesperidin.

46. PABA (Para-aminobenzoic Acid)

FACTS:

Water soluble, one of the newer members of the B-complex family.

Usually measured in milligrams (mg.).

Can be synthesized in the body.

No RDA has yet been established.

Helps form folic acid and is important in the utilization of protein.

Has important sun-screening properties.

Helps in the assimilation—and therefore the effectiveness—of pantothenic acid.

In experiments with animals, it has worked with pantothenic acid to restore gray hair to its natural color.

WHAT IT CAN DO FOR YOU:

Used as an ointment, it can protect against sunburn.
Reduce the pain of burns.
Keep skin healthy and smooth.

Help in delaying wrinkles.
Help to restore natural color to your hair.

DEFICIENCY DISEASE:

Eczema. (For deficiency symptoms, see section 127.)

BEST NATURAL SOURCES:

Liver, brewer's yeast, kidney, whole grains, rice, bran, wheat germ, and molasses.

SUPPLEMENTS:

30 to 100 mgs. are often included in good B-complex capsules as well as high-quality multivitamins.

Available in 30- to 1,000-mg. strengths in regular and time-release form.

Doses most often used are 30 to 100 mg. three times a day.

TOXICITY:

No known toxic effects, but long-term programs of high dosages are not recommended.

Symptoms that might indicate an oversupply of PABA are usually nausea and vomiting.

(See section 290, "Cautions.")

ENEMIES:

Water, sulfa drugs, food-processing techniques, alcohol, estrogen. (See section 250.)

PERSONAL ADVICE:

Some people claim that the combination of folic acid and PABA has returned their graying hair to its natural color. It has worked on animals, so it is certainly worth a try for anyone looking for an alternative to hair dye. For this purpose, 1,000 mg. (time release) daily for six days a week is a viable regimen.

If you tend to burn easily in the sun, use PABA as a protective ointment unless you are sensitive to this product.

Many Hollywood celebrities I know use PABA to prevent wrinkles. It doesn't eliminate them, but it certainly seems to keep them at bay for some people.

If you are taking penicillin, or any sulfa drug, your PABA intake should be increased through natural foods or supplements.

47. Vitamin T

There is very little known about this vitamin, except that it helps in blood coagulation and the forming of platelets. Because of these attributes it is important in warding off certain forms of anemia and hemophilia. No RDA has been established, and there are no supplements for the public on the market. It is found in sesame seeds and egg yolks, and there is no known toxicity.

48. Vitamin U

Even less is known about vitamin U than vitamin T. It is reputed to play an important role in healing ulcers, but medical opinions vary on this. It is found in raw cabbage and no known toxicity exists.

49. Any Questions About Chapter III?

I live in Los Angeles and hear a lot about environmental pollution. I also hear a lot about how I need to take antioxidants. Could you tell me what antioxidants are and if I really need them?

You really need them. Let me begin by saying that if you live in *any* major urban area today, you're breathing polluted air. Every year 200 million tons of potentially dangerous pollutants are released into the atmosphere.

With each breath you subject your lungs and body to a wide range of pollutants, and no part of you is immune. Antioxidants—beta carotene, vitamins C, E, and selenium, are nutrients that are capable of protecting other substances from oxidation. In other words, the free radicals (uncontrolled oxidations that damage cells) that are formed when we inhale pollutants are kept in check by antioxidants.

Beta Carotene protects mucous membranes of mouth, nose, throat, and lungs. It also helps protect vitamin C from oxidation, which allows your C to work better.

Vitamin C fights bacterial infections and reduces the effects of allergy-producing substances. It also protects vitamins A, E, and some of the B complex from oxidation.

Vitamin E protects vitamins B and C from oxidation. It has the ability to unite with oxygen and prevent it from being converted into toxic peroxides. It acts as an antipollutant for the lungs. It has also been shown as a significant protective factor (along with the other antioxidants) against ischemic heart disease.

Selenium and vitamin E must both be present to correct a deficiency in either. The levels of both selenium and vitamin E in the blood of people in various cities has been found to bear a direct relationship to cancer and ischemic heart disease mortality. The higher the levels, the lower the death rate—and vice versa.

And a powerful new antioxidant called pycnogenol that has been found to be significantly more effective than vitamin E and vitamin C as a free radical scavenger. Helpful in reducing free-radical damage shown to lead to such diseases as cancer, heart disease, arthritis and accelerated ageing, among others.

I've read that diets high in broccoli, brussels sprouts, and carrots can help reduce the risk of cancer, but I just hate these vegetables. What vitamins can I take instead?

You can get concentrated forms of cruciferous (cabbage, broccoli, brussels sprouts, cauliflower) and carotene-rich (spinach and carrots) vegetables in tablet form. I'd advise taking these supplements daily. Since they are made from vegetables that are picked ripe, carefully washed, and quickly dehydrated without cooking—as well as being fortified with vitamins A, C, and E, beta-carotene and selenium—they'll provide you with optimal nutritional value.

Can you tell me how choline is helpful in the treatment of Alzheimer's disease?

Alzheimer's disease, which is a slow loss of mental faculties, seems to be caused by a depletion in central nervous system reserves of the neurotransmitter acetylcholine (not by a virus or aluminum, as previously suspected).

It has been found that patients with Alzheimer's syndrome are not only deficient in acetylcholine, but also the enzyme that catalyzes its production—choline acetyltransferase. Ingestion of more choline can apparently prevent existing acetylcholine from being broken down. Phosphatidyl cholene, a new and more potent form of this, is now recommended.

There is still no specific treatment for the disease, but it's been found that certain medications might worsen a patient's condition. For example, hypnotics such as *flurazepam* (DALMANE), drugs for heart disease, and those given for intestinal cramping.

What sort of vitamin is beta carotene? And why is there no RDA for it?

I'll answer the second part first. The reason there is no RDA for it is because it is not in itself a vitamin. Only after it's inside your body does it transform into vitamin A. Beta carotene comes, primarily, from yellow and orange plant sources (carrots, pumpkins, sweet potatoes, cantaloupe) and has been found to be significantly helpful in the prevention of heart disease and many cancers. Levels decrease with old age, but beta carotene can also be unnecessarily depleted by dieting, smoking and heavy drinking.

IV

Your Mineral Essentials

50. Calcium

FACTS:

There is more calcium in the body than any other mineral.

Calcium and phosphorus work together for healthy bones and teeth.

Calcium and magnesium work together for cardiovascular health.

Almost all of the body's calcium (two to three pounds) is found in the bones and teeth.

20 percent of an adult's bone calcium is reabsorbed and replaced every year. (New bone cells form as old ones break down.)

Calcium must exist in a two-to-one relationship with phosphorus. (Two parts calcium to one part phosphorus.)

In order for calcium to be absorbed, the body must have sufficient vitamin D.

For adults, 800 to 1,200 mg. is the RDA.

Calcium and iron are the two minerals most deficient in the American woman's diet.

WHAT IT CAN DO FOR YOU:

Maintain strong bones and healthy teeth.

Keep your heart beating regularly.

Alleviate insomnia.

Help metabolize your body's iron.

Aid your nervous system, especially in impulse transmission.

DEFICIENCY DISEASE:

Rickets, osteomalacia, osteoporosis—commonly known as brittle bones. (See section 127 for symptoms.)

BEST NATURAL SOURCES:

Milk and milk products, all cheeses, soybeans, sardines, salmon, peanuts, walnuts, sunflower seeds, dried beans, kale, broccoli, collard greens.

SUPPLEMENTS:

Most often available in 250- to 500-mg. tablets.

Bonemeal, formerly one of the most popular supplements, is no longer recommended because of its possible high lead content. (You can check with the manufacturer for an analysis.) But calcium gluconate (a vegetarian source) or calcium lactate (a milk sugar derivative) are definitely lead-free and easy to absorb.

The best form is chelated calcium tablets.

Many good multivitamin and mineral preparations include calcium.

When combined with magnesium, the ratio should be twice as much calcium as magnesium. Dolomite is a natural form of calcium and magnesium, and no vitamin D is needed for assimilation. Five dolomite tablets are equivalent to 750 mg. of calcium. Unfortunately, dolomite, like bonemeal, has been found to have a high lead content, and at this writing is not recommended as a supplement—unless a complete analysis of the product can be provided by the manufacturer.

TOXICITY:

Excessive daily intake of over 2,000 mg. might lead to hypercalcemia. (See section 290, "Cautions.") Overly high intakes may also cause constipation and increase the risk of urinary tract infections.

ENEMIES:

Large quantities of fat, oxalic acid (found in chocolate, spinach, Swiss chard, parsley, beet greens, and rhubarb), and phytic acid (found in grains) are capable of preventing proper calcium absorption.

PERSONAL ADVICE:

If you are afflicted with backaches, chelated calcium, or calcium citrate supplements might help.

Menstrual-cramp sufferers can often find relief by increasing their calcium intake.

If you enjoy chewing on chicken or turkey drumsticks, you're in luck. The tips of poultry leg bones are high in calcium.

If you're taking daily doses of 1,500 mg. calcium, and are prone to urinary trace infections, I'd advise taking your supplements with cranberry juice. This juice coats the bacteria and helps stop it from sticking to the urinary tract.

Teenagers who suffer from "growing pains" will usually find that they disappear with an increase in calcium consumption.

Hypoglycemics could use more calcium. (I recommend calcium citrate for best absorption, in doses of 1,000–1,500 mg. daily.)

If you consume lots of soft drinks, be aware that, because they're high in phosphorus, you may be depleting your body of calcium and increasing your chances of osteoporosis.

Calcium works best with vitamins A, C, D; iron, magnesium, and phosphorus. (Too much phosphorus, as I've mentioned above, can deplete calcium.)

New studies have shown that a combination of calcium, magnesium, vitamin D and the trace mineral boron (3 mg. per day) may help prevent osteoporosis.

51. Chlorine

FACTS:

Regulates the blood's alkaline-acid balance.
Works with sodium and potassium in a compound form.
Aids in the cleaning of body wastes by helping the liver to function.
No dietary allowance has been established, but if your daily salt intake is average, you are getting enough.

WHAT IT CAN DO FOR YOU:

Aid in digestion.
Help keep you limber.

DEFICIENCY DISEASE:

Loss of hair and teeth.

BEST NATURAL SOURCES:

Table salt, kelp, olives.

SUPPLEMENTS:

Most good multimineral preparations include it.

TOXICITY:

Over 15 g. can cause unpleasant side effects.
(See section 290, "Cautions.")

PERSONAL ADVICE:

If you have chlorine in your drinking water, you aren't getting all the vitamin E you think. (Chlorinated water destroys vitamin E.)
Anyone who drinks chlorinated water should be well advised to eat yogurt—a good natural way to replace the intestinal bacteria the chlorine destroys.

52. Chromium

FACTS:

Works with insulin in the metabolism of sugar.
Helps bring protein to where it's needed.
No official dietary allowance has been established, but 50–200 mcg. is the tentatively recommended adult intake.
As you get older, you retain less chromium in your body.

WHAT IT CAN DO FOR YOU:

Aid growth.
Help prevent and lower high blood pressure.
Work as a deterrent for diabetes.

DEFICIENCY DISEASE:

A suspected factor in arteriosclerosis and diabetes.

BEST NATURAL SOURCES:

Calves' livers, wheat germ, brewer's yeast, chicken, corn oil, clams.

SUPPLEMENTS:

May be found in the better multimineral preparations. (Glucose tolerance factor and chromium picolinate are the preferred forms.)

TOXICITY:

No known toxicity.
(See section 290, "Cautions.")

PERSONAL ADVICE:

If you are low in chromium (a hair analysis can show this—see section 126), you might try a zinc supplement. For some reason, chelated zinc seems to substitute well for deficient chromium.

The best assurance of an adequate chromium intake is a varied diet that provides a sufficient intake of other essential nutrients.

53. Cobalt

FACTS:

A mineral that is part of vitamin B12.
Usually measured in micrograms (mcg.).
Essential for red blood cells.
Must be obtained from food sources.
No daily allowance has been set for this mineral, and only very small amounts are necessary in the diet (usually no more than 8 mcg.).

WHAT IT CAN DO FOR YOU:

Stave off anemia.

DEFICIENCY DISEASE:

Anemia.

BEST NATURAL SOURCES:

Meat, kidney, liver, milk, oysters, clams.

SUPPLEMENTS:

Rarely found in supplement form.

TOXICITY:

No known toxicity.
(See section 290, "Cautions.")

ENEMIES:

Whatever is antagonistic to B12.

PERSONAL ADVICE:

If you're a strict vegetarian, you are much more likely to be deficient in this mineral than someone who includes meat and shellfish in his or her diet.

54. Copper

FACTS:

Required to convert the body's iron into hemoglobin.

Can reach the bloodstream fifteen minutes after ingestion.

Makes the amino acid tyrosine usable, allowing it to work as the pigmenting factor for hair and skin.

Present in cigarettes, birth-control pills, and automobile pollution.

Essential for the utilization of vitamin C.

The RDA has not been established by the National Research Council, but 1.5–3 mg. for adults is what is currently recommended.

WHAT IT CAN FOR YOU:

Keep your energy up by aiding in effective iron absorption.

DEFICIENCY DISEASE:

Anemia, edema, skeletal defects and possibly rheumatoid arthritis.

NATURAL FOOD SOURCES:

Dried beans, peas, whole wheat, prunes, organ meats, shrimp, and most seafood.

SUPPLEMENTS:

Usually available in multivitamin and mineral supplements in 2-mg. doses.

TOXICITY:

Rare. (See section 290, ''Cautions.'')

ENEMIES:

Not easily destroyed.

PERSONAL ADVICE:

As essential as copper is, I rarely suggest special supplementation. An excess seems to lower zinc level and produces insomnia, hair loss, irregular menses, and depression.

If you eat enough whole-grain products and fresh green leafy vegetables, or organ meats, you don't have to worry about your copper intake.

Cooking or storing acidic foods in copper pots can add to your daily intake.

55. Fluorine

FACTS:

Part of the synthetic compound sodium fluoride (the type added to drinking water) and calcium fluoride (a natural substance).

Decreases chances of dental caries, though too much can discolor teeth.

No RDA has been established, but most people get about 1 mg. daily from fluoridated drinking water. (1.5–4 mg. is suggested by the National Academy of Sciences-National Research Council.)

WHAT IT CAN DO FOR YOU:

Reduce tooth decay.
Strengthen bones.

DEFICIENCY DISEASE:

Tooth decay.

BEST NATURAL SOURCE:

Fluoridated drinking water, seafood, and tea.

SUPPLEMENTS:

Not ordinarily found in multimineral supplements.
Available in prescription multivitamins for children in areas without fluoridated water.

TOXICITY:

20 to 80 mg. per day.
(See section 290, "Cautions.")

ENEMIES:

Aluminum cookware.

PERSONAL ADVICE:

Don't take additional fluoride unless it is prescribed by a physician or dentist.
The fluoride content of food is increased significantly if it's cooked in fluoridated water or a Teflon™-treated utensil.

56. Iodine (Iodide)

FACTS:

Two-thirds of the body's iodine is in the thyroid gland.
Since the thyroid gland controls metabolism, and iodine influences the thyroid, an undersupply of this mineral can result in slow mental reaction, weight gain, and lack of energy.
The RDA, as established by the National Research Council, is 150 mcg. for adults (1 mcg. per kilogram of body weight) and 175 to 200 mcg. for pregnant and lactating women respectively.

WHAT IT CAN DO FOR YOU:

Help you with dieting by burning excess fat.
Promote proper growth.
Give you more energy.

Improve mental alacrity.
Promote healthy hair, nails, skin, and teeth.

DEFICIENCY DISEASE:

Goiter, hypothyroidism.

BEST NATURAL SOURCES:

Kelp, vegetables grown in iodine-rich soil, onions, and all seafood.

SUPPLEMENTS:

Available in multimineral and high-potency vitamin supplements in doses of 0.15 mg.
Natural kelp is a good source of supplemental iodine.

TOXICITY:

No known toxicity from natural iodine, though intakes above 2 mg. are not recommended and iodine as a drug can be harmful if prescribed incorrectly. (See section 290, "Cautions.")

ENEMIES:

Food processing, nutrient-poor soil.

PERSONAL ADVICE:

Aside from kelp, and the iodine included in multimineral and vitamin preparations, I don't recommend additional supplements unless you're advised by a doctor to take them.

If you use salt and live in the Midwest, where iodine-poor soil is common, make sure the salt is iodized.

If you are inclined to eat excessive amounts of raw cabbage, you might *not* be getting the iodine you need, because there are elements in the cabbage that prevent proper utilization of the iodine. This being the case, you might consider a kelp supplement.

57. Iron

FACTS:

Essential and required for life, necessary for the production of hemoglobin (red blood corpuscles), myoglobin (red pigment in muscles), and certain enzymes.

Iron and calcium are the two major dietary deficiencies of American women.

Only about 8 percent of your total iron intake is absorbed and actually enters your bloodstream.

An average 150-pound adult has about 4 g. of iron in his or her body. Hemoglobin, which accounts for most of the iron, is recycled and reutilized as blood cells are replaced every 120 days. Iron bound to protein (ferritin) is stored in the body, as is tissue iron (present in myoglobin) in very small amounts.

The RDA, according to the National Research Council, is 10 to 15 mg. for adults, and 30 mg. for pregnant women. Nursing mothers' RDA is the same as for non-pregnant women (15 mg.).

In one month, women lose almost twice as much iron as men.

Copper, cobalt, manganese, and vitamin C are necessary to assimilate iron.

Iron is necessary for proper metabolization of B vitamins.

WHAT IT CAN DO FOR YOU:

Aid growth.
Promote resistance to disease.
Prevent fatigue.
Cure and prevent iron-deficiency anemia.
Bring back good skin tone.

DEFICIENCY DISEASE:

Iron-deficiency anemia. (For deficiency symptoms, see section 127.)

BEST NATURAL SOURCES:

Pork liver; beef kidney, heart, and liver; farina, raw clams, dried peaches, red meat, egg yolks, oysters, nuts, beans, asparagus, molasses, oatmeal.

SUPPLEMENTS:

The most assimilable form of iron is hydrolyzed-protein chelate, which means organic iron that has been processed for fastest assimilation. This form is nonconstipating and easy on sensitive systems.

Ferrous sulfate, inorganic iron, appears in many vitamin and mineral supplements and can destroy vitamin E (they should be taken at least eight hours apart). Check labels; many drugstore formulas contain ferrous sulfate.

Supplements with organic iron—ferrous gluconate, ferrous fumerate, ferrous citrate, or ferrous peptonate—do not neutralize vitamin E. They are available in a wide variety of doses, usually up to 320 mg.

TOXICITY:

Rare in healthy, normal individuals. Excessive doses, though, can be a hazard for children. A dose of 3 g. can be lethal for a 2-year-old child. (See section 290, "Cautions.") Individuals with idiopathic hemochromatosis are genetically at risk from iron overload.

ENEMIES:

Phosphoproteins in eggs and phytates in unleavened whole wheat reduce iron availability to body.

PERSONAL ADVICE:

If you are a woman, I recommend a chelated or hemoglobin iron supplement. Check the label on your multivitamin or mineral preparation and see what you are already getting and guide yourself accordingly. (Remember, if the iron in your preparation is ferrous sulfate, you're losing your vitamin E.)

If you're on the anti-inflammatory drug Indocin, or take aspirin on a daily basis, you probably need more iron.

Keep your iron supplements out of the reach of children.

Coffee drinkers, as well as tea drinkers, be aware that if you consume large quantities of either beverage you are most likely inhibiting your iron absorption.

If you are pregnant, check with your doctor before taking iron or iron-fortified vitamin supplements. (Iron poisoning has been found in children whose mothers have taken too many pills during pregnancy.)

58. Magnesium

FACTS:

Necessary for calcium and vitamin-C metabolism, as well as that of phosphorus, sodium, and potassium.

Measured in milligrams (mg.).

Essential for effective nerve and muscle functioning.

Important for converting blood sugar into energy.

Known as the antistress mineral.

Alcoholics are usually deficient.

Adults need 250 to 350 mg. daily. For pregnant and lactating women, the recommendation according to the National Research Council is 300 to 355 mg.

The human body contains approximately 21 g. of magnesium.

WHAT IT CAN DO FOR YOU:

Aid in fighting depression.

Promote a healthier cardiovascular system and help prevent heart attacks.

Keep teeth healthier.

Help prevent calcium deposits, kidney and gallstones.

Bring relief from indigestion.

Combined with calcium can work as a natural tranquilizer.

DEFICIENCY DISEASE:

(For deficiency symptoms, see section 127.)

BEST NATURAL SOURCES:

Unmilled grains, figs, almonds, nuts, seeds, dark-green vegetables, bananas.

SUPPLEMENTS:

Chelated magnesium and calcium in perfect balance (half as much magnesium as calcium) is a fine supplement.

Available in multivitamin and mineral preparations.

Can be purchased as magnesium oxide. 250-mg. strength equals 150 mg. per tablet.

Commonly available in 133.3-mg. strengths and taken four times a day.

Supplements of magnesium should not be taken after meals, since the mineral does neutralize stomach acidity.

TOXICITY:

Large amounts, over an extended period of time, can be toxic if your calcium and phosphorus intakes are high or if you have impaired kidney function. (See section 290, "Cautions.")

ENEMIES:

Diuretics, alcohol. (See section 250.)

PERSONAL ADVICE:

If you are a drinker, I suggest you increase your intake of magnesium.

If your daily workouts are exhausting, you probably need more magnesium.

Women who are on the pill or taking estrogen in any form would be well advised to eat more magnesium-rich foods. (Keep in mind that meat, fish, and dairy products are relatively poor sources.)

If you are a heavy consumer of nuts, seeds, and green vegetables, you probably get ample magnesium—as does anyone who lives in an area with hard water.

Magnesium works best with vitamin A, calcium, and phosphorus.

Keep in mind that because magnesium turns on the enzymes that use vitamins B1, B2, and B6, a deficiency of the mineral can cause symptoms associated with an insufficiency of B vitamins—usually convulsions.

59. Manganese

FACTS:

Helps activate enzymes necessary for the body's proper use of biotin, B1, and vitamin C.

Needed for normal bone structure.

Measured in milligrams (mg.).

Important in the formation of thyroxin, the principal hormone of the thyroid gland.

Necessary for the proper digestion and utilization of food.

No official daily allowance has been established, but 2 to 5 mg. is the National Research Council's recommended average adult requirement.

Important for reproduction and normal central nervous system function.

WHAT IT CAN DO FOR YOU:

Help eliminate fatigue.
Aid in muscle reflexes.
Help prevent osteoporosis.
Improve memory.
Reduce nervous irritability.

DEFICIENCY DISEASE:

Ataxia.

BEST NATURAL SOURCES:

Whole-grain cereals, nuts, green leafy vegetables, peas, beets.

SUPPLEMENTS:

Most often found in multivitamin and mineral combinations in dosages of 1 to 9 mg.

TOXICITY:

Rare, except from industrial sources. (See section 290, "Cautions.")

ENEMIES:

Large intakes of calcium and phosphorus will inhibit absorption, as can the fiber and phytic acid contained in bran and beans.

PERSONAL ADVICE:

If you suffer from recurrent dizziness, you might try adding more manganese to your diet.

I advise absent-minded people, or anyone with memory problems, to make sure they are getting enough of this mineral.

Heavy milk drinkers and meat eaters need increased manganese.

60. Molybdenum

FACTS:

Aids in carbohydrate and fat metabolism.

A vital part of the enzyme responsible for iron utilization.

No dietary allowance has been set, but the estimated daily intake of 75 to 250 mcg. has generally been accepted as the adequate human requirement.

WHAT IT CAN DO FOR YOU:

Help in preventing anemia. Promote general well-being.

DEFICIENCY DISEASE:

None known.

BEST NATURAL SOURCES:

Dark-green leafy vegetables, whole grains, legumes.

SUPPLEMENTS:

Not ordinarily available.

TOXICITY:

Rare, but 5 to 10 mg. a day can be considered toxic. (See section 290, "Cautions.")

PERSONAL ADVICE:

As important as molybdenum is, there seems no need for supplementation unless all the food you consume comes from nutrient-deficient soil.

61. Phosphorus

FACTS:

Present in every cell in the body.

Vitamin D and calcium are essential to proper phosphorus functioning.

Calcium and phosphorus should be balanced two to one to work correctly (twice as much calcium as phosphorus).

Involved in virtually all physiological chemical reactions.

Necessary for normal bone and tooth structure.

Niacin cannot be assimilated without phosphorus.

Important for heart regularity.

Essential for normal kidney functioning.

Needed for the transference of nerve impulses.

The RDA is 800 to 1,200 mg. for adults, the higher levels for pregnant and lactating women.

WHAT IT CAN DO FOR YOU:

Aid in growth and body repair.

Provide energy and vigor by helping in the metabolization of fats and starches.

Lessen the pain of arthritis.
Promote healthy gums and teeth.

DEFICIENCY DISEASE:

Rickets, pyorrhea.

BEST NATURAL SOURCES:

Fish, poultry, meat, whole grains, eggs, nuts, seeds.

SUPPLEMENTS:

Bonemeal is a fine natural source of phosphorus. (Make sure vitamin D has been added to help assimilation, *and that the bonemeal is lead-free*!)

TOXICITY:

No known toxicity. (See section 290, "Cautions.")

ENEMIES:

Too much iron, aluminum, and magnesium can render phosphorus ineffective.

PERSONAL ADVICE:

When you get too much phosphorus, you throw off your mineral balance and decrease your calcium. Our diets are usually high in phosphorus—since it does occur in almost every natural food—and therefore calcium deficiencies are frequent. Be aware of this and adjust your diet accordingly.

If you're over forty, you should cut down on your weekly meat consumption and eat more leafy vegetables and drink milk. The reason for this is that after forty our kidneys don't help excrete excess phosphorus, and calcium is again depleted. Be on the lookout for foods preserved with phosphates and consider that as part of your phosphorus intake.

62. Potassium

FACTS:

Works with sodium to regulate the body's water balance and normalize heart rhythms. (Potassium works inside the cells, sodium works just outside them.)

Nerve and muscle functions suffer when the sodium-potassium balance is off.

Hypoglycemia (low blood sugar) causes potassium loss, as does a long fast or severe diarrhea.

No dietary allowance has been set, but 1,600 to 2,000 mg. is considered a sufficient daily intake for healthy adults.

Both mental and physical stress can lead to a potassium deficiency.

WHAT IT CAN DO FOR YOU:

Aid in clear thinking by sending oxygen to brain.
Help dispose of body wastes.
Assist in reducing blood pressure.
Aid in allergy treatment.

DEFICIENCY DISEASE:

Edema, hypoglycemia. (For deficiency symptoms, see section 127.)

BEST NATURAL SOURCES:

Citrus fruits, cantaloupe, tomatoes, watercress, all green leafy vegetables, mint leaves, sunflower seeds, bananas, potatoes.

SUPPLEMENTS:

Available in most high-potency multivitamin and multimineral preparations.

Inorganic potassium "salts" are the sulfate (alum), the chloride, the oxide, and carbonate. Organic potassium refers to the gluconate, the citrate, the fumerate.

Can be bought separately as potassium gluconate, citrate, or chloride in dosages up to nearly 600 mg. (99 mg. elemental potassium.)

TOXICITY:

An intake of 18 g. can cause toxicity. (See section 290, "Cautions.")

ENEMIES:

Alcohol, coffee, sugar, diuretics. (See section 250.)

PERSONAL ADVICE:

If you drink large amounts of coffee, you might find that the fatigue you're fighting is due to the potassium loss you're suffering from.

Heavy drinkers and anyone with a hungry sweet tooth should be aware that their potassium levels are probably low.

If you have low blood sugar, you are likely to be losing potassium while retaining water. And if you take a diuretic, you'll lose even more potassium! Watch your diet, increase your green vegetables, and take enough magnesium to regain your mineral balance.

Losing weight on a low-carbohydrate diet might not be the only thing you're losing. Chances are your potassium level is down. Watch out for weakness and poor reflexes.

63. Selenium

FACTS:

Vitamin E and selenium are synergistic. This means that the two together are stronger than the sum of the equal parts.

Both vitamin E and selenium are antioxidants, preventing or at least slowing down aging and hardening of tissues through oxidation.

Males appear to have a greater need for selenium. Almost half their body's supply concentrates in the testicles and portions of the seminal ducts adjacent to the prostate gland. Also, selenium is lost in the semen.

The official dietary allowance for this mineral, established only recently, is 50 mcg. for women, 70 mcg. for men, 65 mcg. for pregnant women, and 75 mcg. for nursing mothers.

WHAT IT CAN DO FOR YOU:

Aid in keeping youthful elasticity in tissues.
Alleviate hot flashes and menopausal distress.
Help in treatment and prevention of dandruff.
Possibly neutralize certain carcinogens and provide protection from some cancers.

DEFICIENCY DISEASE:

Premature stamina loss; Keshan disease.

BEST NATURAL SOURCES:

Seafood, kidney, liver, wheat germ, bran, tuna fish, onions, tomatoes, broccoli.

SUPPLEMENTS:

Available in small microgram doses—25, 50, 100 and 200 mcg.

Also available combined with vitamin E and other antioxidants.

Natural foods supply sufficient amounts when eaten regularly.

TOXICITY:

Doses of 5 mg. can produce toxic effects.
(See section 290, "Cautions.")

ENEMIES:

Food-processing techniques.

PERSONAL ADVICE:

Selenium was discovered only a little more than twenty years ago. We've just begun to recognize its importance in human nutrition. Until more is known, I advise taking only moderate supplements.

64. Sodium

FACTS:

Sodium and potassium were discovered together and both found to be essential for normal growth.

High intakes of sodium (salt) will result in a depletion of potassium.

Diets high in sodium usually account for many instances of high blood pressure.

There is no official allowance, but the National Research Council's estimated sodium chloride requirement for healthy adults is 500 mg. daily. Sodium aids in keeping calcium and other minerals in the blood soluble.

WHAT IT CAN DO FOR YOU:

Aid in preventing heat prostration or sunstroke.
Help your nerves and muscles function properly.

DEFICIENCY DISEASE:

Impaired carbohydrate digestion, possibly neuralgia.

BEST NATURAL SOURCES:

Salt, shellfish, carrots, beets, artichokes, dried beef, brains, kidney, bacon.

SUPPLEMENTS:

Rarely needed, but if so, kelp is a safe and nutritive supplement.

TOXICITY:

Over 14 g. of sodium chloride daily can produce toxic effects.

(See section 290, "Cautions.")

PERSONAL ADVICE:

If you think you don't eat much salt, see sections 270 and 271 and think again.

If you have high blood pressure, cut down on your sodium intake by reading the labels on the foods you buy. Look for SALT, SODIUM, or the chemical symbol *Na*.

Adding sodium to your diet is as easy as a shake of salt, but subtracting it can be difficult. Avoid luncheon meats, frankfurters, salted cured meats such as ham, bacon, corned beef, as well as condiments—ketchup, chili sauce, soy sauce, mustard. Don't use baking powder or baking soda in cooking.

65. Sulfur

FACTS:

Essential for healthy hair, skin, and nails.

Helps maintain oxygen balance necessary for proper brain function.

Works with B-complex vitamins for basic body metabolism, and is part of tissue-building amino acids.

Aids the liver in bile secretion.

No RDA has been set, but a diet sufficient in protein will generally be sufficient in sulfur.

WHAT IT CAN DO FOR YOU:

Tone up skin and make hair more lustrous.

Help fight bacterial infections.

DEFICIENCY DISEASE:

None known.

BEST NATURAL SOURCES:

Lean beef, dried beans, fish, eggs, cabbage.

SUPPLEMENTS:

Not readily available as a food supplement.
Can be found in topical ointments and creams for skin problems.

TOXICITY:

No known toxicity from organic sulfur, but ill effects may occur from large amounts of inorganic sulfur.
(See section 290, "Cautions.")

PERSONAL ADVICE:

If you're getting enough protein in your daily meals, you are, most likely, getting enough sulfur.
Sulfur creams and ointments have been remarkably successful in treating a variety of skin problems. Check the ingredients in the preparation you are now using. There are many fine natural preparations available at health-food centers.

66. Vanadium

FACTS:

Inhibits the formation of cholesterol in blood vessels.
No dietary allowance set.

WHAT IT CAN DO FOR YOU:

Aid in preventing heart attacks.

DEFICIENCY DISEASE:

None known.

BEST NATURAL SOURCES:

Fish.

SUPPLEMENTS:

Not available.

TOXICITY:

Can easily be toxic if taken in synthetic form.
(See section 290, "Cautions.")

PERSONAL ADVICE:

This is not one of the minerals that needs to be supplemented. A good fish dinner will supply you with the vanadium you need.

67. Zinc

FACTS:

Zinc acts as a traffic policeman, directing and overseeing the efficient flow of body processes, the maintenance of enzyme systems and cells.

Essential for protein synthesis.

Governs the contractibility of muscles.

Helps in the formation of insulin.

Important for blood stability and in maintaining the body's acid-alkaline balance.

Exerts a normalizing effect on the prostate and is important in the development of all reproductive organs.

New studies indicate its importance in brain function and the treatment of schizophrenia.

Strong evidence of its requirement for the synthesis of DNA.

The RDA, as set by the National Research Council, is 12 to 15 mg. for adults (slightly higher allowances for nursing mothers).

Excessive sweating can cause a loss of as much as 3 mg. of zinc per day.

Most zinc in foods is lost in processing, or never exists in substantial amount due to nutrient-poor soil.

WHAT IT CAN DO FOR YOU:

Accelerate healing time for internal and external wounds.
Get rid of white spots on the fingernails.
Help eliminate loss of taste.
Aid in the treatment of infertility.
Help avoid prostate problems.
Promote growth and mental alertness.
Help decrease cholesterol deposits.
Aid in the treatment of mental disorders.

DEFICIENCY DISEASE:

Possibly prostatic hypertrophy (noncancerous enlargement of the prostate gland), arteriosclerosis, hypogonadism.

BEST NATURAL SOURCES:

Meat, liver, seafood (especially oysters), wheat germ, brewer's yeast, pumpkin seeds, eggs, nonfat dry milk, ground mustard.

SUPPLEMENTS:

Available in all good multivitamin and multimineral preparations.

Can be bought as zinc-sulfate, zinc-gluconate or zinc picolinate in doses ranging from 15 to 60 mg. of elemental zinc. Both zinc sulfate and zinc gluconate seem to be equally effective, but zinc gluconate appears to be more easily tolerated.

Chelated zinc and zinc picolinate are the best forms of supplemental zinc.

Zinc is also available in combination with vitamin C, magnesium, and the B-complex vitamins.

TOXICITY:

Virtually nontoxic, except when there is an excessive intake and the food ingested has been stored in galvanized containers. Doses of 2 gm. or more can produce toxic effects. (See section 290, "Cautions.")

PERSONAL ADVICE:

You need higher intakes of zinc if you are taking large amounts of vitamin B6. This is also true if you are an alcoholic or a diabetic.

Men with prostate problems—and without them—would be well advised to keep their zinc levels up.

I have seen success in cases of impotence with a supplement program of B6 and zinc.

Elderly people, concerned about senility, might find a zinc and manganese supplement beneficial.

If you are bothered by irregular menses, you might try a zinc supplement before resorting to hormone treatment to establish regularity.

Remember, if you are adding zinc to your diet, you will increase your need for vitamin A. (Zinc works best with vitamin A, calcium, and phosphorus.)

CAUTION: Megadoses of zinc are suspected of inhibiting immune response, according to new research done at the USDA Nutrition Center at Tufts University.

68. Water

FACTS:

The simple truth is that this is our most important nutrient. One-half to four-fifths of the body's weight is water.

A human being can live for weeks without food, but only a few days without water.

Water is the basic solvent for all the products of digestion. Essential for removing wastes.

There is no specific dietary allowance since water loss varies with climate, situations, and individuals, but under ordinary circumstances six glasses daily is considered healthy. Nursing mothers have increased water requirements because of the amount that's secreted in their milk.

Regulates body temperature.

WHAT IT CAN DO FOR YOU:

Keep all your bodily functions functioning.
Aid in dieting by depressing appetite before meals.
Help prevent constipation.

DEFICIENCY DISEASE:

Dehydration.

BEST NATURAL SOURCES:

Drinking water, juices, fruits, and vegetables.

SUPPLEMENTS:

All drinkable liquids can substitute for our daily water requirements.

TOXICITY:

No known toxicity, but an intake of one and a half gallons (that's sixteen to twenty-four glasses) in about an hour could be dangerous to an adult. It could kill an infant.

PERSONAL ADVICE:

I advise six to eight glasses of water daily, to be drunk a half hour before meals, for anyone who's dieting.

If you're running a fever, be sure to drink lots of water to prevent dehydration and to flush the system of wastes.

Don't drink water from your hot water tap. Hot water dissolves more lead than cold water. And in the morning, always let the water run a few minutes to get the lead out of overnight accumulations.

If you live in an area where there is hard water, you're

probably getting more calcium and magnesium than you think.

SPECIAL WATER CAUTIONS:

If you live in an old home containing lead pipes, have your water analyzed by the local county health department. Water with the wrong PH can dissolve lead from pipes, subjecting children to possible lead poisoning. (Even homes with copper plumbing can have lead-soldered joints that might affect tap water.)

If there are chlorinated solvents or pesticides in your water, they can be absorbed through the skin and are volatile. *Taking a 15-minute shower can be as toxic as drinking 8 glasses of contaminated water!*

All home water filtering systems have drawbacks, and many can be hazardous to your health. For instance:

- Activated carbon filters can become fouled with harmful contaminants if they are not changed on a regular basis.
- Reverse-Osmosis systems, which remove chemicals, but not necessarily inorganic contaminants, must be tested periodically because the filter can be loaded with bacteria without evidencing a reduced flow rate.
- Distillers, which are generally more effective in removing inorganic than organic contaminants, must be descaled regularly. If not, the product water can be *worse* instead of better!

69. Any Questions About Chapter IV?

I'm a 40-year-old woman and drink three glasses of milk every day. Do I still need more calcium?

If that's your sole source of calcium, you do! Three 8-ounce glasses of whole milk give you only 776 mg. of calcium—not enough and certainly not worth the 360 mg. of sodium, 33 mg. of cholesterol, 15 g. of saturated fat, and 577 calories that you also get. Skim, low-fat milk, or buttermilk will lower the amount of calories and fat, but still won't provide you with sufficient calcium. See section 50 for other natural sources.

I've read that chlorinated drinking water can cause cancer. Is this true? If so, why do they chlorinate water?

Unfortunately, chlorination has indeed been linked to a group of cancer-causing chemicals (trihalomethanes) in our water. But according to the Environmental Protection Agency, the risk to the public is far outweighed by the benefits—primarily the prevention of widespread outbreaks of typhoid and other waterborne diseases. Home water-filtering systems can remove chlorine from tap water after bacteria have been killed, but see Section 68 for water cautions to be aware of.

I'm worried about all the pollution in our rivers and streams. How do I know that my tap water is safe to drink?

The best thing to do if you want to find out if there are contaminants in your water is to contact your local water superintendent and ask for the results of water-sampling tests and sanitary surveys. Ask to see the Public Health Service standards, too, so that you'll be able to compare the former with the latter. You can also have your water tested for contaminants at most local hospital laboratories.

Meanwhile, until you are sure that your water is safe, I recommend taking the following emergency measures:

• Let your water run for 3 to 4 minutes before using it. This helps flush out any lead, cadmium, and cobalt that may lodge in your pipes.
• Boil your water (uncovered) for at least 20 minutes before using it. Boiling can kill bacteria and remove some organic chemicals.
• If you're worried about trihalomethanes (which are carcinogens found in chlorinated water), whip your water in a blender for 15 minutes with the top off. Aeration removes chlorine and chlorinated organics.

I get very confused in the supermarket. Is "mineral water" better for me than "spring water?"

Better? Not really. Some bottled "mineral waters" may

actually have fewer dissolved minerals than many city water supplies. In fact, the term "mineral water" is frequently used to describe all bottled water, with the exception of bulk water, club soda, and seltzer. "Spring water" must, under truth-in-labeling laws, come from a spring. But that spring has minerals in it, too. What you want to watch out for are mineral waters without the word "natural" on the label. This means that minerals may have been removed or added—and if you're going to buy a nutrient cocktail, you're better off making it yourself!

I know I need calcium, but I'm allergic to dairy products. Can you recommend alternative dietary sources?

Lots! Orange juice (6 oz.) fortified with calcium will give you approximately 200 mg. A three-ounce can of sardines or salmon (with bones) will give you another 200–300 mg. Tofu, made with calcium sulfate, will also supply calcium (150 mg. per 4-oz. serving) as will almonds, brazil nuts and hazelnuts (approximately 200–300 mg. per cup). You might also want to try "nori" and other seaweeds. They're an acquired taste, but they are high in calcium.

V

Protein—and Those Amazing Amino Acids

70. The Protein Amino Acid Connection

Protein is a life necessity in the diet of man and all animals. Actually, though, it is not protein itself that is required, but the amino acids which are the building blocks of protein.

> If any essential amino acid is low or
> missing, the effectiveness of all
> the others will be proportionately reduced.

Amino acids, which combined with nitrogen form thousands of different proteins, are not only the units from which proteins are formed, but are also the end products of protein digestion.

There are twenty-two known amino acids. Eight of these are called *essential amino acids*. These essential amino acids *cannot*, like the others, be manufactured by the human body and *must* be obtained from food or supplements. A ninth amino acid, histidine, is considered essential only for infants and children.

In order for the body to effectively use and synthesize protein, all the essential amino acids must be present and in the proper proportions. Even the temporary absence of a single essential amino acid can adversely affect protein syn-

THE 22 AMINO ACIDS
(Essential amino acids are marked with asterisks.)

Alanine	*Leucine
Arginine	*Lysine
Asparagine	*Methionine
Aspartic acid	Ornithine
Cysteine	*Phenylalanine
Cystine	Proline
Glutamic acid	Serine
Glutamine	*Threonine
Glycine	*Tryptophan
*Histidine (for infants and children)	*Valine
*Isoleucine	

thesis. In fact, whatever essential amino acid is low or missing will proportionately reduce the effectiveness of all the others.

71. How Much Protein Do You Need, Really?

Everyone's protein requirements differ, depending on a variety of factors including health, age, and size. Actually, the larger and younger you are, the more you need. To estimate your own personal daily recommended allowance, see the chart below.

AGE	1–3	4–6	7–10	11–14	15–18	19 and over
POUND KEY	0.82	0.68	0.55	0.45	0.40	0.36

- Find the pound key under your age group.
- Multiply that number by your weight.
- The result will be your daily protein requirement in grams.

Example: You weigh 100 pounds and are thirty-three years old.
Your pound key is 0.36.
0.36 × 100 = 36g.—your daily protein requirement.

An average minimum protein requirement is around 45 g. a day. That's 15 g. or about half an ounce per meal. Make sure you get enough at breakfast.

72. Types of Protein—What's the Difference?

All proteins are not the same, though they're manufactured from the same twenty-two amino acids. They have different functions and work in different areas of the body.

There are basically two types of protein—complete protein and incomplete protein.

Complete protein provides the proper balance of eight necessary amino acids that build tissue, and is found in foods of animal origin such as meats, poultry, seafood, eggs, milk, and cheese.

Incomplete protein lacks certain essential amino acids and is not used efficiently when eaten alone. However, when it is combined with small amounts of animal-source protein, it becomes complete. It is found in seeds, nuts, peas, grains, and beans.

Mixing complete and incomplete proteins can give you better nutrition than either one alone. A good rice-and-beans dish with some cheese can be just as nourishing, less expensive, and lower in fat than a steak.

73. Protein Myths

A lot of people seem to think that protein is nonfattening. This misconception has frustrated many a determined dieter who forgoes bread but eats healthy portions of steak and wonders where the weight is coming from. The fact is

- 1 g. protein   = 4 calories
- 1 g. carbohydrate = 4 calories
- 1 g. fat   = 9 calories

In other words, protein and carbohydrates have the same gram-for-gram calorie count.

It is also thought that protein can burn up fat. This is another erroneous assumption that leaves dieters staring incomprehensibly at their scales. It just is not true that the more protein you eat the thinner you'll get. And, believe it or not, one homemade beef taco or a slice of cheese pizza will give you more protein than two eggs or four slices of bacon or even a whole cup of milk. (Of course, if the taco or pizza is made with all sorts of additives, you're better off taking a cut in protein and sticking with the eggs.)

74. Protein Supplements

> Two tablespoons of supplement equal
> the protein in a three-ounce steak.

For anyone who isn't able to get his or her daily protein requirement from whole food, protein supplements are helpful. The best formulas are derived from soybeans, egg white, whey, and non-fat milk, which contain all the essential amino acids. They come in liquid and powdered form, are available without carbohydrates or fats, and generally supply about 26 g. of protein an ounce (two tablespoons). That would be about the same amount of protein you get from a three-ounce T-bone.

Supplements can easily be added to beverages and foods. Texturized vegetable protein (TVP) can be added to ground beef to extend and enhance hamburgers, which will be more economical and better for you because of the cut in saturated fat.

75. Amino Acid Supplements

Free-form amino acids are now available in balanced formulas or as individual supplements, because so many have been found to offer specific health-enhancing properties—from improving the immune system to reducing dependence on drugs. (See individual listings, sections 76 through 82.)

It's wise, when taking amino acid supplements, to also take the major vitamins that are involved in their metabolisms, for instance: Vitamins B6, B12, and niacin. And if you're going to take an amino acid formula, make sure it's well-balanced. *Read the label!* For protein synthesis to occur, there must be a balance between "essential" and "nonessential" amino acids, and the essentials in proper proportion to one another. (Lysine should be in a 2:1 ratio to methionine, 3:1 to tryptophan, and so on. When in doubt, ask your pharmacist or consult a reliable nutritionist. Or send a stamped, self-addressed envelope, with your question, to: Amino Acid Research Group, P.O. Box 5277, Berkeley, CA 94705.) What you want is a formula that's modeled after naturally occuring proteins so that you can get the proper therapeutic value.

CAUTION: It's dangerous for any supplement to be used in place of food on a regular basis or taken in megadoses without the advice of a physician. Always keep them out of the reach of children.

76. Let's Talk Tryptophan

Tryptophan is an essential amino acid that's used by the brain—along with vitamin B6, niacin (or niacinamide), and magnesium—to produce serotonin, a neurotransmitter that carries messages between the brain and one of the body's biochemical mechanisms of sleep.

WHAT IT CAN DO FOR YOU:

• Help induce natural sleep.
• Reduce pain sensitivity.
• Act as a non-drug antidepressant.
• Alleviate migraines.
• Aid in reducing anxiety and tension.
• Help relieve some symptoms of alcohol-related body chemistry disorders and aid in control of alcoholism.

BEST NATURAL SOURCES:

Cottage cheese, milk, meat, fish, turkey, bananas, dried dates, peanuts, all protein-rich foods.

SUPPLEMENT GUIDE:

At the time of this writing, L-tryptophan is not available as an over-the-counter supplement in the United States and Canada.

Where it is available, L-tryptophan usually comes in tablets of 250 mg. to 667 mg. strengths. When used as a relaxant, it should be taken during the day between meals, with juice or water—no milk or other protein.

As a sleep inducer, L-tryptophan works best when taken in a 500 mg. dose, along with vitamin B6 100 mg., niacinamide 100 mg., and chelated magnesium 130 mg., 1½ hours before bedtime. (Again, these should be taken with juice or water—no protein.)

Many doctors, including Dr. David Bressler, formerly of the Pain Control Center at the University of Los Angeles, suggest taking an additional tryptophan tablet ½ hour before bedtime to help sleeping all through the night.

CAUTION: Single dosages exceeding 2 grams are not recommended, even though successful tests at the Maryland Psychiatric Research Center have shown that there is no danger of tryptophan addiction or overdose. (Because tryptophan is a natural part of our physical makeup, the body doesn't have to change any function to make use of it as it does with drugs.)

PERSONAL ADVICE AND COMMENTS:

Although the epidemic of the potentially fatal blood disease linked to L-tryptophan was found to be caused by a contamination in batches of the supplement made by a single Japanese manufacturer, at the time of this writing L-tryptophan supplements are still not available over-the-counter in the United States and Canada.

Nonetheless, if you are taking L-tryptophan, be sure that you're also taking a complete balanced B-complex formula (50–100 mg. of B1, B2, and B6) with your morning and evening meals.

You can prolong the relaxant effects of tryptophan by taking it in a 2-to-1 ratio with niacinamide (twice as much tryptophan as niacinamide). Niacinamide has an antidepressant effect of its own. (See section 44.)

77. The Phenomenal Phenylalanine

Phenylalanine is an essential amino acid that is an essential amino acid that is a neurotransmitter, a chemical that transmits its signals between the nerve cells and the brain. In the body it's turned into norepinephrine and dopamine, excitatory transmitters, which promote alertness and vitality. (Do not confuse with DL-phenylalanine; see section 78.) It is also half of the artificial sweetener Aspartame (phenylalanine and aspartic acid) and in virtually all diet soft drinks with the exception of Dr. Pepper, as well as most dietetic foods and medicines.

WHAT IT CAN DO FOR YOU:

- Reduce hunger.
- Increase sexual interest.
- Improve memory and mental alertness.
- Alleviate depression.

BEST NATURAL SOURCES:

All protein-rich foods, bread stuffing, soy products, cottage cheese, dry skim milk, almonds, peanuts, lima beans, pumpkin and sesame seeds.

SUPPLEMENT GUIDE:

Available in 250–500 mg. tablets. For appetite control, tablets should be taken one hour before meals with juice or water (no protein).

For general alertness and vitality, tablets should be taken between meals, but again with water or juice (no protein).

CAUTION: Phenylalanine is contraindicated during pregnancy and for people with PKU (phenylketonuria) or skin cancer.

PERSONAL ADVICE AND COMMENTS:

Before resorting to prescription or recreational drugs, I'd advise giving this natural "upper" a chance. (Keep in mind, though, that it cannot be metabolized if you are deficient in vitamin C.)

Phenylalanine is nonaddictive, *but it can raise blood pressure*! If you are hypertensive or have a heart condition, I'd advise checking with your doctor before using phenylalanine. (In most cases, persons with high blood pressure are able to take phenylalanine *after* meals, but clear it with your doctor first.)

78. DL-Phenylalanine (DLPA)

This form of the essential amino acid phenylalanine is a mixture of equal parts of D (synthetic) and L (natural) phenylalanine. By producing and activating morphine-like hormones called *endorphins*, it intensifies and prolongs the body's own natural pain-killing response to injury, accident, and disease.

Certain enzyme systems in the body continually destroy endorphins, but DL-phenylalanine effectively inhibits these enzymes, allowing the pain-killing endorphins to do their job.

> Many people who do not respond to such
> conventional pain-killers as Empirin
> and Valium *do* respond to DLPA.

People who suffer from chronic pain have lower levels of endorphin activity in their blood and cerebro-spinal fluid. Since DLPA can restore normal endorphin levels, it can thereby assist the body in reducing pain naturally—without the use of drugs.

Moreover, because DLPA is capable of selective pain-blocking, it can effectively alleviate chronic long-term discomfort while leaving the body's natural defense mechanisms for short-term acute pain (burns, cuts, etc.) unhindered.

The effect of DLPA often equals or exceeds that of morphine and other opiate derivatives, but DLPA differs from prescription and over-the-counter medicines in that—

• it is nonaddictive;
• pain relief becomes *more* effective over time (without development of tolerance);
• it has strong antidepressant action;
• it can provide continuous pain relief for up to a month without additional medication;
• it's nontoxic;
• it can be combined with any other medication or therapy to increase benefits without adverse interactions.

WHAT IT CAN DO FOR YOU:

Act as a natural pain-killer for conditions such as whiplash, osteoarthritis, rheumatoid arthritis, lower back pain, migraines, leg and muscle cramps, postoperative pain, and neuralgia.

SUPPLEMENT GUIDE:

DL-phenylalanine is generally available in 375 mg. tablets. Correct dosages vary according to the individual's own experience of pain.

Six tablets per day (two tablets taken approximately 15 minutes before each meal) is the best way to begin a DLPA regimen. Pain relief should occur within the first four days, though it may, in some cases, take as long as three to four weeks. (If no substantial relief is noticed in the first three weeks, double the initial dosage for an additional two to three weeks. If treatment is still not effective, discontinue the regimen. It's been found that 5–15% of users do not respond to DLPA's analgesic properties.)

CAUTION: DLPA is contraindicated during pregnancy and for people with phenylketonuria. Because it elevates blood pressure, people with heart conditions or hypertension should check with a doctor before starting any DLPA regimen. Usually, though, it's allowed if taken *after* meals.

PERSONAL ADVICE AND COMMENTS:

On a DLPA regimen, pain usually diminishes within the first week. Dosages can then be reduced gradually until a minimum requirement is determined. Whatever yours turns out to be, doses should be regularly spaced throughout the day.

Some people require only one week of DLPA supplements a month; others need it on a continuous basis. (I found it interesting to discover that many people who do not respond to such conventional prescription pain-killers as Empirin and Valium *do* respond to DLPA.)

79. Looking at Lysine

This essential amino acid is vital in the makeup of critical body proteins. It's needed for growth, tissue repair, and the production of antibodies, hormones, and enzymes.

WHAT IT CAN DO FOR YOU:

• Help reduce the incidence of and/or prevent herpes simplex infection (fever blister and cold sores).
• Promote better concentration.
• Properly utilize fatty acids needed for energy production.
• Aid in alleviating some fertility problems.

BEST NATURAL SOURCE:

Fish, milk, lima beans, meat, cheese, yeast, eggs, soy products, all protein-rich foods.

SUPPLEMENT GUIDE:

L-lysine is generally available in 500 mg. capsules or tablets. The usual dose is 1–2 daily, half an hour before mealtimes.

PERSONAL ADVICE AND COMMENTS:

If you're often tired, unable to concentrate, prone to bloodshot eyes, nausea, dizziness, hair loss, and anemia, you could have a lysine deficiency.

Older persons, particularly men, require more lysine than younger ones.

Lysine is lacking in certain cereal proteins such as gliadin (from wheat) and zein (from corn). Supplementation of wheat-based foods with lysine improves their protein quality. (See complete and incomplete protein in section 72.)

If you have herpes, lysine supplements in doses of 3–6 grams daily—plus lysine-rich foods—are strongly recommended.

80. All About Arginine

This amino acid is necessary for the normal function of the pituitary gland. Along with ornithine, phenylalanine, and other neuro chemicals, arginine is required for the synthesis and release of the pituitary gland's growth hormone. (See section 81.) The need for arginine is especially great in males, since seminal fluids contain as much as 80% of this protein building-block, and a deficiency could lead to infertility.

WHAT IT CAN DO FOR YOU:

- Increase sperm count in male.
- Aid in immune response and healing of wounds.
- Help metabolize stored body fat and tone up muscle tissue.
- Promote physical and mental alertness.

BEST NATURAL SOURCES:

Nuts, popcorn, carob, gelatin desserts, chocolate, brown rice, oatmeal, raisins, sunflower and sesame seeds, whole wheat bread, and all protein-rich foods.

SUPPLEMENT GUIDE:

L-arginine is available in tablets or powder. It's best taken on an empty stomach (with juice or water) in a 2-gram (2,000 mg.) dose immediately before retiring. Additional benefits—particularly those for muscle-toning—can be gained by taking

2 grams (2,000 mg.) on an empty stomach (with juice or water) one hour prior to engaging in vigorous physical exercise.

CAUTIONS: Do not give to growing children (could cause giantism) or persons with schizophrenic conditions. Arginine supplements—and arginine-rich foods—are contraindicated for anyone who has herpes. Dosages exceeding 20–30 grams daily are not recommended. (Could cause enlarged joints and deformities of bones.)

PERSONAL ADVICE AND COMMENTS:

Arginine is necessary for adults because after the age of 30 there is almost a complete cessation of its secretion from the pituitary gland.

If you notice a thickening or coarsening of your skin, you're taking too much arginine. Several weeks of extremely high doses can cause this side effect, but it is reversible. Just cut back on your intake.

Any physical trauma increases your need for dietary arginine.

L-arginine taken in conjunction with L-ornithine can help stimulate weight loss.

81. Growth Hormone (G.H.) Releasers

Growth Hormone (G.H.) Releasers are nutrients that stimulate the production of growth hormone in the body. The human Growth Hormone is stored in the pituitary gland and the body releases it in response to sleep, exercise, and restricted food intake.

WHAT GROWTH HORMONE CAN DO FOR YOU:

• Help burn fat and convert it into energy and muscle.
• Improve resistance to disease.
• Accelerate wound-healing.
• Aid in tissue repair.

- Strengthen connective tissue for healthier tendons and ligaments.
- Enhance protein synthesis for muscle growth.
- Reduce urea levels in blood and urine.

> By supplementing your diet with the
> amino acids and vitamins that stimulate
> release of growth hormone, production
> can be brought back up to
> young-adult levels.

Important G.H. Releasers are the amino acids ornithine, arginine, tryptophan, glycine, and tyrosine, which work synergistically (more effectively together than separately) with vitamin B6, niacinamide, zinc, calcium, magnesium, potassium, and vitamin C to trigger the nighttime release of growth hormone. Peak secretion of G.H. is reached about 90 minutes after we fall asleep.

Natural growth hormone levels decrease as we grow older. Somewhere around age 50, G. H. production virtually stops completely. But by supplementing your diet with the amino acids and vitamins that stimulate release of growth hormone, production can be brought back up to the levels of a young adult.

THE DYNAMIC AMINO DUO:
ORNITHINE & ARGININE

Ornithine and arginine, two of the amino acids involved in the release of human growth hormone, are among the most popular amino acid supplements today, essentially because they can help you slim down and shape up while you sleep (which is when G.H. is secreted). While some hormones encourage the body to store fat, growth hormone acts as a mobilizer of fat, helping you to not only look trimmer but have more energy as well.

Ornithine stimulates insulin secretion and helps insulin work as an anabolic (muscle-building) hormone, which has increased its use among body builders. Taking extra ornithine will help increase the levels of arginine in your body. (Actually, arginine is constructed from ornithine, ornithine is released from arginine in a continuing cyclic process.)

Because ornithine and arginine are so closely related, the characteristics and cautions for one apply to the other. (See section 80, "All About Arginine.") As a supplement, ornithine works best when taken at the same time and in the same manner as arginine (on an empty stomach, with juice or water—no protein).

82. Other Amazing Amino Acids
GLUTAMINE & GLUTAMIC ACID

Glutamic acid serves primarily as a brain fuel. It has the ability to pick up excess ammonia—which can inhibit high-performance brain function—and convert it into the buffer glutamine. Since glutamine produces marked elevation of glutamic acid, a shortage of the former in the diet can result in a shortage of the latter in the brain.

Aside from improving intelligence (even the IQs of mentally deficient children), glutamine has been shown to help in the control of alcoholism. It has also been found to shorten the healing time for ulcers and alleviate fatigue, depression, and impotence. Most recently it's been used successfully in the treatment of schizophrenia and senility.

L-glutamine (the natural form of glutamine) is available as a supplement in 500 mg. capsules. The recommended dosage is 1–4 grams (1,000–4,000 mg.) daily, in divided doses. (For fatigue, depression, and impotence, the recommended dosage is 500 to 1,000 mg. daily for the first few weeks, 1,200–1,500 mg. for the next few weeks, and finally 2,000 mg. after a month.)

CAUTION: Though glutamine and glutamic acid are not the same as monosodium glutamate (MSG), persons with a sensitivity to the latter could experience an allergic reaction and are advised to consult a physician before using these supplements.

ASPARTIC ACID

Aspartic acid aids in the expulsion of harmful ammonia from the body. (When ammonia enters the circulatory system, it acts as a highly toxic substance.) By disposing of ammonia, aspartic acid helps protect the central nervous system. Recent research indicates that it may be an important factor in increased resistance to fatigue. When salts of aspartic acid were given to athletes, they showed decidedly improved stamina and endurance.

L-aspartic acid (the natural form of aspartic acid) is available as a supplement in 250 mg. and 500 mg. tablets. The usual dosage is 500 mg. 1–3 times daily with juice or water (no protein).

CYSTINE & CYSTEINE

Cystine is the *stable form* of the sulfur-containing amino acid cysteine (an important anti-aging nutrient). The body readily converts one into the other as needed, and the two forms can be considered as a single amino acid in metabolism. When cystine is metabolized, it yields sulfuric acid, which reacts with other substances to help detoxify the system.

Sulfur-containing amino acids, particularly cystine and methionine, have been shown to be effective protectors against copper toxicity. (An excessive accumulation of copper in humans is a sign of Wilson's disease.) Cystine/cysteine can also help "tie up" and protect the body from other harmful metals as well as destructive free radicals that are formed by smoking and drinking. A cysteine supplement (L-cystine) taken daily with vitamin C (three times as much vitamin C as cysteine) is the regimen that's been suggested for smokers and alcohol drinkers. (Supplements need not be taken on an empty stomach.) Recent research also indicates that therapeutic doses of cysteine can offer an important degree of protection against X-ray and nuclear radiation.

CAUTION: Large doses of cysteine/cystine, vitamins C and B1 are not recommended for anyone with diabetes mellitus, and should only be undertaken on the advice of a physician.

(The combination of these nutrients could negate insulin effectiveness.)

METHIONINE

Like cystine, this is another sulfur-containing amino acid. Methionine helps in some cases of schizophrenia by lowering the blood level of histamine, which can cause the brain to relay wrong messages. When combined with choline and folic acid, it has been shown to offer protection against certain tumors.

An insufficiency of methionine can break down the body's ability to process urine and result in edema (swelling due to retention of fluids in tissues) and susceptibility to infection. A methionine deficiency has also been linked to cholesterol deposits, atherosclerosis, and hair loss in laboratory animals.

GLYCINE

Sometimes referred to as the simplest of the amino acids, glycine has been shown to yield quite a few remarkable benefits. It has been found helpful in the treatment of low pituitary gland function, and, because it supplies the body with additional creatine (essential for muscle function), it has also been found effective in the treatment of progressive muscular dystrophy.

Many nutritionally oriented doctors now use glycine in the treatment of hypoglycemia. (Glycine stimulates the release of glucagon, which mobilizes glycogen, which is then released into the blood as glucose.)

Additionally, it is effective as a treatment for gastric hyperacidity (and is included in many gastric antacid drugs). It has also been used to treat certain types of acidemia (low pH of the blood), especially one caused by a leucine imbalance which results in an offensive body and breath odor (a condition formerly treated only by a dietary restriction of leucine).

TYROSINE

Though this is a nonessential amino acid, it's a high-ranking neurotransmitter, and important because of its role in stimulating and modifying brain activity. For instance, in order for phenylalanine to be effective as a mood elevator, appetite depressant, etc. (see section 77), it must first convert into tyrosine. If this conversion does not take place, either because of some enzyme insufficiency or a great need elsewhere in the body for phenylalanine, insufficient quantities of norepinephrine will be produced by the brain and depression will result.

Clinical studies have shown that tyrosine supplementation has helped control medication-resistant depression and anxiety, as well as enable patients taking amphetamines (as mood elevators or diet drugs) to reduce their dosages to minimal levels in a matter of weeks.

Tyrosine has also helped cocaine addicts kick their habit by helping to avert the depression, fatigue, and extreme irritability which accompany withdrawal. A regimen of tyrosine, dissolved in orange juice, taken along with vitamin C, tyrosine hydroxylase (the enzyme that lets the body use tyrosine), and vitamins B1, B2, and niacin seems to work.

83. Any Questions About Chapter V?

I'm prone to convulsions, and my doctor put me on DILANTIN (phenytoin) a year ago. Recently, a friend told me about Taurine, which she said was a nonessential amino acid that was natural and could help me the same way. What I want to know is, if it's nonessential why would I need it? And why would it work?

Let me begin by clearing up a major point of misunderstanding: where amino acids are concerned, nonessential does *not* mean unnecessary. All the amino acids are necessary, it's just that the ones that are deemed essential can't be synthesized by the body in sufficient quantities to promote effective protein synthesis. If these essential ones are not supplied in the diet, *all* amino acids are reduced in the same proportion as the one that's low or missing. As for substituting Taurine for an anticonvulsant medication, that's a decision only your doctor can make. I can say though that Taurine has been shown to be quite successful as an anti-convulsant when taken in combination with glutamic and aspartic acids, but would not recommend undertaking it without consulting a doctor. (For listings of nutritionally oriented doctors in your area, see section 293.)

I've read that exercise stimulates the release of growth hormone. I do at least twenty minutes of dance exercise every day, so does this mean that I probably don't need a G.H. supplement?

On the contrary, you probably do. Only certain exercises, such as weight-lifting, where there is what's known as muscular "peak output" (even briefly sustained), promote a significant release of G.H. Other exercises, even prolonged ones, produce negligible amounts (if any) of growth hormone— unless they are performed with peak muscular effort. In fact, because amino acids are lost through the skin when you sweat, exercise *increases* your need for amino acids that will stimulate growth hormone.

I take DEXATRIM to control my weight. On the label it says that it contains phenylpropanolamine. Is this the same as L-phenylalanine, and are they equally effective?

Phenylpropanolamine (PPA), which is found in many diet pills, is definitely *not* the same as L-phenylalanine. PPA is an appetite depressant (of dubious effectiveness, according to the American Medical Association) with a high incidence of side effects, including adverse interactions with MAO inhibitors and some oral contraceptives. Unlike the amino acid phenylalanine, which stimulates the brain to produce norepinephrine (which has been shown to reduce hunger), and alleviate those down-in-the-dumps diet blues, PPA depletes the brain of norepinephrine—usually in about two weeks— and leaves dieters fatigued and often depressed.

PPA is a poor substitute for a good diet (see sections 125), while L-phenylalanine, which is found naturally in such protein-rich foods as cottage cheese, soy products, almonds, dry skim milk, and many more, can aid in appetite control (while nourishing the brain) if taken one hour before meals with juice or water.

Is there such a thing as an anti-aging amino acid?

As a matter of fact, L-glutathione (GSH) has been called a triple threat anti-aging amino acid. It's actually a tripeptide, synthesized from three amino acids—L-cysteine, L-glutamic acid, and glycine, and it has been shown to act as an antioxidant and deactivate free radicals which speed up the aging process. It is also an anti-tumor agent, a respiratory accelerator in the brain, and has been used to help in the treatment of allergies, cataracts, diabetes, hypoglycemia, and arthritis, as well as in helping to prevent the harmful side effects of high-dose radiation in chemotherapy and X-rays. Additionally, it helps to protect against the harmful effects of cigarette smoke and alcohol.

What is this new amino acid L-carnitine that I have been hearing about?

We're all very excited about it, since recent research has indicated that not only does it play an important role in converting stored body fat into energy, but it can help control hypoglycemia, reduce angina attacks, and benefit patients with diabetes, liver or kidney disease.

It's also being used by athletes, enabling longer periods of intense workouts.

The heart is dependent upon L-carnitine, and a deficiency of this amino acid can cause impairment of heart tissue. The major natural sources are meats and dairy products.

With diseases such as cancer, AIDS, and what-have-you on the rampage these days, is there anything that can be done to improve an individual's immune system?

Fortunately, yes! The answer seems to be Growth Hormone Releasers. (See section 81.)

What happens is that as we get older, our immune system—that ever-ready army of white blood cells (called T-cells because they're under the command of the thymus gland) which are told where and when to attack and what antibodies their cofighters (called B-cells because they're made in the bone marrow) should produce—begins to break down due to the decreasing power and size of the thymus gland. This not only causes an ineffectual defense system, but often danger-ous confusion where the T-cells mistake friends for enemies and attack you, resulting in autoimmune disorders. (It's been suggested that diseases such as multiple sclerosis, myasthenia gravis, and arthritis may be due to this.)

What's been discovered recently, though, is that this is most likely due to a reduced rate of growth hormone, which is produced by the pituitary gland and necessary to the func-tion of the thymus gland and therefore the immune system. But supplements of amino acids (arginine, ornithine, and cysteine), as well as vitamins E, A, C, zinc, selenium, and enzymes such as papain, have been found to work wonders in reversing this degenerative syndrome.

I'm a professional weight lifter and would like to know if there are any legal, natural supplement alternatives to ster-oids?

There certainly are. Branched Chain Amino Acids (BCAAs)—which are comprised of leucine, valine and isoleucine—are natural anabolic muscle-building supple-ments. They regulate how protein is used by the body and play a unique role in protein metabolism in muscles. While all other amino acids are broken down in the liver, BCAAs are oxidized in peripheral muscle.

BCAAs are, in effect, a principal source of calories for human muscle. Intense physical exercise produces a rapid excretion of nitrogen, which causes a decrease in muscle protein synthesis. BCAAs limit this decrease.

During strenuous exercise, such as weight training, the stress on a muscle causes it to break down (catabolism). BCAAs not only act to prevent this, but actually reverse the process. They are, therefore, *anabolic* because they build up muscle.

BCAA facts that can help your work out:

• BCAAs can reduce appetite while preserving basic protein storage in the body.
• One half of your body weight is muscle, and 15–20 percent of muscle is branch chain amino acids.
• 50 percent of ingested BCAA is available to your muscles in one hour, 100 percent in two hours.
• BCAAs produce glycogen, which helps balance insulin secretion.
• BCAAs directly affect muscle and body weight changes, promoting lean muscle distribution.

Supplements should only be taken half an hour before workouts.

QUICK AMINO ACID REFERENCE

ALANINE: Enhances immune system; lowers risk of kidney stones; aids in alleviating hypoglycemia.

ARGININE: Increases sperm count; accelerates wound healing; tones muscle tissue.

ASPARTIC ACID: Enhances immune system; increases stamina and endurance; expels harmful ammonia from the body.

BRANCHED CHAIN AMINO ACIDS (LEUCINE, ISO-LEUCINE, VALINE): (See above.)

CYSTEINE: Helps prevent baldness; alleviates psoriasis; improves condition of hair, skin and nails.

GLUTAMIC ACID AND GLUTAMINE: Help improve brain function; alleviate fatigue; aid in ulcer healing time; act as mood elevators.

HISTIDINE: Helps alleviate rheumatoid arthritis; alleviates stress; aids in improving libido.

LYSINE: Helps improve concentration; enhances fertility; aids in preventing herpes simplex infection.

METHIONINE: Aids in lowering cholesterol; helps in treatment of schizophrenia and Parkinson's disease; may protect against tumors.

ORNITHINE: Works as a muscle building hormone; increases potency of arginine.

PHENYLALANINE: Acts as an anti-depressant; helps suppress appetite; can function in some forms as a natural pain killer.

PROLINE: Aids in wound healing; helps increase learning ability.

SERINE: Helps alleviate pain; can act as a natural anti-psychotic.

THREONINE: Necessary for utilization of protein in diet.

TRYPTOPHAN: Aids in reducing anxiety; helps induce sleep; may help in control of alcoholism.

TYROSINE: Improves sex drive; helps alleviate stress; can act as an appetite suppresant and mood elevator.

VI

Fat and Fat Manipulators

84. Lipotropics—What Are They?

Methionine, choline, inositol, and betaine are all lipotropics, which means their prime function is to prevent abnormal or excessive accumulation of fat in the liver.

Lipotropics also increase the liver's production of lecithin, which keeps cholesterol more soluble, detoxify the liver, and increase resistance to disease by helping the thymus gland carry out its functions.

85. Who Needs Them and Why

We all need lipotropics, some of us more than others. Anyone on a high-protein diet falls into the latter category. Methionine and choline are *necessary* to detoxify the amines that are by-products of protein metabolism.

Because nearly all of us consume too much fat (the average consumption in the United States is now 36 to 42 percent of total calories), and a substantial part of that is saturated fat, lipotropics are indispensable. By helping the liver produce lecithin, they're helping to keep cholesterol from forming dangerous deposits in blood vessels, lessening chances of heart attacks, arteriosclerosis, and gallstone formation as well.

Lipotropics keep cholesterol
moving safely.

We also need lipotropics to stay healthy, since they aid the thymus in stimulating the production of antibodies, the growth and action of phagocytes (which surround and gobble up invading viruses and microbes), and in destroying foreign or abnormal tissue.

86. The Cholesterol Story

Like everything else, there's a good and bad side to fats. The general misconception that all of them are bad for you, prevalent as it may be, simply is not true. And the most maligned of all is cholesterol.

Practically everyone knows that cholesterol can be responsible for arteriosclerosis, heart attacks, a variety of illnesses, but very few are aware of the ways that it is *essential* to health.

At least two-thirds of your body cholesterol is produced by the liver or in the intestine. It is found there as well as in the brain, the adrenals, and nerve fiber sheaths. And when it's good, it's very, very good:

• Cholesterol in the skin is converted to essential vitamin D when touched by the sun's ultraviolet rays.
• Cholesterol aids in the metabolism of carbohydrates. (The more carbohydrates ingested, the more cholesterol produced.)
• Cholesterol is a prime supplier of life-essential adrenal steroid hormones, such as cortisone.
• Cholesterol is a component of every membrane and necessary for the production of male and female sex hormones.

Differences in the behavior of cholesterol depend upon the protein to which it is bound. Lipoproteins are the factors in our blood which transport cholesterol.

Low-density lipoproteins (LDL) carry about 65 percent of blood cholesterol and are the bad guys who deposit it in the

arteries where, joined by other substances, it becomes artery-
blocking plaque.

Very-low density lipoproteins (VLDL) carry only about 15
percent of blood cholesterol but are the substances the liver
needs and uses to produce LDL. The more of them, the more
LDL the liver sends out and the greater your chance of heart
disease.

High-density lipoproteins (HDL) carry about 20 percent of
blood cholesterol and, composed principally of lecithin, are
the good guys whose detergent action breaks up plaque and
can transport cholesterol through the blood without clogging
arteries. (A recent study found that people with big hips and
trim waists have higher HDL cholesterol levels than do those
with potbellies, which might explain why females, on the
average, live eight years longer than males.)

In short: the higher your HDL the lower your chances of
developing heart disease.

> Eggs might not be as bad
> as you thought

It is also worth mentioning that though the egg consumption
in the United States is one-half of what it was in 1945, there
has *not* been a comparable decline in heart disease. And
though the American Heart Association deems eggs hazardous, a diet without them can be equally hazardous. Not only
do eggs have the most perfect protein components of any
food, but they contain lecithin, which aids in fat assimilation.
And, most important, they *raise* HDL levels!

87. Leveling About Cholesterol Levels

When people talk about their "cholesterol levels," they're
referring to the total amount of cholesterol in their blood
(serum cholesterol). The amounts are measured in milligrams
per deciliter; the accepted levels—for *everyone*—should not
exceed 200 mg/dl.

The ratio of HDL (good cholesterol) to LDL (bad cholesterol) is as important as the ratio of HDL to your total cho-

lesterol level. The more HDL you have, therefore, the more protection you have against clogged arteries.

Blood cholesterol tests will usually also measure your levels of *triglycerides*. These fats differ from cholesterol, but there is a connection between them; although you can have high triglyceride levels without high cholesterol (and vice versa), lowering triglyceride levels does seem to help bring down cholesterol.

Keeping your daily fat intake to no more than 30 percent (and preferably 20 percent) of total calories consumed is vital to leveling off elevated cholesterol levels. And no more than 10 percent of that fat should be saturated.

88. Saturated Fat Vs. Unsaturated Fat

Saturated fat comes from animal sources (with a few exceptions, notably coconut and palm oils, and hydrogenated or partially hydrogenated vegetable oils) and *all* animal fats contain cholesterol.

Unsaturated fat (be it mono- or polyunsaturated) comes from vegetable sources—and *no* vegetables or fruits contain cholesterol.

BUT, and this is a big "but," even if foods don't contain cholesterol, that doesn't mean they don't contain fat. Avocados, for instance, are free of cholesterol, but just one used for guacamole will give you more than 30 grams of fat!

89. Foods and Nutrients That Can Lower Your Cholesterol Naturally

- Activated charcoal
- Barley
- Carrots
- Chromium
- Corn bran
- Cruciferous vegetables (broccoli, cauliflower)
- Eggplant
- Evening Primrose Oil
- Fenugreek Seed

- Fiber
- Fish Oils: EPA and DHA (Omega 3 Fatty acids)
- Garlic
- Ginger
- Guar Gum
- Lemon Grass Oil
- Lentils: Pinto beans, Lima beans, Navy beans, Kidney beans
- Monosaturated oils (olive, peanut, canola)
- Niacin
- Oat bran
- Onions
- Pectin (Apples, grapefruit)
- Phytosterols: Beta Sitosterol, Stigmasterol, Campesterol
- Polyunsaturated oils (sunflower, corn, safflower)
- Psyllium husk
- Raw carrots
- Red pepper
- Rice bran
- Soy beans
- Vitamin C
- Vitamin E
- Yogurt

90. Do You Know What's Raising Your Cholesterol?

Many things that you might not be aware of can be raising your cholesterol levels or undermining your efforts to lower them. Here are a few you should think about:

- Smoking
- Caffeine
- Stress
- The pill
- Refined sugar
- Food additives
- Environmental pollutants

If you're watching your cholesterol, you probably know

that turkey is a good dinner choice. Just remember that although three ounces of light-meat turkey has only about 67 mg. of cholesterol, the same amount of dark meat has 75 mg. And a cup of chopped turkey liver has about 830 mg.!

91. Any Questions About Chapter VI?

I'd like to know if there is any difference in being "hyperlipidemic" and "hypercholesterolemic?"

There is, but unfortunately, not much when it comes to being a candidate for coronary heart disease. A person who is "hyperlipidemic" has elevated fats in general in the blood and someone who is "hypercholesterolemic" just has elevated cholesterol levels. It's sort of a semantic moot point where health is concerned.

I'm confused. Some products say "low-fat" and some "low cholesterol." Is there a difference?

You bet there is! In fact, a product that's marked "cholesterol-free" can be loaded with fat! You have to understand that cholesterol and fat are not synonymous. Unlike fat, cholesterol is not used for energy; it's used primarily to transport fat to cells through the body.

What's the difference, as far as lowering cholesterol is concerned, between polyunsaturated and monounsaturated oils?

Polyunsaturated oils (sunflower, corn, safflower, soy) lower both the bad and the good (LDL and HDL) cholesterol. Monounsaturated oils (olive, peanut, canola), on the other hand, not only reduce the bad cholesterol, but raise the good (HDL) levels. Most medical authorities, though, according to Robert E. Kowalski, author of *The 8-Week Cholesterol Cure*, are not ready to commit on which is better and suggest using both.

I've heard that polyunsaturated oils, which I use frequently, can cause cancer. Is there any truth to this?

Perhaps. Studies have found that large amounts of "processed" polyunsaturates in the diet can increase the formation of carcinogens. This seems to happen when vegetable oils are "hydrogenated" to make them into solid shortenings— a process that, in effect, turns unsaturated fats into saturated ones. I'd suggest you supplement your diet with vitamin E (200–400 IU daily) to help prevent lipid peroxidation (fats "rusting" in the body); avoid products containing "hydrogenated" oils; increase your intake of cruciferous vegetables; and alternate your polyunsaturated oils with monounsaturated ones.

Are lipotropics available as supplements, and if so, what's the recommended dosage and are there any special instructions for taking them?

Lipotropics are available as supplements in tablet form. (Usually 3 tablets equal 1,000 mg.—or 1 gram of each lipotropic agent.) The dosage most often recommended is 1–2 tablets taken 3 times daily, *with* food.

Do you consider lipotropic supplements more important for some people than others?

Definitely, especially meat eaters. Lipotropics are the substances which can liquify or homogenize fats. I feel that supplementation is particularly important for anyone on a high-protein diet, the reason being that lipotropics detoxify amines, which are by-products of protein metabolism. Also, anyone worried about gallstone formation would be wise to consider these supplements.

Can you explain, simply, what omega-3 fatty acids are and what they can do for me?

Simply, omega-3 fatty acids are a unique component of fish and fish oils, EPA and DHA (eicosapentaenoic and docosahexaenoic acid) and there are many things that they've been found to do. As for what they can do for you, take your pick. They can:

- help retard atherosclerosis.
- lower LDL cholesterol and triglycerides.
- reduce blood viscosity and help prevent heart attacks and strokes.
- lower blood pressure.
- enhance the immune system.
- alleviate rheumatoid arthritis.
- help protect the body from lupus erythematosus.
- offer protection against migraines and kidney disease.

If you're a vegetarian, omega-3 fatty acids can also be found in vegetable oils such as soybean, canola and flaxseed—but the conversion to EPA and DHA is much slower.

What's the difference between omega-3 and omega-6 fatty acids on a cholesterol-lowering regimen?

Only the omega-3 fatty acids lower triglycerides as well as cholesterol.

I've been using margarine for years because I was told to stay away from saturated fat. Now, I hear that margarine can be worse for me than butter. Is this true?

Not exactly. Let me put it this way: margarine isn't worse for you than butter—but it isn't much better. We all know that saturated fats give an unhealthy boost to cholesterol levels and unsaturated fats don't. But recent studies have shown that when unsaturated fats are "hydrogenated" (a process which solidifies them so they resemble butter at room temperature) they not only continue to raise cholesterol levels, they do something that saturated fats don't—they *lower* the levels of the body's HDL (good cholesterol)!

What's the skinny on these new fake fats?

Pretty thin. The synthetic fat called sucrose polyester (SPE) was designed so that it couldn't be broken down by our body's enzymes and would, therefore, not be absorbed by the body. Great in theory, but this faux oil has not yet been shown to be completely free of side effects and is currently being used in conjunction with other vegetable oils. Admittedly, this does reduce the total grams of fat, but until long-term safety is assured, I'd recommend lowering your fat intake the old-fashioned way—by cutting back on products that contain it.

As for fake fats such as "Simpless," which is a milk and egg white fat substitute used primarily in low calorie frozen desserts, the problem is that it is unstable in heat and, at least at this time, cannot be used in cooked products. Considering most of our fats come from cooked foods, the percentage of fat saved by eating products with this type of fake fat is *not* impressive. What's worse is that these fake fats can lull you into a false sense of low-fat security and get you to indulge in products you ordinarily wouldn't eat—and they don't get you to change your basic fat-eating patterns at all!

VII

Carbohydrates and Enzymes

92. Why Carbohydrates Are Necessary

Carbohydrates, the scourge of misinformed dieters, are the main suppliers of our body's energy. During digestion, starches and sugars, the principal kinds of carbohydrates, are broken down into glucose, better known as blood sugar. This blood sugar provides the essential energy for our brain and central nervous system.

You need carbohydrates in your daily diet so that vital tissue-building protein is not wasted for energy when it might be needed for repair.

> They have the same calories
> as protein.

If you eat too many carbohydrates, more than can be converted into glucose or glycogen (which is stored in liver and muscles), the result, as we know all too well, is fat. When the body needs more fuel, the fat is converted back to glucose and you lose weight.

Don't be too down on carbohydrates. They're as important for good health as other nutrients—and gram for gram they have the same 4 calories as protein. Though no official requirement exists, a minimum of 50 g. daily is recommended to avoid ketosis, an acid condition of the blood that can happen when your own fat is used primarily for energy.

93. The Truth About Enzymes

Enzymes are necessary for the digestion of food, releasing valuable vitamins, minerals, and amino acids which keep us alive and healthy.

Enzymes are catalysts, meaning they have the power to cause an internal action without themselves being changed or destroyed in the process.

Enzymes are destroyed under certain heat conditions.

Enzymes are best obtained from uncooked or unprocessed fruits, vegetables, eggs, meats, and fish.

Each enzyme acts upon a specific food; one cannot substitute for the other. A deficiency, shortage, or even the absence of one single enzyme can mean the difference between sickness and health.

Enzymes that end in -*ase* are named by the food substance they act upon. For example, with phosphorus the enzyme is called phosphatase; with sugar (sucrose) it is known as sucrase.

Pepsin is a vital digestive enzyme that breaks up the proteins of ingested food, splitting them into usable amino acids. Without pepsin, protein could not be used to build healthy skin, strong skeletal structure, rich blood supply, and strong muscles.

Renin is a digestive enzyme which causes coagulation of milk, changing its protein, casein, into a usable form in the body. Renin releases the valuable minerals from milk, calcium, phosphorus, potassium, and iron that are used by the body to stabilize the water balance, strengthen the nervous system, and produce strong teeth and bones.

Lipase splits fat, which is then utilized to nourish the skin cells, protect the body against bruises and blows, and ward off the entrance of infectious virus cells and allergic conditions.

Hydrochloric acid in the stomach works on tough foods such as fibrous meats, vegetables, and poultry. It digests protein, calcium, and iron. Without HC1, problems such as pernicious anemia, gastric carcinoma, congenital achlorhydria, and allergies can develop. Because stress, tension, anger, and anxiety before eating, as well as deficiencies of some vitamins (B complex primarily) and minerals, can all cause a lack of HC1, more of us are short of it than realize it. If you think that you have an overacid problem or heartburn, for which you are dosing yourself with an antacid such as Maalox, Di-Gel, Tums, Rolaids, or Alka-Seltzer, you are probably unaware that *the symptoms of having too little acid are exactly the same as having too much*, in which case the taking of antacids could be the worst possible thing for you to do.

Dr. Alan Nittler, author of *A New Breed of Doctor*, has stated emphatically that everyone over the age of forty should be using a HC1 supplement.

Betaine HC1 and glutamic acid HC1 are the best forms of commercially available hydrochloric acid.

CAUTION: If you have an ulcer condition, consult your doctor before using these supplements.

94. The Twelve Tissue Salts and Their Functions

Tissue salts are inorganic mineral components of your body's tissues. They are also known as Schuessler biochemical cell salts, after Dr. W. H. Schuessler, who isolated them in the late nineteenth century. Dr. Schuessler found that if the body was deficient in any of these salts, illness occurred, and that if the deficiency was corrected, the body could heal itself. In other words, tissue salts are *not a cure*, but merely a remedy.

The twelve tissue salts are:

Fluoride of lime (calc. flour.)—Part of all the connective tissues in your body. An imbalance can be the cause of varicose veins, late dentition, muscle tendon strain, carbuncles, and cracked skin.

Phosphate of lime (calc. phos.)—Found in all your body's cells and fluids, an important element in gastric juices as well as bones and teeth. An imbalance or deficiency can be the cause of cold hands and feet, numbness, hydrocele, sore breasts, and night sweats.

Sulfate of lime (calc. sulf.)—A constituent of all connective tissue in minute particles, as well as in the cells of the liver. An imbalance or deficiency can be the cause of skin eruptions, deep abscesses, or chronic oozing ulcers.

Phosphate of iron (ferr. phos.)—Part of your blood and other body cells, with the exception of nerves. An imbalance or deficiency can be the cause of continuous diarrhea or, paradoxically, constipation. It has also been used as a remedy for nosebleeds and excessive menses.

Chloride of potash (kali. mur.)—Found in lining and under the surface body cells. An imbalance or deficiency can be the cause of granulation of the eyelids, blistering eczema, and warts.

Sulfate of potash (kali. Sulf.)—The cells that form your skin and internal organ linings interact with this salt. An imbalance or deficiency can be the cause of skin eruptions, a yellow coating on the back of the tongue, feelings of heaviness, and pains in the limbs.

Potassium phosphate (kali. phos.)—Found in all your body tissues, particularly nerve, brain, and blood cells. An imbalance or deficiency can be the cause of improper fat digestion, poor memory, anxiety, insomnia, and a faint, rapid pulse.

Phosphate of magnesia (mag. phos.)—Another mineral element of bones, teeth, brain, nerves, blood, and muscle cells. An imbalance or deficiency can be the cause of cramps, neuralgia, shooting pains, and colic.

Chloride of soda (nat. mur.)—Regulates the amount of moisture in the body and carries moisture to cells. An imbalance or deficiency can be the cause of salt cravings, hay fever, watery discharges from eyes and nose.

Phosphate of soda (nat. phos.)—Emulsifies fatty acids and keeps uric acid soluble in the blood. An imbalance or deficiency can be the cause of jaundice, sour breath, an acid or coppery taste in the mouth.

Sulfate of soda (nat. sulf.)—A slight irritant to tissues and functions as a stimulant for natural secretions. An imbalance or deficiency can be the cause of low fevers, edema, depression, and gallbladder disorders.

Silicic acid (silicea)—Part of all connective tissue cells, as well as those of the hair, nails, and skin. A deficiency or imbalance can be the cause of poor memory, carbuncles, falling hair, and ribbed, ingrowing nails. Eating whole-grain products should supply the normal need for this tissue salt.

95. Any Questions About Chapter VII?

My father-in-law suffers terribly from heartburn and takes Maalox so often that it's virtually his dessert after meals. Isn't there some natural alternative?

There sure is, and it tastes a lot better than any chalky liquid. Chewable papaya enzyme tablets, made from nature's "magic melon" fruit, can actually digest 2,230 times their weight of starch. They do this because they contain pepsin and prolase, enzymes which assist in protein digestion and combine with mylase, a potent starch digestive enzyme. (Papain, by the way, is the chief ingredient in meat tenderizers, which work on foods before they even reach your stomach.) The U.S. Department of Agriculture has attested to the fact that papaya contains valuable digestive properties, so your father-in-law would be well-advised (and probably a lot happier) to take one or two of these pleasant-tasting natural tablets after his meals.

I'm on a diet. Am I better off eating pasta or steak?

You're better off eating pasta. Carbohydrates, though they
have the same caloric value as protein, are less fattening than
fat (which steak has a lot of). It works this way: in order to
convert 100 calories of carbohydrates, you use up 25 calories;
in order to convert 100 calories of fat, you use up only 3
calories.

VIII

Other Wonder Workers

96. Acidophilus

Lactobacilus acidophilus, or acidophilus, as it is commonly known, is a source of friendly intestinal bacteria and more effective than yogurt. It is available as acidophilus culture, incubated in soy, milk, or yeast bases.

> Regular use of acidophilus keeps
> the intestines clean.

Many doctors prescribe acidophilus in conjunction with oral antibiotic treatment because antibiotics destroy beneficial intestinal flora, often causing diarrhea as well as an overgrowth of the fungus monilia abricans. This fungus can grow in the intestines, vagina, lungs, mouth (thrush), on the fingers, or under the nails. It will usually disappear after a few days use of generous amounts of acidophilus culture.

Regular use of acidophilus culture keeps the intestines clean. It can eliminate bad breath caused by intestinal putrefaction (the sort resistant to mouthwash or breath spray), constipation, foul-smelling flatulence, and aid in the treatment of acne and other skin problems.

Keep in mind that lactose, complex carbohydrates, pectin, and vitamin C plus roughage encourage additional growth of intestinal flora. This is important since friendly bacteria can

die within five days unless they are continuously supplied
with some form of lactic acid or lactose.

97. Ginseng

It is generally well-accepted that ginseng is a stimulant of
both mental and physical energy. The Chinese have been
using it for nearly five thousand years and still revere it as a
preventive and cure-all. It is a mild laxative and helps the
body pass poisons through more rapidly. Its reputed benefits
include cures for impotence, high and low blood pressure,
anemia, arthritis, indigestion, insomnia, fatigue, hypoglycemia, poor circulation, and more.

Miracles aside, ginseng does help you assimilate vitamins
and minerals by acting as an endocrine-gland stimulant. It is
best to take it on an empty stomach, preferably before breakfast, if you want it to be its most effective.

Vitamin C has been said to neutralize part of ginseng's
value, but there is no real evidence to support this. (If you
take a vitamin-C supplement, the time-release form makes
any counteraction less likely.)

Ginseng is available in capsule form, under names such as
Siberian ginseng, Korean and American ginseng, in 500-mg.
to 650-mg. (10-grain) doses. It can also be purchased as tea,
liquid concentrate, or as ginseng root in a bottle. It is now
considered a class A adaptogen (a non-toxic substance which
increases the resistance of an organism to a wide variety of
stress factors, whether they be physical, chemical, or biological in nature).

98. Alfalfa, Garlic, Chlorophyll, and Yucca

> A natural diuretic

Alfalfa has been dubbed "the great healer" by noted biologist
and author Frank Bouer, who discovered that the green leaves
of this remarkable legume contain *eight* essential enzymes.

Also, for every 100 g., it contains 8,000 IU of vitamin A and 20,000 to 40,000 units of vitamin K, which protects against hemorrhaging and helps in blood-clotting. It is additionally a fine source of vitamins B6 and E, and contains enough vitamin D, lime, and phosphorus to secure strong bones and teeth in growing children.

Many doctors have used alfalfa in treating stomach ailments, gas pains, ulcerous conditions, and poor appetite, because it contains vitamin U, which is also found in raw cabbage and cabbage juice. The latter has frequently been used as an aid in treating peptic ulcers. Alfalfa is also a good laxative and a natural diuretic.

"Russian penicillin"

Garlic contains potassium, phosphorus, a significant amount of B and C vitamins, as well as calcium and protein. In Europe it is respected as a valuable medicine. The Soviets call it "Russian penicillin." In America it is virtually ignored.

Despite its small acceptance here, it does appear to have some amazing properties. Many medical authorities feel that it can reduce high blood pressure by either neutralizing the poisonous substances in the intestines or acting as a vasodilator. F.G. Piotrousky, of the University of Vienna, found that 40 percent of his hypertensive patients had substantially lower blood pressure after they were given garlic.

Garlic has also been found to be effective in lowering cholesterol and cleansing the blood of excess glucose. (Blood sugar ranks with cholesterol as a causative factor in arteriosclerosis and heart attacks.) In addition, it has also been reported to alleviate grippe, sore throat, and bronchial congestion.

The best way to take garlic as a supplement is in the form of aged odorless capsules. These caps contain the valuable garlic and leave no after-odor on the breath. Garlic tablets with parsley (which contains natural chlorophyll) are also available.

Chlorophyll, according to G.W. Rapp in the *American Jour-*

nal of Pharmacy, possesses positive antibacterial action. It also appears to act as a wound-healing agent, and, while stimulating the growth of new tissue, it reduces the hazard of bacterial contamination.

Nature's deodorant, it is used in commercial air fresheners, as a topical body deodorant, and as an oral breath refresher. It is available in tablets and in liquid preparations.

Yucca extract comes from the genus of trees and shrubs belonging to the Liliaceae family. (The Joshua tree is a yucca.) The Indians used the yucca for many purposes and revered it as a plant that guaranteed their health and survival. Dr. John W. Yale, a botanical biochemist, extracted the steroid saponin from the plant and used the extract in a tablet for the treatment of arthritis. The treatment proved safe and effective, the average dose being four tablets daily, and there was no gastrointestinal irritation. Yucca-extract tablets are nontoxic and available in most health-food and vitamin stores.

99. Fiber and Bran

When research appeared in the *Journal of the American Medical Association* indicating that we would all be a great deal healthier and live longer if we ate coarser diets that sent more indigestible dietary fiber through our digestive tracts, a lot of people, wisely, jumped on the fiber bandwagon, though most weren't aware (and still aren't) that all fiber is not the same and that different types perform different functions.

TYPES OF FIBER YOU SHOULD KNOW ABOUT

Cellulose This is found in whole-wheat flour, bran, cabbage, young peas, green beans, wax beans, broccoli, brussels sprouts, cucumber skins, peppers, apples, and carrots.

Hemicelluloses These are found in bran, cereals, whole grains, brussels sprouts, mustard greens, and beet root.

Cellulose and hemicelluloses absorb water and can smooth functioning of the large bowel. Essentially, they "bulk" waste and move it through the colon more rapidly. This not only can prevent constipation, but may also protect against diverticulosis, spastic colon, hemorrhoids, cancer of the colon, and varicose veins.

CAUTION: Increased fiber is contraindicated in certain bowel disorders. A physician should be consulted before starting any high-fiber diet.

   Gums These are usually found in oatmeal and other rolled oat products as well as in dried beans.
   Pectin This is found in apples, citrus fruits, carrots, cauliflower, cabbage, dried peas, green beans, potatoes, squash, and strawberries.

Gums and pectin primarily influence absorption in the stomach and small bowel. By binding with bile acids, they decrease fat absorption and lower cholesterol levels. They delay stomach-emptying by coating the lining of the gut, and by so doing they slow sugar absorption after a meal, which is helpful to diabetics since it reduces the amount of insulin needed at any one time.

CAUTION: Gums and pectin can interfere with the effectiveness of certain anti-fungal medications containing *griseofulvin*, such as Grifulvin V, Grisactin and Fulvicin.

   Lignin This type of fiber is found in breakfast cereals, bran, older vegetables (when vegetables age, their lignin content rises, and they become less digestible), eggplant, green beans, strawberries, pears, and radishes.

Lignin reduces the digestibility of other fibers. It also binds with bile acids to lower cholesterol and helps speed food through the gut.

CAUTION: While it's true that most of us still don't have enough fiber in our diet, too much can cause gas, bloating, nausea, vomiting, diarrhea, and possibly interfere with your body's ability to absorb certain minerals, such as zinc, calcium, iron, magnesium, and vitamin B12, though this is easily prevented by varying your diet along with your high-fiber foods.

100. Kelp

This amazing seaweed contains more vitamins and minerals than any other food. To be more specific, kelp has vitamin B2, niacin, choline, carotin, and algenic acid, as well as twenty-three minerals which range as follows:

Iodine	0.15–0.20%	Magnesium	0.76%
Calcium	1.20%	Sulfur	0.93%
Phosphorus	0.30%	Chlorine	12.21%
Iron	0.10%	Copper	0.0008%
Sodium	3.14%	Zinc	0.0003%
Potassium	0.63%	Manganese	0.0008%

Plus traces of: barium, boron, chromium, lithium, nickel, silver, titanium, vanadium, aluminum, strontium, and silicon.

Because of its natural iodine content, kelp has a normalizing effect on the thyroid gland. In other words, thin people with thyroid trouble can gain weight by using kelp, and obese people can lose weight with it.

Homeopathic physicians use kelp for obesity, poor digestion, flatulence, and obstinate constipation; and, for the past several years, one of the most widespread fads has been the kelp, lecithin, vinegar, and B6 diet. (See section 260.)

101. Yeast

> One of the richest sources of
> organic iron

It's known as nature's wonder food, and it does a lot to deserve its reputation. Yeast is an excellent source of protein and a superior source of the natural B-complex vitamins. It is one of the richest sources of organic iron and a gold mine of minerals, trace minerals, and amino acids. It has been known to help lower cholesterol (when combined with lecithin), help reverse gout, and ease the aches and pains of neuritis.

There are various sources of yeast:

Brewer's yeast (from hops, a by-product of beer), sometimes called nutritional yeast.

Torula yeast grown on wood pulp used in the manufacture of paper. Or from blackstrap molasses.

Whey, a by-product of milk and cheese (best-tasting and most potent nonyeast product).

Liquid yeast from Switzerland and Germany, fed on herbs, honey malt, and oranges or grapefruit.

Avoid live baker's yeast! Live yeast cells deplete the B vitamins in the intestines and rob your body of all vitamins. In nutritional yeast, these live cells are heat-killed, thus preventing that depletion.

Yeast has all the major B vitamins (except B12), which can be especially bred into it. It contains sixteen amino acids, fourteen or more minerals, and seventeen vitamins (except for A, E, and C). It can be considered a whole food.

Because yeast, like other protein foods, is high in phosphorus, it is advisable when taking it to add extra calcium to the diet. Phosphorus, though a coworker of calcium, can take calcium out of the body, leaving a deficiency. The remedy is simple: increase your calcium (calcium lactate assimilates well in the body). *B-complex vitamins should be taken together with yeast to be more effective. Together they work like a powerhouse.*

Yeast can be stirred into liquid, juice, or water and taken between meals. Many people who feel fatigued take a tablespoon or more in liquid and feel a return of energy within minutes, and the good effects last for several hours. Yeast can also be used as a reducing food. Stir into liquid and drink just before a meal. It takes the edge off a large appetite and saves you a lot in calories.

102. Any Questions About Chapter VIII?

What's the scoop on spirulina? Is it some sort of wonder drug?

It's not a drug at all. Spirulina is a natural, easily assimilated complete protein. (It's known as spirulina plankton or blue green algae.) It's nature's highest source of chlorophyll pigment, rich in such chelated minerals as iron, calcium, zinc, potassium, and magnesium, a fine source of vitamin A and B-complex vitamins, and it contains phenylalanine, which acts on the brain's appetite center to decrease hunger pangs —while also keeping your blood sugar at the proper level.

And if you'd like to slim down, this is a wonderful aid for weight reduction. Take three 500 mg. tablets ½ hour before meals. Once the dosage begins to work, decrease to two or one tablet before meals.

Are there any new "wonder workers" available as supplements that haven't been publicized?

Yes, there are. And my pick for the most impressive among them is shark cartilage. It's now available as a food supplement in powdered capsules and oils and, aside from exhibiting no adverse side effects, it's been found to boost the immune system (and is currently being investigated as a preventive for AIDS). It's also been shown to provide immunity to carcinogens, help prevent osteoarthritis, inflammation, scleroderma—and last, but far from least, this anti-tumor substance has also been found to enhance sexuality!

What is the recommended daily amount of fiber?

The recommended intake of fiber for adults is 30 grams a day. (The National Cancer Institute suggests 35 grams.) Although fiber, which comes mainly from plant foods, does not itself provide nutrients, it does affect the way our bodies absorb them. And, as far as helping to prevent a wide variety of diseases goes, every gram counts!

CAUTION: When reaching for that high-fiber cereal, be sure to check the fat content. Many cereals high in fiber are also high in fat. Being nutritionally forewarned helps being nutritionally forearmed!

I've been told about an algae (not spirulina) that's supposed to have amazing health and healing properties. Have you heard of it and can you tell me what it is?

I have, and it's "chlorella." Chlorella (the emerald algae) has been touted as the perfect whole food. Aside from being a complete protein and containing all the B vitamins, vitamin C, vitamin E and the major minerals (with zinc and iron in amounts large enough to be considered supplementary), it has been found to improve the immune system, improve digestion, detoxify the body, accelerate healing, protect against radiation, aid in the prevention of degenerative diseases, help in treatment of *candida albicans*, relieve arthritis pain and, because of its nutritional content, aid in the success of numerous weight loss programs.

It is available in tablets, powder and water soluble extracts (which contain the highest concentrations of Chlorella Growth Factor [CGF]). Be aware, though, that although chlorella products are widely available, they differ depending on the particular strain of chlorella used.

The average dosage is: 5–8 tablets 3 times daily. I'd suggest starting with only 1 tablet 3 times daily and working up, just to make sure you have no allergic reactions. Possible adverse reactions include: gas, bloating, bowel irregularity, nausea, green stools and mild skin breakouts or eczema. (These reactions, unless severe, are not unusual and should clear up in a few days. If not, discontinue supplementation and consult a nutritionally oriented doctor. See section 293.)

Dr. David Steenblock, author of *Chlorella, Natural Medicinal Algae*, has found that for detoxification purposes, chlorella is best taken on an empty stomach; however, because it is a food, it can also be taken with other foods as well as medications.

A lot of the guys who work out at my gym have mentioned "cytochrome C." Can you tell me about it?

With pleasure. This simple compound of amino acids and iron has become known as one of the foremost aerobic energy enhancers. It increases muscle performance, acts as a carrier of oxygen to the mitochondria (the cell powerhouse of skeletal muscle), and is an essential part of the metabolic process that makes prolonged exercise possible. In actively working muscles, the aerobic process of energy production is dependent on cytochromes. If this system becomes ineffective, the muscle cell metabolism switches to an alternate aerobic pathway that produces lactic acid. As the lactic acid builds, muscle fatigue ensues and thus reduces working endurance.

Cytochrome C is available in supplement form and highly recommended if you want to get the best results from any aerobic exercise.

I know that bran is good for me. I just don't know which bran is best.

It depends on what you're looking for nutritionally. The following bran name guide may help:

Barley bran is high in soluble fiber and helpful in lowering cholesterol.

Corn bran is high in insoluble fiber and may be helpful in reducing the risk of colon cancer.

Oat bran is high in soluble fiber and helpful in lowering cholesterol. (In fact, studies have shown that just 2 ounces daily can help reduce cholesterol levels by 7 to 10 percent!)

Rice bran is high in soluble fiber and may be helpful in lowering cholesterol. (It's similar to oat bran in nutritional benefits, but less of it is needed to produce the same results.

Two tablespoons rice bran will give you as much soluble fiber as one half cup oat bran.)

Wheat bran is high in insoluble fiber and may be helpful in reducing the risk of colon cancer.

For natural sources of these types of fiber—and cautions—see section 99.

IX

Herbs and Folk Remedies

103. What You Should Know About Natural Remedies

Just because herbs are natural doesn't mean that they can be used indiscriminately. Before trying any herbal remedy, be sure you know what it does, how to prepare and use it—and what cautions or side effects you should be aware of.

> Never try any natural or herbal remedy
> without knowing what it does, how it should
> be prepared and taken, what cautions should
> be observed, and what its possible side effects
> could be!

As a rule, few medical problems occur from ingesting herbal remedies, but the potential for an allergic or toxic response is always there.

IMPORTANT: If you are now taking any drugs, or have any medical problems it's wise to consult a nutritionally oriented physician who is aware of herb-drug interactions, as well as any potentially dangerous side effects.

104. Basil

Sweet basil is a plant that can be used as a poultice to draw poison from the skin. It's frequently used to alleviate bee stings and to draw underskin pimples to a head.

105. Echinacea

This herb has been found to help protect healthy cells from viral and bacterial attack by stimulating activity of the immune system in general and T-cells—which attack pathogens and toxins—in particular.

106. Saw-Palmetto (berries)

Saw-Palmetto berries are helpful in the treatment of chronic cystitis and in the prevention of genito-urinary tract infections.

107. Poke Weed

This is a root that's used primarily to treat arthritis pain. It's also an ingredient in creams that help fight fungal infections.

108. Aconite

Small amounts of a fluid extract of the root of this plant mixed in a cup of warm water have been reported to successfully reduce pain, fever, inflammation of the stomach, and heart palpitations.

CAUTION: This is one of the few herbs where misuse can cause a particularly dangerous side effect: heart failure.

109. Aloe Vera

The aloe vera plant contains a wound-healing substance called Aloe Vera Gel, a mixture of antibiotic, astringent, and co-agulating agents.

Taken internally, it works as a mild laxative. One table-spoon taken at regular intervals (preferably on an empty stomach) totaling a pint a day, can help in the treatment of stomach ulcers.

External uses of Aloe Vera Gel are many:

• It acts as an immediate and effective wound-healer, aiding in the treatment of burns, insect stings, and poison ivy. Split a leaf and apply pulp directly to the injured area, or soak cloth with Aloe Vera Gel and bind on.
• Aloe Vera Gel ointments, creams, and lotions can prevent blistering and peeling from sunburn.
• It can help soften corns and calluses on the feet.
• Applied to the face and throat, it can soften skin and hold aging lines in check.
• It can alleviate the pain and itching of hemorrhoids and bleeding piles.
• It can be used as an effective hair-conditioner.

CAUTION: As an ointment it can cause hives, rashes, itching and other allergic reactions in sensitive individuals—and can be extremely dangerous if taken internally by pregnant women.

110. Anise (seed)

This is a natural diuretic and gastric stimulant and is often used to relieve flatulence. It's also been used in home remedies as a treatment for dry cough.

111. Astragalus

This herb has been found to alleviate fatigue and lessen the frequency of colds. It's an immune system booster that improves resistance to viruses and bacterial infections and also accelerates healing. It works best with zinc and vitamins A and C.

112. Blessed Thistle

Often used as an appetite stimulant and in the treatment of digestive problems, it can reduce fevers and break up congestion.

CAUTION: In high doses, this can cause burns of the mouth and esophagus, as well as diarrhea.

113. Chamomile

This plant has antispasmodic and gastric-stimulant properties, and is usually taken internally for migraines, gastric cramps, and anxiety. Externally it's used as a treatment for wounds, skin ulcers, and conjunctivitis.

CAUTION: May cause severe allergic reactions—including fatal shock—in individuals with hay fever, or those sensitive to ragweed, asters, and related plants.

114. Comfrey

When used in teas, comfrey has been found to alleviate stomach ailments, coughs, diarrhea, arthritis pain, liver and gallbladder conditions.

CAUTION: A possible side effect of using this herb is that it can reduce your absorption of iron and vitamin B12.

115. Juniper (berries)

These are often used as a stomach tonic, can act as appetite and digestion enhancers, as well as a diuretic and a disinfectant of the urinary tract.

CAUTION: Excessive ingestion of the berries, or beverages and tonics containing them, can cause hallucinations.

116. Licorice

An effective restorer of membrane and tissue function, it is also a hormone balancer, an intestinal secretion stimulant, a respiratory stimulant, and a laxative.

CAUTION: High blood pressure and cardiac arrhythmias are possible side effects of licorice. (American manufactured licorice, the sort used in candy, is a synthetic flavoring and does not have these potential side effects—of course, it also doesn't offer any of the benefits.)

117. Evening Primrose Oil

As a dietary supplement, Evening Primrose Oil can help lower blood cholesterol, lower blood pressure, help in weight reduction, relieve premenstrual pain, improve eczema, aid in the treatment of moderate cases of rheumatoid arthritis, slow progression of multiple sclerosis, help hyperactive children, improve acne (when taken with zinc), and help build stronger fingernails.

The active ingredient in Evening Primrose Oil is Gamma linolenic acid (GLA), which is needed for the body to produce hormonelike compounds called prostaglandins (PGs), vital for good health. In other words, a deficiency of the former can result in impaired production of the latter and adversely affect your physical well-being.

118. Parsley (seeds and leaves)

A diuretic and gastric stimulant, parsley is used medicinally to treat coughs, asthma, amorrhea, dysmenorrhea, and conjunctivitis.

119. Pennyroyal

This herb, often referred to as "lung mint," is used as an inhalant in treating colds; it's also used as a tea for curing headaches, menstrual cramps, and pain.

CAUTION: Pennyroyal can induce abortion and should therefore NEVER be used during pregnancy.

120. Peppermint (leaves)

An antispasmodic, tonic, and stimulant, peppermint has been used to treat nervousness, insomnia, cramps, dizziness, and coughs. (For headaches, you might want to try a strong cup of peppermint tea, then lie down for 15 to 20 minutes. It usually works as effectively as aspirin—and there are NO side effects.)

121. Rosemary (leaves)

Used externally in an ointment, these can soothe rheumatism aches, sprains, wounds, bruises, and eczema. Taken internally, in the proper preparation, rosemary can relieve flatulence, colic, and stimulate bile release from the gallbladder.

CAUTION: Rosemary can be toxic in large quantities.

122. Thyme

A natural antiseptic deodorant, thyme—applied externally in compresses—can be an effective liniment for wounds; internally it can act as an antidiarrhetic, relieve gastritis cramps, as well as soothe bronchitis and laryngitis.

123. Dangerous Herbs

The following herbs can be hazardous to your health and should not be brewed in teas or used in other fashion because of their potential toxicity.

NOTE: Since many herbs have several common names, the botanical name of the plant is given in italics.

ARNICA, WOLF'S BANE, LEOPARD'S BANE, MOUNTAIN TOBACCO (*ARNICA MONTANA*)
  Arnica is an irritant and can produce violent toxic gastroenteritis, intense muscular weakness, nervous disorders, and death.
BELLADONNA, DEADLY NIGHTSHADE (*ATROPA BELLADONNA*)
  Poisonous. Contains toxic alkaloids.
BITTERSWEET, DULCAMARA, WOODY or CLIMBING NIGHTSHADE (*SOLANUM DULCAMARA*)
  Poisonous.

BLOODROOT, SANGUINARIA, RED PUCCOON (*SAN-GUINARIS CANADENSIS*)
Contains the poisonous alkaloid sanguinarine, among others.

BROOM-TOPS, SCOPARIUS, SPARTIUM, IRISH BROOM, SCOTCH BROOM, BROOM (*CYTISUS SCO-PARIUS*)
Contains toxic sparteine and other harmful alkaloids.

AESCULUS, BUCKEYES, HORSE CHESTNUT (*AES-CULUS HIPPOCASTERANNUM*)
A poisonous plant which contains a toxic coumarin substance.

CALAMUS, SWEET FLAG, SWEET ROOT, SWEET CANE, SWEET CINNAMON (not to be confused with the bark used as a popular spice) (*ACORUS CALAMUS*)
Oil of Calamus is a carcinogen (a cancer-causing agent).

HELIOTROPE (*HELIOTROPIUM EUROPAEUM*)
This plant is poisonous and also contains alkaloids that cause liver damage. (It should not be confused with garden heliotrope, whose botanical name is *Valeriana officinalis*, and safe.)

HEMLOCK, CONIUM, SPOTTED HEMLOCK, SPOTTED PARSLEY, ST. BENNET'S HERB, SPOTTED COW-BANE, FOOL'S PARSLEY (*CONIUM MACULATUM*)
Contains poisonous alkaloids. It's often mistaken for water hemlock (*Cicuta maculata*) and hemlock spruce (*Tsuga canadensis*)

HENBANE, HYOSCYAMUS, HOG'S BEAN, POISON TOBACCO, DEVIL'S EYE (*HYOSCYAMUS NIGER*)
Poisonous. Contains dangerously toxic alkaloids.

JALAP ROOT, JALAP, TURE JALAP, VERA CRUZ JA-LAP, HIGH JOHN ROOT, JOHN CONQUEROR, ST. JOHN THE CONQUEROR ROOT (*EXAGONIUM PURGA, IPOMOEA JALAPA*, and *IPOMOEA PURGA*)
This is a twining Mexican vine known by many different names, but it can be extremely dangerous. The drug is a potent cathartic, and its extreme purgative action can result in life-threatening excessive bowel movements.

JIMSON WEED, DATURA, STRAMONIUM, APPLE OF PERU, JAMESTOWN WEED, THORNAPPLE, TOLGUACHA (*DATURA STRAMONIUM*)

This is a poisonous plant which contains stropine, hyoscyamine, and scopolamine, drugs that are illegal (for good reason) for nonprescription use.

LILY OF THE VALLEY, CONVALLARIA, MAY LILY (*CONVALLARIA MAJALIS*)

A poisonous plant which contains cardiac toxins.

LOBELIA, INDIAN TOBACCO, WILD TOBACCO, ASTHMA WEED, EMETIC WEED (*LOBELIA INFLATA*)

A poisonous plant that is often unwisely used as an emetic. Overdoses of extracts from the plant's leaves or fruit produce severe vomiting, sweating, paralysis, rapid but feeble pulse, and—more often than not—collapse, coma, and death.

MANDRAKE, MANDRAGORA, EUROPEAN MANDRAKE (*MANDRAGORA OFFICINARUM*)

A poisonous narcotic similar to belladonna.

MAY APPLE, MANDRAKE, PODOPHYLLUM, AMERICAN MANDRAKE, DEVIL'S APPLE, UMBRELLA PLANT, VEGETABLE CALOMEL, WILD LEMON, VEGETABLE MERCUTY (*PODOPHYLLUM PELATUM*)

A poisonous plant with complex toxic constituents.

MISTLETOE, VISCUM, AMERICAN MISTLETOE (*PHORADENDRON FLAVESCENS* and *VISCUM FLAVESCENS*)

Contains toxic amines. Consider it poisonous.

MISTLETOE, VISCUM, JUNIPER MISTLETOE (*PHORADENDRON JUNIPERINUM*)

This particular mistletoe may or may not be poisonous, but too little is known about it for any wise person to use it for anything but holding up at Christmas time and kissing beneath.

MISTLETOE, VISCUM, EUROPEAN MISTLETOE (*VISCUM ALBUM*)

This branch of mistletoe definitely contains toxic amines and is considered poisonous.

MORNING GLORY (*IPOMOEA PURPUREA*)

The seeds of this particular morning glory do contain amides of lysergic acid, but with a potency much less than that of LSD. Anyone planning to take a "trip" on them will be in for an unpleasant and potentially dangerous surprise, since the seeds also contain a very unhealthy purgative resin.

PERIWINKLE, VINCA, GREATER PERIWINKLE, LESSER PERIWINKLE (*VINCA MAJOR* and *VINCA MINOR*)

Keep these in your garden and out of your system. They contain toxic alkaloids that can cause adverse neurological actions and injure the liver and kidneys.

SASSAFRAS

A "blood purifier" that's carcinogenic and can damage the liver.

SPINDLE-TREE (*EUONYMUS EUROPAEUS*)

An extremely violent purgative.

TONKA BEAN, TONCO BEAN, TONQUIN BEAN (*DIPTERYX ODORATA, COUMAROUNA ODORATA, DIPTERYX OPPOSITIFOLIA*, and *COUMAROUNA OPPOSITIFOLIA*)

The active constituent of these seeds is coumarin, which the FDA has prohibited marketing as a food or food additive, after having been found to cause extensive liver damage, growth retardation, and testicular atrophy when used in the diet of experimental animals. (Check the labels on your OTC medicines!)

WAHOO BARK, EUONYMUS, BURNING BUSH (*EUONYMUS ATROPURPUREUS*)

Often used as a laxative, but though its poisonous qualities have not been thoroughly identified, it's best to play it safe and keep away from it.

WHITE SNAKEROOT, SNAKEROOT, RICHWEED (*EUPATORIUM RUGOSUM, E. OGERATOIDES*, and *E. URTICAEFOLIUM*)

This poisonous plant contains a toxic, unsaturated alcohol. It causes "trembles" in livestock and can engender milk sickness in humans who ingest milk, butter, and possibly meat from animals who have eaten this plant.

WORMWOOD, ABSINTHIUM, ABSINTH, MADDER-WORT, WERMUTH, MUGWORT, MINGWORT, WARMOT, MAGENKRAUT, HERBA ABSINTHII, (*ARTEMISIA ABSINTHIUM*)

Oil of wormwood is an active narcotic poison. It is used to flavor an alcoholic liqueur—*absinthe*—which is now illegal in America because its use can damage the nervous system.

YOHIMBE (*CORYNANTHE YOHIMBI* and *PAUSINYS-TALIA YOHIMBE*)

Not an herb to play around with. It contains the toxic alkaloid yohimbine.

124. Any Questions About Chapter IX?

Does dill have any nutritive or health-giving properties?

It does indeed. It can improve appetite and digestion and also act as a diuretic. Furthermore, chewing the seeds can help eliminate bad breath.

Is it true that flaxseed is a laxative?

It can act as one. The seeds are bulk formers. Flaxseed can be eaten raw or cooked (it's great in soups), and one tablespoon daily has been found to prevent constipation in adults. Flaxseed oil is also one of the richest sources of omega-3 fatty acids, helpful in reducing cholesterol and alleviating arthritis pain.

Are there any herbs that are okay under ordinary circumstances, but might be contraindicated during pregnancy or for breast-feeding?

Well, for one, goldenseal should be avoided during pregnancy and lactation. (Berberine, the alkaloid in goldenseal, is quite similar to morphine.) Also to be avoided are caffeine-containing herbs, such as guarans and kola nuts.

Laxatives, be they natural or manufactured, should not be taken during the first few months of pregnancy, as they could cause miscarriage. (Buckthorn, rhubarb, and senna are natural laxatives.) Strong sedative herbs like skullcap and valerian are not advisable, nor are strong spices such as capsicum and horseradish. Emetics, such as lobelia, can be dangerous early in pregnancy and in the last trimester.

Though garlic and onions are great for many things, it might be wise to avoid them if you're either pregnant or nursing, especially during the latter, as they have been known to pass through the breast milk and produce colic in infants.

My husband has liver problems and hates doctors. I've been told about a plant extract called "milk thistle." Can you tell me something about it?

I can tell you that the fruit of milk thistle contains silymarin, which is one of the most potent liver-protecting substances, and that silymarin has been shown to help in the treatment of chronic hepatitis, cirrhosis, and a variety of other liver diseases.

I can also tell you that some of the extracts are based in alcohol and *should be avoided by anyone with liver problems*.

The standard dose, according to Michael T. Murray, author of *PSA Textbook of Natural Medicine* and *The 21st Century Herbal*, is 70–150 mg. three times a day. But before your husband starts a regimen using silymarin, he should definitely consult a nutritionally oriented doctor (see section 293).

What are "adaptogens?" And are they available as supplements?

Adaptogens are a rare group of plants that seem to be able to use their properties within the body—where the body actually needs them—to help protect it from physical, emotional and environmental stresses (including radiation and chemical poisons).

Among other reported benefits of adaptogens are: increased immunity defenses; enhanced energy; accelerated healing from respiratory infections; improved nerve functions; blood-pressure and blood-sugar normalizing effects.

One of the most highly touted for its health benefits is Suma (*Pfaffia paniculata martius kuntze*), often called "Brazilian ginseng."

Although unrelated to ginseng, Suma (a member of the amaranth family) has been found to contain numerous vitamins, minerals, amino acids and other healing elements, including germanium (an immune cell activator), allantoin (a wound healer) and sitosterol and stigmasterol (two vegetable hormones that have been found to reduce blood cholesterol and increase—when needed—the body's natural estrogen.)

Supplements are available in pill form and as teas.

What is "germanium"? Is it an herb or a mineral—and what are its natural sources?

Germanium is what is known as a trace element (Ge-132). According to Dr. Parris M. Kidd, director of the Germanium Institute of North America, it has the ability to restore and stimulate immune function, supplement tissue oxygen (important for diets high in unsaturated fats, which—although cholesterol-lowering—deplete oxygen), help inhibit tumor development and alleviate major diseases.

It is found in trace amounts in garlic, ginseng, sushi, chlorella, pearl barley, and comfrey.

My niece is very much into alternative healing therapies, and she suggests I take an herb called Dong Quai for my hot flashes, as opposed to a drug. I know nothing about Dong Quai. What do you think?

I think Dong Quai (*Angelica sinensis*) is a terrific herb and has been shown to be quite effective in alleviating menopausal hot flashes, as well as vaginal dryness and depression. It potentiates the effectiveness of female (as well as male) sex hormones, and helps the body to maximize utilization of existing hormones. For instance, during menopause, it assists the transition of estrogen production from the ovaries to the adrenal glands.

As to whether it would be better for you than a drug, I suggest you consult with your doctor or a nutritionally oriented physician (see section 293). If you do decide to use it, be aware that it works best in combination with vitamins E, B6, and zinc.

What can you tell me about an herb called Pau D'Arco?

I can tell you that I think its uses in alternative therapies are just beginning. Pau D'Arco (Tabebuia impetiginosa) has been found to be quite effective in inhibiting the growth of Candida Albicans (see section 217). It is also effective in treating allergies where symptoms of bronchial asthma, eczema and sinus congestion exist. And, last but far from least, it is systemically helpful after long-term antibiotic therapy, immunosuppressant therapy and steroidal anti-inflammatory therapy.

For best results, Pau D'Arco should be taken in conjunction with vitamins A, C, potassium, magnesium and digestive enzymes.

X

How to Find out What Vitamins You Really Need

125. What Is A Balanced Diet and Are You Eating It?

A balanced diet is something easily found in books and rarely on the table. Though nutrients are widely scattered all through our food supply, soil depletion, storage, food processing, and cooking destroy many of them. Still, there are enough left to make balancing meals important. After all, supplements cannot work without food, and the better the food you eat, the more effective your supplements will be. Unfortunately, no possible "balanced" diet is likely to meet nutritional needs today.

Nevertheless, to know whether or not you are balancing your meals, you should become familiar with the basic food groups, and the recommended number of portions that should be eaten from them each day. Serving sizes should be individually determined; smaller amounts for less active people, larger amounts for teenagers and people who do physically strenuous work. Keep in mind that as you get older your metabolic rate slows and your energy needs decrease.

PLEASE NOTE: At the time of this writing, a new food pyramid is being designed to replace the former "four basic food groups" circle and recommended dietary guidelines. In it, the suggested servings per day of grains, breads, cereals, vegetables and fruits have been significantly increased while servings of dairy and meat products have been decreased. They are now as follows:

GRAIN GROUP

Whole or enriched grains, bread, hot or cold cereals, pasta, rice.
6–11 servings per day

VEGETABLE GROUP

Dark-green, leafy, yellow or orange vegetables.
3–5 servings per day

FRUIT GROUP

Citrus fruits, tomatoes, or others rich in vitamin C.
2–4 servings per day

DAIRY GROUP

Milk, cheese, yogurt, foods made from milk.
2–3 servings per day

MEAT GROUP

Beef, veal, pork, lamb, fish, poultry, liver, eggs, meat substitutes.
2–3 servings per day

FATS, OILS, SWEETS

Use sparingly

The recommended servings, as outlined by the National Research Council, are still designed to supply 1,200 calories. You are expected to adjust the size of the servings to suit your own individual growth, weight, and energy needs.

126. How To Test for Deficiencies

If you're wondering whether or not you need vitamin or mineral supplementation, your best bet would be to contact a nutritionally oriented doctor. (See section 293.) Other than that, there are a variety of "indicator" tests that should tell you enough to point you in the right supplement direction.

Dr. John M. Ellis has devised a quick early-warning test for B6 (pyridoxine) deficiency. Extend your hand, palm up, then try to bend the two joints in your four fingers (not the knuckles of your hand), until your fingertips reach your palm. (This is not a fist, only two joints are bent.) Do this with both hands. If it is difficult, if finger joints don't allow tips to reach your palm, a pyridoxine deficiency is likely.

Betty Lee Morales, the late well-known nutritionist, stated that urine is a fair indicator of the B vitamins in your body. Since B vitamins are water soluble and lost each day through excretion, when your body demands more your urine will be light in color. When the urine is dark, your B demands are less. (NOTE: Many drugs, illnesses, and foods also alter urine color. This should be taken into consideration.)

Hair analyses, where a tablespoon of hair clipped from the back of the neck is sent to a laboratory to check for abnormally high toxic mineral levels, have recently become a subject of controversy regarding their reliability. Hair analysts say that hair can serve as a permanent record of nutrient consumption and toxic exposure, since substances entering the hair stay there until the hair falls out. Their detractors, on the other hand, say that there are too many factors besides what we eat and drink that can influence the content of hair (dyes, shampoos, colorings, waving lotions, pool chemicals, etc.) to provide a reliable analysis.

As of this writing, the controversy has not been resolved either way. So my advice, once again, is to check with a nutritionally oriented doctor (see section 293) before investing in an analysis on your own.

Probably the best indicator of any vitamin or mineral deficiency is your body—and the way that it's feeling.

127. Possible Warning Signs

A body in need of vitamins usually lets you know about it sooner or later. It's unlikely that any of us will come down with scurvy before realizing we need vitamin C, but more often than not our bodies are giving us clues that we just don't recognize. With the price of medical insurance rising daily, paying attention to your nutritional warning system is about the best and cheapest insurance around. Here are a few common symptoms that you might be ignoring—and shouldn't.

The supplements recommended are not intended as medical advice, only a guide in working with your doctor.

NOTE: MVP stands for Mindell Vitamin Program (or Most Valuable Player in the nutrition game). It consists of a high potency multiple vitamin with chelated minerals, preferably time release; a vitamin C, 1,000 mg. with bioflavonoids, rutin, hesperidin, and rose hips, with time release; and a high potency chelated multiple mineral supplement.

POSSIBLE DEFICIENCY   ARE YOU EATING ENOUGH?

SYMPTOM: *Appetite Loss*

Protein	Meat, fish, eggs, dairy products, soybeans, peanuts
Vitamin A	Fish, liver, egg yolks, green leafy or yellow vegetables
Vitamin B1	Brewer's yeast, whole grains, meat (pork or liver), nuts, legumes, potatoes
Vitamin C	Citrus fruits, tomatoes, potatoes, cabbage, green peppers
Biotin	Brewer's yeast, nuts, beef liver, kidney, unpolished rice
Phosphorus	Milk, cheese, meat, poultry, fish, cereals, nuts, legumes
Sodium	Beef, pork, sardines, cheese, green olives, corn bread, sauerkraut
Zinc	Vegetables, whole grains, wheat bran, wheat germ, pumpkin seeds, sunflower seeds

POSSIBLE DEFICIENCY ARE YOU EATING ENOUGH?

RECOMMENDED SUPPLEMENT: 1 B complex, 50 mg.,
taken with each meal
1 B12, 2,1000 mcg. (time
release) with breakfast
1 organic iron complex
tablet (containing
vitamin C, copper, liver,
manganese, and zinc to
help assimilate iron)

SYMPTOM: *Bad breath*

Niacin   Liver, meat, fish, whole grains,
legumes

RECOMMENDED SUPPLEMENT: 1–2 tbsp. acidophilus
liquid (flavored) 1–3
times daily
1 chlorophyll tablet or
capsule 3 times daily
1 chelated zinc 50 mg. tab
daily
1–2 multiple digestive
enzyme tabs 1–3 times
daily

SYMPTOM: *Body odor*

B12   Yeast, liver, beef, eggs, kidney
Zinc   Vegetables, whole grains, wheat
bran, wheat germ, pumpkin seeds,
sunflower seeds

RECOMMENDED SUPPLEMENT: 1–2 tbsp. acidophilus
liquid (flavored) 1–3
times daily

POSSIBLE DEFICIENCY   ARE YOU EATING ENOUGH?

---

1 chlorophyll tablet or
capsule 3 times daily
1 chelated zinc 15–50 mg.
tab daily
1–2 multiple digestive
enzyme tabs 1–3 times
daily

SYMPTOM: *Bruising easily* (when slight or minor injuries
produce bluish, purplish discoloration of skin)

Vitamin C   Citrus fruits, tomatoes, potatoes,
                       cabbage, green peppers
Bioflavonoids   Orange, lemon, lime, tangerine,
                       peas

RECOMMENDED SUPPLEMENT: 1 C complex, 1,000 mg.
                         (time release) with
                         bioflavonoids, rutin, and
                         hesperidin A.M. and
                         P.M.

SYMPTOM: *High cholesterol*

B complex Inositol   Yeast, brewer's yeast, dried lima
                       beans, raisins, cantaloupe

RECOMMENDED SUPPLEMENT: 1 tbsp. lecithin granules 3
                         times daily (used on
                         salads or on cottage
                         cheese)
                         or
                         3 1,200 mg. caps lecithin
                         3–4 times daily

SYMPTOM: *Constipation*

B complex   Liver, beef, cheese, pork, kidney

POSSIBLE DEFICIENCY ARE YOU EATING ENOUGH?

RECOMMENDED SUPPLEMENT: 8–10 glasses of water daily
1 tbsp. acidophilus liquid 3
   times daily
3–9 bran tabs daily
3 tbsp. bran daily

SYMPTOM: *Diarrhea*

Vitamin K   Yogurt, alfalfa, soybean oil, fish-
                     liver oils, kelp
Niacin   Liver, lean meat, brewer's yeast,
                     wheat germ, peanuts, dried
                     nutritional yeast, white meat of
                     poultry, avodado, fish, legumes,
                     whole grain
Vitamin F   Vegetable oils, peanuts, sunflower
                     seeds, walnuts

RECOMMENDED SUPPLEMENT: 1 g. potassium divided
                              over 3 meals
                            As a preventive 1–2 tbsp.
                              acidophilus liquid
                              (flavored) 3 times daily

SYMPTOM: *Dizziness*

Manganese   Nuts, green leafy vegetables, peas,
                     beets, egg yolks
B2 (Riboflavin)   Milk, liver, kidney, yeast, cheese,
                     fish, eggs

RECOMMENDED SUPPLEMENT: 50–100 mg. niacin 3 times
                              a day
                            200 IU dry vitamin E 1–3
                              times a day

POSSIBLE DEFICIENCY   ARE YOU EATING ENOUGH?

SYMPTOM: *Ear noises*

Manganese	Nuts, green leafy vegetables, peas, beets, egg yolks
Potassium	Bananas, watercress, all leafy green vegetables, citrus fruits, sunflower seeds

RECOMMENDED SUPPLEMENT: 50–100 mg. niacin 3 times a day
400 IU dry vitamin E 1–3 times a day
50 mg. zinc daily

SYMPTOM: *Eye problems* (night blindness, inability to adjust to darkness, bloodshot eyes, inflammations, burning sensations, sties)

Vitamin A	Fish, liver, egg yolks, butter, cream, green leafy or yellow vegetables
B2 (Riboflavin)	Milk, liver, kidney, yeast, cheese, fish, eggs

RECOMMENDED SUPPLEMENT: 10,000 IU Beta carotene 1–2 times daily
100 mg. B complex (time release), 1 in A.M. and P.M.
500 mg. vitamin C with bioflavonoids, rutin, and hesperidin, 1 in A.M. and P.M.
400 IU vitamin E (dry), 1 in A.M. and P.M.

POSSIBLE DEFICIENCY ARE YOU EATING ENOUGH?

SYMPTOM: *Fatigue* (lassitude, weakness, no inclination
            for physical activity)

Zinc	Vegetables, whole-grain products, brewer's yeast, wheat bran, wheat germ, pumpkin and sunflower seeds
Carbohydrates	Cellulose
Protein	Meat, fish, eggs, dairy products, soybeans, peanuts
Vitamin A	Fish, liver, egg yolks, butter, cream, green leafy or yellow vegetables
Vitamin B complex	Yeast, brewer's yeast,
PABA	dried lima beans, raisins, cantaloupe
Iron	Wheat germ, soybean flour, beef, kidney, liver, beans, clams, peaches, and molasses
Iodine	Seafoods, dairy products, kelp
Vitamin C	Citrus fruits, tomatoes, potatoes, cabbage, green peppers
Vitamin D	Fish-liver oils, butter, egg yolks, liver, sunshine

RECOMMENDED SUPPLEMENT: 1 B complex, 100 mg.
                                (time release), 2 times
                                daily
                           1 2,000-mcg. B12 A.M.
                                and P.M.
                           1 50-mg. B15 with each
                                meal
                           MVP, 1 A.M. and P.M.

SYMPTOM: *Gastrointestinal problems* (gastritis, gastric
            ulcers, gallbladder, digestive disturbances)

Vitamin B1 (thiamin) Brewer's yeast, whole grains, meat

POSSIBLE DEFICIENCY   ARE YOU EATING ENOUGH?

	(pork or liver), nuts, legumes, potatoes
Vitamin B2 (riboflavin)	Milk, liver, kidney, yeast, cheese, fish, eggs
Folic acid (folacin)	Fresh green leafy vegetables, fruit, organ meats, liver, dried nutritional yeast
PABA	Yeast, brewer's yeast, dried lima beans, raisins, cantaloupe
Vitamin C	Citrus fruits, tomatoes, potatoes, cabbage, green peppers
Chlorine	Kelp, rye flour, ripe olives, sea greens
Pantothenic acid	Yeast, brewer's yeast, dried lima beans, raisins, cantaloupe

RECOMMENDED SUPPLEMENT: 10,000 IU Beta carotene 1–2 times daily

100 mg. B complex (time release), 1 A.M. and P.M.

Multiple minerals, 1 A.M. and P.M.

Betaine HC1 500 mg. ½ hour before meals with glass of water

Multiple digestive enzyme ½ hour after meals with glass of water

Fresh-squeezed cabbage juice, 1 glass after meals

SYMPTOM: *Hair problems*
   1. DANDRUFF (loose flakes —dry or yellow and greasy— which fall from scalp)

POSSIBLE DEFICIENCY   ARE YOU EATING ENOUGH?

Vitamin B12 (cyanocobalamin)	Liver, beef, pork, organ meats, eggs, milk and milk products
Vitamin F	Vegetable oils, peanuts, sunflower seeds, walnuts
Vitamin B6	Dried nutritional yeast, liver, organ meats, legumes, whole-grain cereals, fish
Selenium	Bran, germ of cereals, broccoli, onions, tomatoes, and tuna

RECOMMENDED SUPPLEMENT: 100 mcg. selenium twice
daily
1 MVP A.M. and P.M.
3 vitamin F caps 3 times
daily with meals

SYMPTOM: *Hair problems*
2. DULL, DRY, BRITTLE,
OR GRAYING HAIR

Vitamin A complex PABA	Yeast, brewer's yeast, dried lima beans, raisins, cantaloupe
Vitamin F	Vegetable oils, peanuts, sunflower seeds, walnuts
Iodine	Seafoods, iodized salt, dairy products

RECOMMENDED SUPPLEMENT: 3 vitamin-F caps with each
meal
3–6 lecithin caps with each
meal
1 MVP A.M. and P.M.

SYMPTOM: *Hair problems*
3. LOSS OF HAIR

POSSIBLE DEFICIENCY   ARE YOU EATING ENOUGH?

Biotin	Brewer's yeast, nuts, beef liver, kidney, unpolished rice
Inositol	Unrefined molasses and liver, lecithin, unprocessed whole grains, citrus fruits, brewer's yeast
Chlorine	Sodium chloride (table salt)
B complex with C and folic acid	Yeast, brewer's yeast, dried lima beans, raisins, cantaloupe, citrus fruits, green peppers, tomatoes, cabbage, potatoes, fresh green leafy vegetables, fruit, organ meats, liver, dried nutritional yeast

RECOMMENDED SUPPLEMENT: 1,000 mg. choline and
                                            inositol daily
                                      multiple mineral daily
                                    Cysteine 1 g. daily
                                    Vitamin C 3,000 mg. daily
                                    B complex 100 mg. (time
                                            release) A.M. and P.M.

SYMPTOM: *Heart palpitation*

Vitamin B12 (cobalamin, cyancobalamin)	Yeast, liver, beef, eggs, kidney

RECOMMENDED SUPPLEMENT: 1 MVP A.M. and P.M.
                                    100 mg. vitamin B
                                            complex (time release)
                                            A.M. and P.M.
                                    100 mg. niacin 1–3 times
                                            daily
                                    3 caps lecithin 3 times
                                            daily

SYMPTOM: *High blood pressure*

POSSIBLE DEFICIENCY   ARE YOU EATING ENOUGH?

Choline	Egg yolks, brain, heart, green leafy vegetables, yeast, liver, wheat germ

RECOMMENDED SUPPLEMENT: Lecithin granules, 3 tbsp. daily or 3 caps 3 times daily
1 MVP A.M. and P.M.
Start with 100 IU vitamin E and work up to higher strengths. (See section 39.)
1–3 kelp tabs daily
1 odorless garlic capsule 3 times daily

SYMPTOM: *Infections* (high susceptibility)

Vitamin A (carotene)	Fish, liver, egg yolks, butter, cream, green leafy or yellow vegetables
Pantothenic acid	Yeast, brewer's yeast, dried lima beans, raisins, cantaloupe

RECOMMENDED SUPPLEMENT: 1–2 tbsp. acidophilus 3 times daily
Vitamin A up to 10,000 IU every other day for duration of infection
1 MVP A.M. and P.M.
(2–5 g. vitamin C for duration of infection)

SYMPTOM: *Insomnia*

Potassium	Bananas, watercress, all leafy green vegetables, citrus fruits, sunflower seeds

POSSIBLE DEFICIENCY	ARE YOU EATING ENOUGH?
B complex	Yeast, brewer's yeast, dried lima beans, raisins, cantaloupe
Biotin	Brewer's yeast, nuts, beef liver, kidney, unpolished rice
Calcium	Milk and milk products, meat, fish, eggs, cereal products, beans, fruit, vegetables

RECOMMENDED SUPPLEMENT: 2 g. tryptophan ½ hr. before bedtime (see section 76)
Vitamin B6 100 mg., niacinamide 100 mg., & chelated calcium & magnesium ½ hr. before bedtime
1 MVP A.M. and P.M.

SYMPTOM: *Loss of smell*

Vitamin A	Fish, liver, egg yolks, butter, cream, green leafy or yellow vegetables
Zinc	Vegetables, whole grains, wheat bran, wheat germ, pumpkin and sunflower seeds

RECOMMENDED SUPPLEMENT: 50 mg. chelated zinc 3 times daily (cut back to 1–2 daily when condition improves)

SYMPTOM: *Memory loss*

B1 (thiamine)	Brewer's yeast, whole grains, meat (pork or liver), nuts, legumes, potatoes

POSSIBLE DEFICIENCY   ARE YOU EATING ENOUGH?

RECOMMENDED SUPPLEMENT:	L-glutamine, 500 mg. 3 times daily 50 mg. B complex A.M. and P.M. Choline, 2 g. daily in divided doses

---

SYMPTOM: *Menstrual problems*

B12	Yeast, liver, beef, eggs, kidney

RECOMMENDED SUPPLEMENT:	7–10 days before period: 1 MVP A.M. and P.M. 100 mg. B6 3 times daily 100 mg. B complex (time release) A.M. and P.M. Evening Primrose oil, 500 mg. 3 times daily 500 mg. magnesium & ½ as much calcium once daily

---

SYMPTOM: *Mouth sores and cracks*

Vitamin B12 (riboflavin)	Milk, liver, kidney, yeast, cheese, fish, eggs
Vitamin B6 (pyridoxine)	Dried nutritional yeast, liver, organ meats, legumes, whole-grain cereals, fish

RECOMMENDED SUPPLEMENT:	50 mg. B complex 3 times daily with meals 1 MVP A.M. and P.M.

SYMPTOM: *Muscle cramps* (general muscle weakness, tenderness in calf, night cramps, charley horse)

Vitamin B1	Brewer's yeast, whole grains, meat

POSSIBLE DEFICIENCY	ARE YOU EATING ENOUGH?
(thiamin)	(pork or liver), nuts, legumes, potatoes
Vitamin B6 (pyridoxine)	Dried nutritional yeast, liver, organ meats, legumes, whole-grain cereals, fish
Biotin	Brewer's yeast, nuts, beef liver, kidney, unpolished rice
Chlorine	Sodium chloride (table salt)
Sodium	Beef, pork, sardines, cheese, green olives, corn bread, sauerkraut
Vitamin D (calciferol)	Fish-liver oils, butter, egg yolks, liver, sunshine

RECOMMENDED SUPPLEMENT: 400 IU vitamin E (dry) 3
times daily
Chelated calcium &
magnesium, 3 tabs 3
times daily
100 mg. niacin 3 times
daily

SYMPTOM: *Nervousness*

Vitamin B6 (pyridoxine)	Dried nutritional yeast, liver, organ meats, legumes, whole-grain cereals, fish
Vitamin B12 (cyanocobalamin)	Yeast, liver, beef, eggs, kidney
Niacin (nicotinic acid, niacinamide)	Liver, meat, fish, whole grains, legumes
PABA	Yeast, brewer's yeast, dried lima beans, raisins, cantaloupe
Magnesium	Green leafy vegetables, nuts, cereals, grains, seafoods

RECOMMENDED SUPPLEMENT: Stress B with C 1–3 times
daily (50 mg. of all B
vitamins)

POSSIBLE DEFICIENCY   ARE YOU EATING ENOUGH?

	3 chelated calcium and magnesium tabs 3 times daily
	1 MVP A.M. and P.M.

SYMPTOM: *Nosebleeds*

Vitamin C	Citrus fruits, tomatoes, potatoes, cabbage, green peppers
Vitamin K	Yogurt, alfalfa, soybean oil, fish-liver oils, kelp
Bioflavonoids	Orange, lemon, lime, tangerine peels

RECOMMENDED SUPPLEMENT: 1,000 mg. vitamin C with 50 mg. rutin, hesperidin, and 500 mg. bioflavonoids (time release) A.M. and P.M.

SYMPTOM: *Retarded growth*

Fat	Meat, butter
Protein	Meat, fish, eggs, dairy products, soybeans, peanuts
Vitamin B2 (riboflavin)	Milk, liver, kidney, yeast, cheese, fish, eggs
Folic acid	Fresh green leafy vegetables, fruit, organ meats, liver, dried nutritional yeast
Zinc	Vegetables, whole grains, wheat bran, wheat germ, pumpkin and sunflower seeds
Cobalt	Liver, kidney, pancreas, and spleen (organ meats)

RECOMMENDED SUPPLEMENT: 1 MVP A.M. and P.M.

POSSIBLE DEFICIENCY ARE YOU EATING ENOUGH?

SYMPTOM: *Skin problems*

1. ACNE (face blemishes, thickened skin, blackheads, whiteheads, red spots)

Water-solubilized vitamin A — Fish, liver, egg yolks, butter, cream, green leafy or yellow vegetables

Vitamin B complex — Yeast, brewer's yeast, dried lima beans, raisins, cantaloupe

RECOMMENDED SUPPLEMENT:

1 multiple vitamin-mineral (low in iodine) daily

1–2 400 IU vitamin E (dry) daily

25,000 IU Beta carotene, 1–2 tabs daily 6 days a week

50 mg. chelated zinc once daily with food

1–2 tbsp. acidophilus liquid 3 times daily or 3–6 caps 3 times daily

(Iodine worsens acne, so eliminate all processed foods—high in iodized salt—from your diet)

---

2. DERMATITIS (skin inflammation)

Vitamin B2 (riboflavin) — Milk, liver, kidney, yeast, cheese, fish, eggs

Vitamin B6 (pyridoxine) — Dried nutritional yeast, liver, organ meats, legumes, whole-grain cereals, fish

POSSIBLE DEFICIENCY   ARE YOU EATING ENOUGH?

Biotin	Brewer's yeast, nuts, beef liver, kidney, unpolished rice
Niacin (nicotinic acid, niacinamide)	Liver, meat, fish, whole grains, legumes

RECOMMENDED SUPPLEMENT: 1 multiple vitamin-mineral (low in iodine) daily
1–2 400 IU vitamin E (dry) daily
25,000 IU Beta carotene 1–2 tabs daily 6 days a week
50 mg. chelated zinc once daily with food
1–2 tbsp. acidophilus liquid 3 times daily or 3–6 caps 3 times daily

---

3. ECZEMA (rough, dry, scaly skin, redness and swelling, small blisters)

Fat	Meat, butter
Vitamin A (carotene)	Fish, liver, egg yolks, butter, cream, green leafy or yellow vegetables
Vitamin B complex	Yeast, brewer's yeast,
Inositol	dried lima beans, raisins, cantaloupe
Copper	Organ meats, oysters, nuts, dried legumes, whole-grain cereals
Iodine	Seafoods, iodized salt, dairy products

RECOMMENDED SUPPLEMENT: 1 multiple vitamin-mineral (low in iodine) daily

POSSIBLE DEFICIENCY   ARE YOU EATING ENOUGH?

	1–2 400 IU vitamin E (dry) daily
	25,000 IU Beta carotene, 1–2 tabs daily 6 days a week
	50 mg. chelated zinc once daily with food
	1–2 tbsp. acidophilus liquid 3 times daily or 3–6 caps 3 times daily

SYMPTOM: *Slow-healing wounds and fractures*

Vitamin C	Citrus fruits, tomatoes, potatoes, cabbage, green peppers

RECOMMENDED SUPPLEMENT:	50 mg. zinc once daily 400 IU dry vitamin E 3 times daily 1 MVP A.M. and P.M.

SYMPTOM: *Softening of bones and teeth*

Vitamin D (calciferol)	Fish-liver oils, butter, egg yolks, liver, sunshine
Calcium	Milk and milk products, meat, fish, eggs, cereal products, beans, fruit, vegetables

RECOMMENDED SUPPLEMENT:	1,000–1,500 mg. calcium, 500 mg. magnesium divided over 2 meals daily

SYMPTOM: *Tremors*

Magnesium	Green leafy vegetables, nuts, cereals, grains, seafoods

POSSIBLE DEFICIENCY ARE YOU EATING ENOUGH?

RECOMMENDED SUPPLEMENT: B complex and 50 mg. B6
3 times daily
1,000 mg. calcium, 500
mg. magnesium divided
over 3 meals daily

SYMPTOM: *Vaginal itching*

Vitamin B2   Milk, liver, kidney, yeast, cheese,
fish, eggs

RECOMMENDED SUPPLEMENT: 2 tbsp. acidophilus 3 times
daily or 3–6 caps 3–4
times daily
(Acidophilus or vinegar
douche can also help.)

SYMPTOM: *Water retention*

Vitamin B6   Dried nutritional yeast, liver, organ
meats, legumes, whole-grain
cereals, fish

RECOMMENDED SUPPLEMENT: 100 mg. B6 3 times daily

SYMPTOM: *White spots on nails*

Zinc   Vegetables, whole grains, wheat
bran, wheat germ, pumpkin and
sunflower seeds

RECOMMENDED SUPPLEMENT: 50 mg. zinc 3 times daily
Stress B with C 1–2 times
daily
1 multiple mineral 2 times
daily

128. Cravings—What They Might Mean

Cravings, which can sometimes mean allergies, are more often nature's way of letting you know that you're not getting enough of certain vitamins or minerals. Frequently these specific hungers develop because overall diet is inadequate.

Some of the most common cravings are:

Peanut Butter   This is definitely among the top ten, and it's not at all surprising. Peanut butter is a rich source of B vitamins. If you find yourself dipping into the jar often, it might be because you're under stress and your ordinary B intake has become insufficient. Since 50 g. of peanut butter—a third of a cup—is 284 calories, you'll find it easier on your waistline to take a B-complex supplement if you do not want to gain weight.

Bananas   When you catch yourself reaching for this fruit again and again, it could be because your body needs potassium. One medium banana has 555 mg. People taking diuretics or cortisone (which rob the body of needed potassium) often crave bananas.

Cheese   If you're more a cheese luster than a cheese lover, there's a good chance that your real hunger is for calcium and phosphorus. (If it's processed cheese that you've been snacking on, you've been getting aluminum and salt, too, without knowing it.) For one thing, you might try eating more broccoli. That's high in calcium and phosphorus, and a lot lower in calories than cheese.

Apples   An apple a day doesn't necessarily keep the doctor away, but it offers a lot of good things that you might be missing in other foods—calcium, magnesium, phosphorus, potassium—and is an excellent source of cholesterol-lowering pectin! If you have a tendency to eat a lot of saturated fat, it could account for your apple cravings.

Butter   Most often vegetarians crave butter because of their own low-saturated-fat intake. Salted butter, on the other hand, might be craved for the salt alone.

Cola   The craving for cola is most often a sugar hunger and an addiction to caffeine. (See section 240.) The beverage has no nutritive value.

Nuts If you're a little nutty about nuts, you probably could use more protein, B vitamins, or fat in your diet. If it's salted nuts you favor, you could be craving the sodium and not the nuts. You'll find that people under stress tend to eat more nuts than relaxed individuals.

Ice cream High as ice cream is in calcium, most people crave it for its sugar content. Hypoglycemics and diabetics have great hungers for it, as do people asking to recapture the security of childhood.

Pickles If you're pregnant and want pickles, you're probably after the salt. And if you're not pregnant and crave pickles, the reason is most likely the same. (Pickles also contain a substantial amount of potassium.)

Bacon Cravings for bacon are usually because of its fat. People on restricted diets are most susceptible to greasy binges. Unfortunately, saturated fat is not bacon's only drawback. Bacon is very high in carcinogenic nitrites. If you do indulge in bacon, be sure you're ingesting enough vitamin C and A, D, and E to counteract the nitrites.

Eggs Aside from the protein (two eggs give you 13 g.), sulfur, amino acids, and selenium protein, egg lovers might also be seeking the yolk's fat content or, paradoxically, its cholesterol-and-fat-dissolving choline.

Cantaloupe Just because you like its taste might not be the only reason you crave this melon. Cantaloupe is high in potassium and vitamin A. In fact, a quarter of a melon has 3,400 IU vitamin A. Since the melon also offers vitamin C, calcium, magnesium, phosphorus, biotin, and inositol, it's not a bad craving to give in to. There's only about 60 calories in half a melon.

Olives Whether you crave them green or black, you're likely to be after the salt. People with underactive thyroids are most often the first to reach for them.

Salt No guesswork here, it's the sodium you're after. Cravers quite possibly have a thyroid iodine deficiency or low sodium Addison's disease. Hypertensives often crave salt, and shouldn't.

Onions Cravings for spicy foods can sometimes indicate problems in the lungs or sinuses.

Chocolate   Definitely one of the foremost cravings, if not *the* foremost. Chocoholics are addicted to the caffeine as well as the sugar. (There are 5 to 10 mg. of caffeine in a cup of cocoa.) If you want to kick the chocolate habit, try carob instead. (Carob, also called St. John's Bread, is made from the edible pods of the Mediterranean carob tree.)

Milk   If you're still craving milk as an adult, you might need a calcium supplement. Then again, it might be the amino acids—such as tryptophan, leucine, and lysine—that your body needs. Nervous people often seek out the tryptophan in milk, since it has a very soothing effect.

Chinese food   Of course it's delicious, but often it's the monosodium glutamate in the food that fosters the craving. People with salt deficiencies usually go all out for Chinese food. (MSG can cause a histamine reaction in some individuals. Headaches and flushing may occur. Most Chinese restaurants will now prepare your food without MSG if you request it.)

Mayonnaise   Since this is a fatty food, it is often craved by vegetarians and people who have eliminated other fats from their diet.

Tart fruits   A persistent craving for tart fruits can often indicate problems with the gallbladder or liver.

Paint and dirt   Children have a tendency to eat paint and dirt. Frequently this is an indication of a calcium or vitamin-D deficiency. A hard reevaluation of your child's diet is essential, and a visit to your pediatrician is recommended. This craving for non-food items is known as Pica. It's a condition also experienced by pregnant women, who should be aware that ingesting such substances can harm fetal development.

129. Getting the Most Vitamins from Your Food

Eating the right foods doesn't necessarily mean that you're getting the vitamins they contain. Food processing, storing, and cooking can easily undermine the best nutritious intentions. To get the most from what you eat (not to mention what you spend) keep the following tips in mind.

- Wash but don't soak fresh vegetables if you hope to benefit from the B vitamins and C they contain.
- Forgo convenience and make your salads when you're ready to eat them. Fruits and vegetables cup up and left to stand lose vitamins.
- Use a sharp knife when cutting or shredding fresh vegetables, because vitamins A and C are diminished when vegetable tissues are bruised.
- If you don't plan to eat your fresh fruit or vegetables for a few days, you're better off buying flash-frozen ones. The vitamin content of good frozen green beans will be higher than those fresh ones you've kept in your refrigerator for a week.
- Store frozen meat at 0 degrees F. or lower immediately after purchase to prevent loss of quality and bacterial growth.
- Outer green leaves of letture, though coarser than inner ones, have higher calcium, iron, and vitamin A content.
- Don't thaw your frozen vegetables before cooking.
- Broccoli leaves have a higher vitamin A value than the flower buds or stalks.
- There are more vitamins in converted and parboiled rice than in polished rice, and brown rice is more nutritious than white.
- Frozen foods that you can boil in their bags offer more vitamins than the ordinary kind, and all frozen foods are preferable to canned ones.
- Cooking in copper pots can destroy vitamin C, folic acid, and vitamin E.
- Stainless steel, glass, and enamel are the best utensils for retaining nutrients while cooking. (Iron pots can give you the benefit of that mineral, but they will shortchange you on Vitamin C.)
- The shortest cooking time and the smallest amount of water are the least destructive to nutrients.
- Milk in glass containers can lose riboflavin, as well as

vitamins A and D, unless kept out of the light. (Breads exposed to light can also lose these nutrients.)
• Well-browned, crusty, or toasted baked goods have less thiamine than others.
• Bake and boil potatoes in their skins to get the most vitamins from them.
• Use cooking water from vegetables to make soups, juices from meats for gravies, and syrups from canned fruits to make desserts.
• Refrain from using any baking soda when cooking vegetables if you want to benefit from their thiamine and vitamin C.
• Store vegetables and fruits in the refrigerator as soon as you bring them home from the market.

BUT DID YOU KNOW: When your grocer sprays water on vegetables to keep them looking fresh, it benefits you as well as him. Broccoli, for instance, when sprayed with a fine mist of water, keeps almost twice as much of its vitamin C as it would if it weren't sprayed. Considering that broccoli is a cruciferous, cancer-fighting vegetable, this is something you'll want to look for when making your selection.

130. Any Questions About Chapter X?

I feed my children what I think is a pretty well-balanced diet. But they're teenagers and when they're out they often have burgers, hot dogs, shakes, and that sort of junk food. Are these really bad for them?

Well, ounce for ounce, munch for munch, and sip for sip, the bad far outweighs the good. For instance, a fast-food burger can supply 44 percent of a teenage boy's requirement for protein. But when you consider that a Big Mac, for example, is also supplying 591 calories, 33 grams of fat, 6 *grams* of sugar, and 963 mg. of sodium (a Burger King Whopper has *1,083 mg. of sodium*), you have to admit that's an awfully high nutritional price to pay for protein. No one needs all that salt (see section 269).

As for hot dogs, there's very little good to say about them. They're a high-fat, low-protein meat, and usually contain sodium or potassium nitrite. Nitrites combine with substances called amines, commonly found in foods, and form nitrosamines, which have been found to be carcinogenic (cancer-causing).

Shakes, which do contain milk or a milk product, also contain 8 to 14 teaspoons of sugar and 276 to 685 mg. of salt. Your kids could blend one up at home for half the price, calories, sugar, and salt—and double the nutritional value. Passing this information along to your children might be a good way to get them to pass up those fast-food places.

Very often I experience a sort of hot, burning feeling on my tongue and lips. It doesn't seem to be related to any foods I've eaten. Could it indicate a vitamin deficiency?

It's very possible. The feeling of having a burning tongue or lips has in many instances been linked to a vitamin B1 (thiamine) deficiency. I'd suggest increasing your intake of whole wheat, oatmeal, bran, vegetables, and brewer's yeast, along with taking a balanced vitamin B complex, 100 mg., 3 times a day.

My mother has a craving for ice. Not just on hot days, but all the time. She chews cubes as if they were candy. Could this sort of craving have anything to do with a dietary deficiency?

If your mother is often tired, her craving for ice might indicate an iron deficiency (which can cause a low-grade anemia). You might try encouraging her to add more iron-rich foods to her diet (liver, dried peaches, red meat, oysters, asparagus, oatmeal) and to take an organic iron supplement, 50–100 mg. 1 to 3 times a day.

I'm 42 years old and am developing yellowish growths around my eyes. Is there some vitamin or nutrient that's missing from my diet that could be causing this?

More likely those growths are cholesterol deposits, which can occur when the body is trying to rid itself of excess cholesterol. This sort of condition tends to run in families and could possibly indicate that you're in the high-risk heart disease percentile. See section 89 for how to reduce cholesterol. Also, increase your intake of vitamin B, chromium, and zinc, in foods and supplements.

How long does orange juice retain its vitamin C?

For commercial orange juice, the vitamin C lifespan is about one week from the time you've opened the container. For fresh-squeezed juice kept refrigerated in a sealed container, the lifespan of vitamin C is about three weeks.

Do you lose more or less nutrients by microwaving food?

As a rule, less. Microwaving requires minimum cooking time and minimum water.

I've heard that microwaving can add carcinogens to food. Is this true? And if so, why aren't there widespread warnings about it?

Microwaving itself does not add carcinogens to foods. What you probably heard about were the narrow strips of plastic and aluminum, known as "heat susceptors," that are used by manufacturers to crisp microwavable foods such as pizza, fish sticks, french fries, popcorn, and the like. These plastic and aluminum strips have the potential to break down under high heat and release chemicals, including the carcinogen benzene, into food. Whether this is actually happening and if there is any danger to consumers is currently being investigated by the Food and Drug Administration. But until the FDA verdict is reached, I'd advise you to keep the amount of crunchy microwavable foods you eat to a minimum.

XI

Read the Label

131. The Importance of Understanding What's On Labels

All too often people buy supplements and never even look at the labels. They ask a clerk for a multivitamin and take what they are given, not realizing that they might be getting shortchanged on the vitamin content. All multivitamins differ in amounts included, and the most expensive tablet is not necessarily the best. The only way to be sure you're getting the B6, folacin, or C that you need is to read the small print on the label. Also, if you have any allergies, it's wise to check what else you're getting with your supplement. (See section 21.)

If there are words on the label that you don't understand, ask the pharmacist or vitamin clerk to explain them. If they can't, buy your supplements where someone can. And above all, remember to check the dosage you're getting. If you've been instructed to take vitamin E four times a day, it's unlikely that you want 400 IU. Vitamins and minerals come in different strengths. Be sure you're getting what you ask for—and need. Not understanding labels can often negate a lot of vitamin benefits.

132. How Does That Measure Up?

> IU, RE, MG, MCG—a little
> can mean a lot.

The terminology for measuring vitamin activity is not as confusing as you might think. Fat-soluble vitamins (A, E, D, and K) are usually measured in International Units (IU). But a few years ago, an expert committee of the Food and Agriculture Organization/World Health Organization (FAO/WHO) decided to change this order of measurement for vitamin A. Instead of using International Units, they proposed that vitamin A be evaluated in terms of retinol equivalents (RE), that is, the equivalent weight of retinol (vitamin A1, alcohol) *actually absorbed and converted.*

Retinol equivalents come out to about five times less than International Units (IU). Recommended allowances of 5,000 IU for a male between the ages of twenty-three and fifty would only be 1,000 RE; 4,000 IU for similarly aged females would only be 800 RE.

Most other vitamins and minerals are measured in milligrams (mg.) and micrograms (mcg.). If you know that 1 g. equals .035 ounce, that it takes 28.35 g. to equal 1 ounce (and 1 fluid ounce equals 2 tablespoons), you'll have a better idea of just how much—or rather, how little—it takes for vitamins and minerals to do their job. The following table is a handy guide to refer to:

WHAT'S WHAT IN WEIGHTS AND MEASURES

Metric Measure

1 kilogram equals 1,000 grams
1 gram equals 1,000 milligrams
1 milligram equals 1/1,000th part of a gram
1 microgram equals 1/1,000 part of a milligram
1 gamma equals 1 microgram

Avoirdupois Weight

16 ounces equal 1 pound
7,000 grains equal 1 pound
453.6 grams equal 1 pound
1 ounce av. equals 437.5 grains
1 ounce av. equals 28.35 grams

Conversion Factors

1 gram equals 15.4 grains
1 grain equals 0.085 grams (85 milligrams)
1 ounce apothecary equals 31.1 grams
1 fluid ounce equals 29.8 cc.
1 fluid ounce equals 480 minims

Liquid Measure

1 drop equals 1 minim
1 minim equals 0.06 cc.
15 minims equal 1.0 cc.
4 cc. equal 1 fluid dram
30 cc. equal 1 fluid ounce

Household Measure

1 teaspoon equals 4 cc. equals 1 fluid dram
1 tablespoon equals 15 cc. equals ½ fluid ounce
½ pint equals 240 cc. equals 8 fluid ounces

Abbreviations

AMDR	Adult Minimum Daily Requirement
USP Unit	United States Pharmacopia
IU	International Unit
MDR	Minimum Daily Requirement
mg.	milligram
mcg.	microgram
g.	gram
gr.	grain

133. Breaking the RDA Code

Many people are bewildered by the variances between vitamin standards listed as RDA, U.S. RDA, and MDR. It becomes much less confusing when you understand that they are not the same thing.

RDA (Recommended Dietary Allowances) came into being in 1941, when the Food and Nutrition Board of the National Research Council of the Academy of Sciences was established by the government to safeguard public health. The RDA are not formulated to cover the needs of those who are ill—they are not therapeutic and are meant strictly for healthy individuals—nor do they take into account nutrient losses that occur during processing and preparation. They are *estimates* of nutritional needs necessary to ensure satisfactory growth of children and the prevention of nutrient depletion in adults. *They are not meant to be optimal intakes, nor are they recommendations for an ideal diet.* They are not average requirements but recommendations intended to meet the needs of those *healthy* people with the highest requirements.

U.S. RDA (U.S. Recommended Daily Allowances) were formulated by the Food and Drug Administration (FDA) to be used as the *legal* standards for food labeling in regard to nutrient content. (The RDA were used as the basis for the U.S. RDA.) Serving size, number of servings per container, calories and ten nutrients (protein, carbohydrate, fat, vitamin A, vitamin C, thiamin, riboflavin, niacin, calcium, and iron) must be listed on food labels. Information about sodium, cholesterol, and saturated and unsaturated fat is optional at this writing, but expected to become a legal requirement soon. (U.S. RDA percentages for vitamins D, E, B6, phosphorus, iodine, magnesium, zinc, copper, biotin, and pantothenic acid remain optional.)

Because the U.S. RDA are based on the highest values of the RDA, the former is frequently higher than the basic needs of most healthy people, though very few individuals today fall into that hypothetical category. Stress and illness, past or present, affect everyone's nutritional requirements differently. Just because a product claims to provide 100 percent of the U.S. RDA for a nutrient doesn't necessarily mean that *you* are getting it, or that it's a sufficient amount for *your* individual needs. As far as I and many other leading nutritionists are concerned, the RDA and the U.S. RDA are woefully inadequate. Nonetheless, you will find them listed in sections 26–67 in the facts section for each vitamin and mineral.

134. What To Look For

When buying minerals, look for *chelated* on the label. Only 10 percent of ordinary minerals will be assimilated by the body, but when combined with amino acids in chelation, the assimilation is three to five times more efficient.

Hydrolyzed means water dispersible. *Hydrolyzed protein-chelate* means the supplement is in its most easily assimilated form.

Predigested protein is protein that has already been broken down and can go straight to the bloodstream.

Cold pressed is important to look for when buying oil or oil capsules. It means vitamins haven't been destroyed by heat and that the oil, extracted by cold-pressed methods, remains polyunsaturated.

135. Any Questions About Chapter XI?

What are emulsifiers?

Emulsifiers are used to homogenize ingredients which do not normally mix well. Lecithin and pectin, which are natural and safe, are commonly used, but unfortunately they're not used exclusively. Polysorbate 60 (which the FDA still has under investigation), locust bean (on the FDA list of additives requiring further study for mutagenic, reproductive, and teratogenic effects), and carrageenan (another being studied all too slowly by the FDA), among others, are still being used.

Though these are at present generally recognized as safe (GRAS) I personally prefer and recommend products without them.

Are the dyes used in vitamin coatings natural or artificial, and how can I tell?

Regrettably, a lot of synthetic vitamins use coal-tar dyes in their coatings—and keep it a secret. (In other words, there's no mention on the label.) These dyes are not necessarily harmful, but they can cause allergic reactions. My advice is to play it safe and buy natural vitamins that have no artificial adulterants—and *say so*!

Are calories counted differently in foreign countries?

Most foreign countries use the metric system, and the energy value of food is measured in units called *joules*, our kilocalories, better known as calories. Four of our calories are the equivalent of 17 joules. In other words, a joule is slightly more than four times a calorie.

When dealing with vitamin A, how do you convert IUs into mgs. or mcgs.?

There are no rigid conversions, but 1 IU vitamin A = 0.3 mcg. Retinol and 1 IU Beta carotene = 0.1 mcg. Retinol.

XII

Your Special Vitamin Needs

136. Selecting Your Regimen

We all know that not everyone has the same metabolism, but we often forget that this also means that not everyone requires the same vitamins. In the following sections I have outlined a number of personalized regimens for a variety of specialized needs. Look them all over and see which ones best fit your own special situation. If you fall under more than one category, adjust the combined regimens so that you are not double-dosing yourself, only adding the additional vitamins.

You will notice that in many cases I advise what I call an MVP, a Mindell Vitamin Program (which can make you an MVP—a Most Valuable Player in the nutrition game). This basic vitamin trio is my foundation for general good health.

MVP MINDELL VITAMIN PROGRAM

• High-potency multiple vitamin with chelated minerals (time release preferred)
• Vitamin C, 1,000 mg. with bioflavonoids, rutin, hesperidin, and rose hips
• High-potency chelated multiple minerals

> IMPORTANT NOTE: Before starting any program, you should check "Cautions" (section 290) and with a nutritionally oriented doctor. *The regimens in this book are not prescriptive nor are they intended as medical advice.*

137. Women

12–18	Multiple vitamin and mineral Vitamin C, 500 mg. with rose hips Vitamin E, 200 IU (dry form) 1 of each with breakfast
19–50	MVP (see section 136) Vitamin E, 400 IU (dry form) 1 of each with breakfast, and again with evening meal if necessary
Also:	3 RNA-DNA 100 mg. tablets daily 3 SOD tablets (see section 279) daily (take for only 6 days a week) Magnesium, 1,000 mg. and calcium 500 mg. daily Iron, 15–50 mg. daily 1 multiple digestive enzyme when needed Stress B complex A.M. and P.M. if stress conditions exist
50+	MVP (see section 136) Vitamin E, 400 IU (dry form) 1 of each with breakfast, and again at evening meal 3 RNA-DNA 100 mg. tablets daily 1–3 multiple digestive enzymes daily

138. Men

11–18	Multiple vitamin and mineral Vitamin C, 500 mg. with rose hips Vitamin E, 400 IU (dry form) 1 of each with breakfast

19–50   MVP (see section 136)

Vitamin E, 400 IU (dry form)

1 of each A.M. and P.M.

3 RNA-DNA 100 mg. tablets daily

3 SOD tablets (see section 279) daily (take for only 6 days a week)

Zinc, 15–50 mg. daily

Lecithin granules, 2 tbsp. or 9 capsules daily

Stress B complex A.M. and P.M. if needed

50+   MVP (see section 136)

Vitamin E, 400 IU (dry form)

1 of each twice a day

3 RNA-DNA 100 mg. tablets daily

3 SOD tablets (see section 279) (take for only 5 days a week)

1–3 multiple digestive enzymes daily

139. Infants

1–4   One good-tasting chewable multiple vitamin daily (check label to see that all the primary vitamins are included); there should be no artificial color, flavors, or sugar (sucrose) added. (Liquid vitamins are available for very young children. Remember to check with your pediatrician before making any supplement choice.)

140. Children

4–12   Growing children need a stronger multiple vitamin containing minerals, especially calcium and iron, for normal growth. The tablet should also be high in B complex and vitamin C (50 percent of American children do not even get the RDA for vitamin C). One daily is sufficient (check label to be sure there is no artificial color, flavor, or sugar—sucrose—added).

141. Pregnant Women

The right vitamins are essential at this time:

A good high-potency multiple vitamin and mineral rich in
vitamins A, B6, B12, C, and folic acid.
Multiple chelated minerals, rich in calcium (2 tablets should
equal 1,000 mg. calcium and 500 mg. magnesium)
1 of each twice daily
Also, folic acid, 800 mg. 3 times a day

142. Nursing Mothers

The same supplements recommended for pregnant women
plus additional vitamins A, B6, B12, and C. Your body and
your baby need the best nourishment you can give them.

143. Runners

During the first fifteen to twenty minutes of running, you
burn up almost only glucose. The body then comes in with
fats (lipids) for energy (in utilizing lipids for energy, a compound called acegyl-coenzyme-A is formed). If there are only
animal fats present, the compound forms slowly and energy
is insufficient. If polyunsaturates are present, on the other
hand, the compound forms quickly. Increase your intake of
polyunsaturates—seeds, peanuts—and antioxidants, such as
vitamins A, C, E, and selenium, to avoid free radical reactions.

A good supplement program would be:

Multiple vitamin with chelated minerals
Vitamin C complex, 1,000 mg.
Stress B complex with zinc
1 of each 2–3 times a day
Also, vitamin E, 400 IU A.M. and P.M. and 1 multiple chelated
mineral tablet daily.
Cytochrome-C and inosine, plus octacosanol with pangamic
acid 1–3 times day.

144. Joggers

The nutritional needs of joggers are the same as those for runners. Just remember: for highest energy keep polyunsaturates in mind.

145. Executives

With tension and stress an accepted part of your daily life, and energy a necessity, you need a vitamin regimen that won't let you down. Many high-level executives I know use this one:

MVP (see section 136) A.M. and P.M.
Stress B complex A.M. and P.M.
Lecithin granules, 2 tbsp. or 3 capsules with each meal
B15, 50 mg. 1–3 times daily

If you're in a hurry in the morning, you might want to try my high-energy breakfast drink:

RECIPE:

2 tbsp. protein powder	3 ice cubes
1 tbsp. natural yeast	2 tbsp. fresh fruit,
2 tbsp. lecithin granules	honey, or fructose

Mix in blender at high speed for one minute.

146. Students

Eating on the run, skipping breakfast, and not getting enough rest is a way of life for most students. And as if this isn't bad enough for good health, student diets usually consist of mostly starches and carbohydrates. If you're in this category, be aware that these factors, as well as your constant stress situations at school, are taking their toll. A good supplement program would be:

MVP (see section 136)
Dry vitamin E, 400 IU
Stress B complex with zinc

1 of each with breakfast and dinner
Choline, 500 mg. 2 times daily

Also, you might improve your work performance by increasing your intake of choline-rich foods. (See section 37.)

147. Senior Citizens

The nutritional needs of senior citizens may vary widely, depending on the individual. As a general rule, however, if you're over sixty-five, you need extra minerals, especially calcium, magnesium, and iron, as well as extra vitamins such as B complex and C. Vitamin E can help alleviate poor circulation, which is often responsible for leg cramps. And don't forget about fiber. If chewing is a problem, high-fiber foods can be ground to convenient sizes and textures and are just as effective. Also, sweets should be discouraged; there is a high incidence of sugar diabetes among older people.

A good supplement regimen would be:

Multiple vitamin and mineral
Rose hips vitamin C, 500 mg. with bioflavonoids
Multiple chelated mineral tablet
Vitamin E 200–400 IU
1 of each with breakfast and dinner

(See section 250 for drug, food, and nutrient interactions that can cause malabsorption and other problems.)

148. Athletes

Athletes have very demanding nutritional needs. The prime nutritional requirement for performance is energy, and high-energy—as opposed to ''quick energy'' foods—should be eaten. If you're involved in action sports, you need a diet with more complex carbohydrates and protein than someone involved in a low energy sport. Then again, even golf can become a high-energy game when carried on intensively for a long time. Keep in mind that excess amounts of glucose, sugar, honey or hard candy tend to draw fluid into the gastrointestinal tract. This can add to dehydration problems in endurance performance. A thirst-quenching tart drink of frozen or canned fruit juice is the best quick-energy beverage.

For supplements, I recommend:

Multiple vitamin and chelated minerals
Stress B complex
Vitamin C complex, 1,000 mg.
Vitamin E, 400–1,000 IU
Multiple chelated minerals
1 of each with breakfast, lunch, and dinner
Cytochrome-C and inosine
Vitamin B15, 50 mg.
Octacosonal
All 1–3 times day

A protein supplement is also a good idea.

149. Body Builders

If you work out with weights, being on the right diet is as important as your warm-ups and cool-downs. In fact, without combining them, you may wind up with bulging muscles that will be layered with fat and won't do much for your overall shape.

While it's true that protein builds and repairs muscles, it is complex carbohydrates that supply energy for the continuous and repeated muscular contractions that occur during prolonged exercise. For best results, I'd advise getting 80 to 90 percent of your calories from complex carbohydrates and no more than 10 percent from meat protein. You might also want to try Branched Chain Amino Acids (see section 83) which are natural anabolic muscle builders.

My supplement suggestion:

• MVP, A.M. and P.M.
• Stress B complex with zinc 1–3 times daily
• Vitamin E (dry form) 400–800 IU 1–3 times daily
• Cytochrome-C, inosine, and octacosanol, 1,000 mcg. 1–3 times daily

OPTIONAL: Branched Chain Amino Acids (BCAA) 600 mg.
For heavy workout 4–6, take ½ hour before workout
For moderate workout 3–4, take ½ hour before workout
For light workout 1–2, take ½ hour before workout

150. Night Workers

The Center for Research on Stress and Health at the Stanford Research Institute has found that "the rotating shift exacts a heavy physical and emotional toll from workers." When eating and sleeping patterns are disrupted, so are the body's biological rhythms, and it takes "three to four weeks for the circadian rhythms to become synchronized." If you change from day to night shifts, often, your body is under much stress, your chances of illness are greater, and your risk of ulcers is high. I feel that supplements are essential:

MVP (see section 136).
1 vitamin D, 400 IU with largest meal

151. Truck Drivers

Tension, stress, and a diet that is all too often high in greasy foods are important reasons for considering the following supplements:

MVP (see section 136)
Lecithin granules, 3 tbsp. or 12 capsules daily
1 B complex, 100 mg.

152. Dancers

Dancers have energy requirements that rank with those of athletes, but because of weight restrictions they cannot consume the same amount of carbohydrates. Good supplements are indispensable, as most dancers will tell you. I suggest:

MVP (see section 136).
(Be sure to take the multiple mineral twice daily.)
1 balanced calcium and magnesium supplement daily
B15, 50 mg. 3 times daily

153. Construction Workers

One out of every four workers is exposed to substances considered hazardous, according to the National Institute of Occupational Safety and Health (NIOSH). Construction workers are particularly vulnerable. Depending upon the sort of construction you're doing and where you're doing it, you're exposed to a variety of harmful conditions from general pollution to inhaling lead oxide, which can happen if you're soldering scrap metal or plastics. In any event, a diet rich in antioxidants such as vitamins A, C, and E will help detoxify your body. The following supplements are recommended:

MVP (see section 136)
B complex, 100 mg. twice daily
Vitamin E, 400–1,000 IU daily.

154. Gamblers

If you're a gambler, I don't have to tell you about your stress, sleep, and dietary needs. I'm sure you're aware that all three are higher than average. What you might not realize, though, is that you could be in need of vitamin-D supplementation because of lack of sunlight. For best performance at any table, I suggest the following supplements:

MPV (see section 136) A.M. and P.M.
Dry vitamin E, 400–1,000 IU daily
Vitamin D, 400 IU if necessary
Stress B complex with zinc

155. Salespersons

The daily grind of having to deal with the public cannot be underestimated. Whether you're selling automobiles, books, exercise machines, or food, doing it on the road or from behind a counter, the emotional and physical stress on your body is great. And because appearances are often as important as products in your line of work, you'd be wise to pack the right supplements along with your samples. You'll be happily surprised with the results.

MVP (see section 136)
Stress B complex 3 times daily (with each meal)
Vitamin E, 400 IU A.M. and P.M.

156. Actors—Stage, Screen, Radio and TV Performers

There's not an actor I know who doesn't need a B-vitamin supplement. The stress and tension of performing is an occupational given. And if you're like most theatrical performers, dieting is the only form of eating you know, too often denying you necessary vitamins. A helpful supplement scenario would be:

MVP (see section 136) A.M. and P.M.
Stress B complex with zinc A.M. and P.M.
Vitamin E, 400 IU twice daily.

157. Singers

Like actors, singers are also under high levels of stress, whether performing or rehearsing. If you worry about laryngitis, or other throat infections, it's advisable to keep your vitamin-C levels high at all times. Time-release vitamin C is your best choice.

MVP (see section 136) A.M. and P.M.
Additional vitamin C, 1,000 mg. A.M. and P.M. when necessary.

158. Doctors and Nurses

If you work with illness, you need all the protection you can get. Long hours, stress, and germs themselves, all contribute to your need for vitamin and mineral supplementation.

MVP (see section 136) A.M. and P.M.
Stress B complex twice daily
Extra vitamin C to ward off infections.

159. Handicapped

If you're disabled, your needs for vitamins are usually increased. More often than not, if one part of your body is not functioning properly, another part is working twice as hard —and needs nourishment. Helpful basic supplements would be:

1 B complex, 50 mg. A.M. and P.M.
1 high-potency multiple mineral twice daily

160. Golfers

As much as you enjoy it, golfing takes a lot out of you. The stress and tension of the game can use up B vitamins at a rapid clip. The right supplements might not get you down into the seventies, but they can help you stay energetic throughout the game.

MVP (see section 136) A.M. and P.M.
Stress B complex with zinc A.M. and P.M.

161. Tennis Players

If you play tennis often, you might look good on the outside, but be a nutritional mess inside. I've found that far too many tennis buffs skip meals, or eat only protein—both bad habits. A demanding game like tennis requires that you serve yourself all the vitamins you need.

MVP (see section 136) A.M. and P.M.
Stress B complex A.M. and P.M.
Extra calcium to prevent muscle fatigue, 750 mg. 1–3 times
    daily
Vitamin B15, 500 mg. 1–3 times daily
Vitamin E (dry form), 400–800 IU daily
Wheat-germ oil

162. Racketball Players

Few sports require as intense physical stamina as racketball, so if you intend to play it on a regular basis (or even on an occasional lunch hour), you'd better be prepared to not only meet your opponent, but the nutritional challenge as well.

MVP (see section 136) A.M. and P.M.
Cytochrome-C, inosine, and octacosanol, 1,000 mcg. 1–3 times daily
Vitamin E (dry form), 400 IU daily
Stress B complex with zinc, 1–3 times daily

163. Teachers

School days are as stressful for teachers as they are for students, if not more so. To keep your energy and spirits up, a good vitamin program is important.

MVP (see section 136) A.M. and P.M.
Stress B complex with zinc, twice daily

164. Smokers

Every cigarette you smoke destroys about 25 to 100 mg. of vitamin C. Also, lung cancer risks aside, you're more prone to cardiovascular and pulmonary disorders than nonsmokers. Without going into the long list of deleterious effects cigarettes can have, I feel confident in telling smokers that they need all the nutritional help they can get, especially from antioxidants such as vitamins A, C, E, and selenium.

MVP (see section 136) A.M. and P.M.
Vitamin C, 2,000 mg. A.M. and P.M.
Dry vitamin E, 400–800 IU daily
Selenium 100 mcg. daily
Beta carotene 25,000 IU daily

165. Drinkers

Alcoholism is the chief cause of vitamin deficiency among civilized people with ample food supplies. If you're a heavy drinker, the alcohol you consume usually takes the place of needed protein, or, in some cases, prevents absorption or proper storage of ingested vitamins.

MVP (see section 136) A.M. and P.M.
B complex, 100 mg. twice daily (especially needed are B1,
    B6, and folic acid)
Dry vitamin E, 400–800 IU daily

166. Excessive TV Watchers

Just because you spend a lot of time relaxing in front of your
set doesn't mean you're not in need of extra vitamins. For
the eyestrain it's more than likely that you need additional
vitamin A. And if you rarely get to see the light of day, you
might need vitamin D also.

MVP (see section 136) with food
Beta carotene, 10,000 IU with breakfast (take for 5 days,
    stop for 2)
Vitamin D, 400 IU 5 days a week if necessary

167. Travelers On The Go

The stresses of travel, though they often go unnoticed, can
be significant. If you're heading to warm or tropical places,
be sure that the vitamins you take are in opaque containers
and that you keep them in a cool place, not out in the sun.
If you're headed for chillier environs, be sure to bring along
plenty of vitamin C and take it with all your meals, not just
breakfast and dinner. And if you're traveling to foreign ports,
keep in mind that acidophilus (3 capsules or 2 tablespoons
liquid) 3 times a day is a good diarrhea preventive.

MVP (see section 136) A.M. and P.M.
Vitamin E (dry form) 400 IU 1–2 times daily
Stress B complex, 50 mg. 2–3 times daily

168. Any Questions About Chapter XII?

Are foreign vitamins different?

Vitamins the world over are the same, only dosages vary.
The metric system is used internationally for measurement,
and nutrients are measured by weight. (See section 132 for
a better understanding of what equals what.)

My obstetrician doesn't say too much to me, except "Take your vitamins." Since you're a pharmacist as well as a nutritionist, could you tell me what drugs or medicines could be dangerous to me and my baby?

I'd feel safest in saying all of them—unless specifically prescribed by your doctor. No drug—whether it's OTC (over-the-counter) or prescription, alcohol, nicotine, or caffeine—should be considered safe during pregnancy. Most drugs can cross the placenta and thus affect fetus as well as mother. Considering that the major stages in an embryo's development occur during life's first few weeks, if you're even *thinking* about being a mother, check with your doctor before taking any medication.

Are older people subject to any specific nutrient deficiencies?

As a general rule, they are. Aside from the fact that they consume more drugs than any other age group, they usually suffer from subclinical nutritional deficiencies because of their lifestyle and marginal intakes of key nutrients due to malabsorption, poor teeth, loneliness and other social problems.

Their most common nutrient deficiencies are folic acid, calcium, vitamin B12, vitamin D, and vitamin C. Also, because older people have a tendency to take stimulant laxatives on a regular basis, they lose large amounts of vitamins A, D, E, and K as well as calcium and potassium. (See section 250 for other drug-related vitamin deficiencies.)

I'm a 35-year-old woman and I work out daily. And I mean WORK OUT—weights, Nautilus, the whole nine yards. I know I must need more of certain nutrients than ordinary people do. But what are they?

They are vitamin A, vitamin B6, vitamin C; calcium (for optimal protein utilization), magnesium (lost through workout sweating and essential for muscle relaxation), and branched-chain amino acids (for repair and reconstruction). For extended energy to keep you going through workouts, some nutrients and foods are better than others. For instance: soy beans would be better for you than peas; whole wheat spaghetti better than white; beets preferable to carrots; grapefruit better than oranges, apples or bananas.

XIII

The Right Vitamin at the Right Time

169. Special Situation Supplements

Your body's vitamin needs are not always the same, and special situations require special food regimens and supplements. What follows is a list of such situations, most of them temporary, with supplement suggestions. For foods that offer specific vitamins and minerals, see sections 26 through 68. Once again, this information is not prescriptive. (See section 136 for MVP.)

170. Acne

This scourge of teenage years has been treated in a variety of ways, from X-rays to tetracycline, with only varying degrees of success. I encourage more natural treatment of the condition, and have been delighted by the results.

Multiple vitamin with minerals, but low in iodine (iodine can worsen acne conditions) 1 daily
Vitamin E (dry form), 400 IU 1–2 times daily
Beta carotene, 25,000 IU 1–2 times daily
Zinc, 50 mg. chelated, 1 tablet daily with a meal
Acidophilus liquid, 1–2 tbsp. 3 times daily, or 3–6 capsules 3 times daily.
Cysteine, 1 g. daily half an hour before meals with vitamin C, 1,000 mg. 3 times daily

Eliminate all processed foods. They are usually high in salt that has been iodized. (CAUTION: If you are taking a prescription medication for acne, do NOT take extra Vitamin A unless advised by your doctor.)

171. Athlete's Foot

Vitamin-C powder or crystals applied directly to the affected areas seems to help this fungus infection. Keep your feet dry, and out of shoes as much as possible, until the infection clears. Tea tree oil applied to the affected area can help as well.

172. Bad Breath

Along with proper brushing and flossing, you might try:

MVP (see section 136)
1 chlorophyll tablet or capsule 1–3 times daily
3 acidophilus capsules 3 times daily, or 1–2 tbsp. flavored acidophilus
Zinc, 50 mg. daily

173. Baldness or Falling Hair

There are no guarantees, but many people report a definite diminution of hair loss with this regimen:

Stress B complex twice daily
Choline and inositol, 1,000 mg. of each daily
Daily jojoba oil scalp massage and shampoo
A multiple-mineral formula with 1,000 mg. calcium and 500 mg. magnesium, 1 daily
Cysteine, 1,000 mg. daily
Vitamin C, 1,000 mg. 3 times daily

174. Bee Stings

The best thing to do about bee stings is try to avoid them. Vitamin B1 (thiamine) has been shown to be a fairly good insect repellant. Taken three times daily, 100 mg. B1 creates a smell at the level of your skin that insects do not like. If you're too late with the B1 and do get stung, 1,000 mg. vitamin C could help ease allergic reactions.

175. Bleeding Gums

The most effective vitamin therapy for bleeding gums is 1,000 mg. vitamin C complex, with bioflavonoids, rutin, and hesperidin, taken three times a day.

176. Broken Bones

If you've ever broken a bone, you know how frustrating it is waiting for it to mend. That feeling can be alleviated, and bone-healing accelerated, by increasing your calcium and vitamin-D intakes. Daily doses of 1,000–1,500 mg. calcium and 400–500 IU vitamin D are good.

177. Bruises

Vitamin C complex, 1,000 mg. with bioflavonoids, rutin, and hesperidin, taken three times daily will help prevent capillary fragility, those black-and-blue marks that occur when the tiny blood vessels beneath the skin rupture.

178. Burns

The most important thing to do with a burn is to put cold water on it immediately. To effectively stimulate wound-healing, 50 mg. zinc daily has been found useful and is worth trying. Vitamin C complex, 1,000 mg. with bioflavonoids, taken in the morning and evening is recommended to prevent infections. Vitamin E, 1,000 IU used orally and topically can help prevent scarring. Aloe vera gel or ointment is great first aid for minor burns.

179. Cold Feet

If you're embarrassed by wearing socks to bed all the time, you could try a good multimineral supplement with iodine twice a day, along with kelp tablets. The cold feet could be due to the fact that your thyroid glands are not producing enough thyroxin. Niacin and vitamin E can also help circulation.

180. Cold Sores and Herpes Simplex

Few things are more annoying than cold sores. The best supplement remedy I've discovered is:

Vitamin C complex, 1,000 mg. with bioflavonoids A.M. and P.M.
Lactobacillus acidophilus, 3 capsules 3 times a day
Vitamin-E oil, 28,000 IU applied directly to affected area
Lysine, 3 g. (3,000 mg.) daily (in divided doses) between meals (with water or juice—no protein)
As a preventive: Lysine, 500 mg. daily (with water or juice —no protein)
Vitamin C, 1,000 mg. A.M. and P.M.

181. Constipation

Everyone is bothered by constipation at some time or other. Usually this is due to a lack of bulk in the diet or because of certain medications, such as codeine. Harsh laxatives can rob the body of nutrients, as well as cause rebound constipation and laxative dependency, so natural remedies should be your first choice.

1 rounded teaspoon psyllium fiber (if not allergic to it) in juice or non-fat milk works wonders.
1 tbsp. acidophilus liquid 3 times daily
A vegetable laxative and sugar-free stool softener for a short time if necessary.
8–10 glasses of water daily (and a little exercise wouldn't hurt)

182. Cuts

Vitamin C complex, 1,000 mg. with bioflavonoids twice daily, along with 50 mg. zinc and 400 IU vitamin E.

183. Dry Skin

Vitamin-E (dry form) oil seems to work wonders when applied to dry skin, as do oils rich in vitamins A and D. As a dietary supplement, I recommend 200–400 IU vitamin E daily and 10,000 IU vitamin A (take for 5 days and stop for 2). I also recommend an MVP (see section 136) and omega-3 fatty acids, 1–3 capsules three times a day. (See section 91 for the complete lowdown on omega-3 fatty acids.)

If you don't want to take fish oils (omega-3 fatty acids are marketed primarily as EPA [eicosapentaenoic and docosahexaenoic acid]), other natural sources of omega-3 fatty acids are flaxseed oil, pumpkin oil, canola oil, and soy oil (1–2 teaspoons added to a salad dressing should help). Significant amounts are also found in English walnuts, Navy bean, kidney beans, soy beans and Great Northern beans.

184. Hangovers

To prevent them, take 1 B complex, 100 mg., before going out, 1 again while you're drinking, and another right before going to bed. (Alcohol destroys B complex.) Cysteine, 500 mg. with vitamin C, 1,500 mg., can help, too.

185. Hay Fever

Stress can cause hay fever attacks to worsen. If you're one of the many who suffer, you might find relief with 1 stress B complex twice daily, pantothenic acid 1,000 mg. three times daily, and the same dose of vitamin C, which has evidenced effective antihistamine properties.

186. Headaches

A surprisingly effective vitamin-mineral regimen for headaches is:

100 mg. niacin 3 times daily
100 mg. stress B complex (time release) twice daily
Calcium and magnesium (twice as much calcium as magnesium is the proper ratio), which are nature's tranquilizers

187. Heartburn

Over-the-counter antacids, such as Gelusil, Winger, Kolantyl, Maalox, Di-Gel, Rolaids, contain aluminum, which disturbs calcium and phosphorus metabolism. You'll probably be better off taking 5 lead-free bonemeal tablets daily (with food), multiple digestive enzymes one to three times daily, chewable papaya, and drinking fluids before or after meals, *not* during.

188. Hemorrhoids

Just about half the people over fifty are afflicted by hemorrhoids. Improper diet, lack of exercise, and straining at stool are all contributing factors. And coffee, chocolate, cola, and cocoa are accessories to the discomfort by promoting anal itching. If you're bothered by hemorrhoids, 1 tablespoon of unprocessed bran three times a day is helpful, along with 1,000 mg. vitamin C complex twice a day for healing membranes, and 3 acidophilus capsules three times a day (or 1 to 2 tablespoons of acidophilus liquid one to three times a day). Vitamin E oil, 28,000 IU per ounce, can be applied to affected area with a cotton swab.

189. Insomnia

Barbiturates, such as phenobarbital, Seconal, Nembutal, and Butisol, are strong sedatives and hypnotics that are too often prescribed for insomnia. Aside from being habit-forming and dangerous if mixed with other drugs, these barbiturates can also cause low calcium levels.

Tryptophan, on the other hand, is a natural amino acid that is essential to our bodies, and can help induce sleep.

An effective insomnia program:

1 chelated calcium and magnesium tablet 3 times daily and 3 tablets a half-hour before bedtime

Vitamin B6, 100 mg., and niacinamide 100 mg. work together to produce the brain chemical serotonin, which is essential for restful REM sleep.

Milk, as you know, is a fine natural source of calcium and tryptophan. Turkey is a good source of tryptophan. Therefore, an open-face turkey sandwich and a glass of warm milk before bedtime could be the sleep remedy of your life.

190. Itching

As an antihistamine, two 1,000-mg. vitamin-C tablets (time release) in the morning and in the evening, with food, might be helpful. I would also recommend a stress B complex with breakfast and dinner, 1,000 mg. pantothenic acid one to three times daily, and vitamin-E cream (20,000 IU per ounce) applied to afflicted area three times daily.

191. Jet Lag

So your plane from London lands at 9 A.M. and you're supposed to be at a meeting at 10 A.M. No problem, except for the fact that as far as your body is concerned, it's still only 4 A.M. and you should be asleep. Your best bet is to help your system catch up with your schedule by giving it the vitamins it needs.

Stress B complex (time release) A.M. and P.M. (start while still on the plane).

MVP with food, twice during flights of 5 or more hours
Vitamin E, 400 IU twice daily

If you're feeling run-down, as well as tired, be sure to take additional vitamin C.

NOTE: Intestinal gas expands at high altitudes, so pass on the beans and other gas-inducing foods right before and during the flight if you want to feel fit on arrival. Also, keep in mind that alcohol destroys vitamin B complex, which is one of the best jet-lag fighters around.

192. Leg pains

Increase your calcium. Try 1 chelated calcium and magnesium tablet with breakfast and dinner, along with a chelated multiple mineral. Vitamin E has been reported quite helpful in cases of charley horse. The most common doses for it are 400 to 1,000 IU vitamin E one to three times daily.

193. Menopause

Because of the risks that have recently been brought to light about estrogens, many women have been seeking other ways to relieve the discomforts of menopause. A good number of menopausal women have found that 200–400 IU vitamin E (mixed tocopherols) with selenium one to three times a day does indeed alleviate hot flashes. If you're at that time of life, MVP and a 600-mg. stress B complex twice a day also seem to help. Ginseng, 500 mg. A.M. and P.M.; calcium (500 mg.) and magnesium (250 mg.) 3 times daily. And for soothing, mood-elevating drinks, chamomile-based and passion flower (passiflora) teas.

194. Menstruation

Between the cramps and the bloating, menstruation is for most women a monthly annoyance. But this annoyance can dwindle down to a mere distraction once the discomfort is alleviated.

Vitamin B6, 50 mg. 3 times daily (most effective as a natural diuretic)
B complex, 100 mg. (time release) A.M. and P.M.
MVP
Evening Primrose Oil, 500 mg., 3 times daily

195. Motion Sickness

This is one condition where remedies are most effective if taken beforehand. Vitamins B1 and B6 are the nutrients of choice (in fact, many prenatal antinausea preparations contain vitamin B6). Taking 100 mg. B complex the night before you leave and the morning of your trip has been found to be effective by many queasy travelers.

Ginger root capsules taken 3 times daily work also!

196. Muscle Soreness

For that ache-all-over feeling after a workout, or just general muscle soreness, I've seen many people find relief with vitamin E, 400 to 800 IU taken one to three times daily. A chelated multiple mineral in the morning and at night also has helped.

197. The Pill

If you take oral contraceptives, not only are you more vulnerable than other women to blood clots, strokes, and heart attacks, but you're also more likely to be deficient in zinc, folic acid, vitamins C, B6, and B12 (which accounts for much nervousness and depression among pill-takers.)

Supplements are important:

MVP
Zinc, 50 mg. chelated, 1 tablet daily
Folic acid, 800 mcg. 1–3 times daily
B12, 2,000 mg. (time release or sublingual), A.M.
B6, 150 mg. 1–3 times daily

198. Poison Ivy

Vitamin-E oil or aloe vera gel applied externally can help healing. Two 1,000-mg. vitamin C complex (time release) taken A.M. and P.M. along with vitamin E, 400 to 1,000 IU, should alleviate the itching.

199. Polyps

These small annoying growths should definitely be seen by a doctor, and in most instances surgical removal is necessary. But as far as supplements go, Dr. Jerome J. DeCosse, professor and chairman of surgery at the Medical College of Wisconsin, used 3,000 mg. vitamin C (time release) daily on patients with polyps, and had noteworthy success with the treatment.

200. Postoperative Healing

After surgery, your body needs all the nutritional support it can get.

Vitamin E, 200–400 IU (dry form), 3 times daily
2 vitamin C complex, 1,000 mg. with bioflavonoids, hesperidin, and rutin A.M. and P.M.
High-potency multiple vitamin with chelated minerals A.M. and P.M.
High-potency multiple chelated mineral tablet A.M. and P.M.
Beta carotene, 25,000 IU daily
Chelated zinc, 15–50 mg. daily
This regimen can be used for 2 weeks before and 1 month after surgery.

201. Prickly Heat

Much like itching, prickly heat seems to respond to the antihistamine properties of vitamin C. (See section 190 for regimen.)

202. Prostate Problems

Chronic prostitis, where inflammation of the gland is often combined with infection, has been found to respond to treatment with zinc. (The prostate gland normally contains about ten times more zinc than any other organ in the body.) In many cases, symptoms have completely disappeared.

MVP
Chelated zinc, 50 mg. 3 times daily
Vitamin F or pumpkin seed capsules 3 caps 3 times daily

203. Psoriasis

Though many jokes have been made about this disease, it is no laughing matter to the millions who suffer from it. No one treatment has been found to be totally effective, but the following has met with much success:

MVP
Beta carotene, 25,000 IU daily
B complex, 100 mg. (time release) A.M. and P.M.
Rose hips vitamin C, 1,000 mg. A.M. and P.M. (this is in
    addition to the vitamin C called for in the MVP)
Vitamin E (dry form), 200–400 IU 3 times daily
3 vitamin-F or lecithin capsules 3 times daily
Selenium, 100 mcg. daily
Increase protein (preferably animal source)

204. Stopping Smoking

It's no mean feat to stop smoking, and your body knows it.
Those withdrawal symptoms are real. For the irritability that
occurs, take 1 B complex, 100 mg. (time release), with the
evening meal, and cysteine, 1,000 mg. daily. And don't
forget your MVP, and a dry vitamin E, 400 IU daily.

205. Sunburn

A good sunscreening preparation should always be used before exposing yourself to the sun's ultraviolet rays for any
length of time. What most people don't realize is that the sun
actually burns the skin, and bad burns can break the skin and
leave it vulnerable to infection.

It it's too late for preventives, try this:

Aloe vera gel applied 3–4 times daily
A PABA cream or vitamin-E cream (20,000 IU) also applied
    3–4 times daily
MVP
Additional vitamin C, 1,000 mg. A.M. and P.M. until burn
    heals

206. Teeth Grinding

People are usually unaware of grinding their teeth. It occurs
more often in children than adults, and most often during
sleep. MVP; B complex, 100 mg. A.M. and P.M.; and a few
bonemeal tablets nightly before sleep can help.

207. Varicose Veins

Age, lack of exercise, and chronic constipation are contributing factors to varicose veins. Watching your diet and exercising regularly can do a lot toward preventing them. MVP with an extra 1,000 mg. vitamin C complex twice daily has been found to help, along with 400 to 800 IU vitamin E.

208. Vasectomy

Men with vasectomies are more susceptible to infections and would be wise to take an additional 1,000 mg. vitamin C complex daily, along with regular MVP diet supplementation. Extra zinc, 15–50 mg. every day, is also a good idea.

209. Warts

They don't come from handling frogs, but they do seem to effectively disappear when treated with vitamin-E oil. The most successful regimen appears to be 28,000 IU vitamin E applied externally one to two times daily and 400 IU vitamin E (dry form) taken internally three times a day. Vitamin C complex, 1,000–2,000 mg. daily, can help build up the body's immunity and possibly prevent warts from occurring at all.

210. Any Questions About Chapter XIII?

You talk about digestive enzymes being helpful for heartburn. What are they and what do they do?

Enzymes, which can be purchased as supplements, can help your own digestive system assimilate the foods you eat. *Bromelain*, for instance, is a digestive enzyme from pineapple. *Cellulase* is an aid to digesting vegetable matter and breaking down food fiber. *Hydrochloric acid (HCl)* works in the stomach on tough foods, such as fibrous meats, vegetables, and poultry. (Betaine HCL is the best form available.) *Lipase* assists in fat digestion and *mylase* dissolves thousands of times its own weight in starches so you can more easily assimilate them. *Papain* is a protein-digesting enzyme (from papaya), and *prolase* is a concentrated protein-digesting enzyme derived from papain. (See section 187).

Is there a specific reason for your recommending ginseng in the treatment of menopause?

Definitely. Since estrogen replacement began in the 1960s, it has been linked to a 35% increase in uterine cancer. Ginseng contains estriol, an anticarcinogenic (cancer-fighting) variant of estrogen.

CAUTION: If you are using a nicotine gum to help you quit smoking, be aware that colas and coffee may be undermining your efforts. Studies done by the University of Kentucky and the National Institute on Drug Abuse's Addiction Research Center have found that consuming coffee, cola or acidic drinks before chewing nicotine gum *significantly inhibits its absorption*!

XIV

Getting Well and Staying That Way

211. Why You Need Supplements During Illness

During illness the body is under stress. Cells are destroyed, exhausted adrenal glands deprived of nutrients are unable to function properly, and the body's stress-fighting team of vitamin C, B6, folic acid, and pantothenic acid is severely depleted, zinc and vitamin C are also needed in greater amounts.

Because we require these vitamins to effectively utilize other nutrients and to keep our metabolism functioning all the time, our need for them is obviously increased when we're ill. And since we know that fever and stress rob our body of its most essential nutrients, the importance of supplements is self-evident.

Again, the following regimens are not intended as medical advice, only as a guide in working with your doctor.

212. Allergies

Allergies come in all shapes and sizes, with all sorts of symptoms, and you can contract them for just about anything. Nonetheless they take their nutritional toll, and supplements can help.

MVP (see section 136) A.M. and P.M.

Vitamin B complex, 100 mg. 3 times daily
Pantothenic acid, 1,000 mg. A.M. and P.M.

If you have an allergy, it would be a good idea to take a hard look at your present diet. Many allergies are caused by MSG, food coloring, additives, and preservatives.

213. Arthritis

Thousands of people suffer from this painful chronic condition. Because it puts so much stress on the body, vitamin-mineral supplementation is really essential.

MVP (see section 136)
Extra vitamin C, 1,000 mg. 1–3 times a day (if you're taking lots of aspirin, you're losing vitamin C)
B complex, 100 mg. 1–3 times a day
B12, up to 2,000 mcg. daily
Niacin up to 1 g. daily
1–3 yucca tabs 3 times daily
Pantothenic acid, 100 mg. 3 times daily
2–3 EPA capsules 2–3 times daily
1–3 alfalfa tabs 3 times daily
Copper, 2 mg. daily
Germanium, 50 mg., 1–3 times daily

214. Asthma

Asthma is a chronic allergic condition that affects the bronchial tubes. When an attack occurs, the muscle tissue of the tubes constricts spasmodically, squeezing the air passages and causing labored breathing and a feeling of suffocation. Allergies, heredity, and emotional stress have all been implicated as contributing factors to asthmatic conditions, but many nutrients have been found to provide remarkable natural relief.

MVP (see section 136) A.M. and P.M.
Extra vitamin C, 1,000 mg. 1–3 times daily
(CAUTION: Vitamin C that's buffered with calcium as-

corbate can interfere with the action of tetracyclines. A sodium ascorbate form of vitamin C can be used with tetracyclines, but not if you are on a sodium-restricted diet or taking steroids.)

Evening Primrose Oil, 2 500 mg. capsules, 3 times daily for 3 to 4 months; then 1 tablet 3 times daily. (If you are taking steroids, you won't benefit from EPO, because steroids interfere with EPO's action.)

Vitamin B15, 50 mg., 1 tablet daily for one month, then twice daily for the second month, and 3 times daily in the third month.
(Severe cases may require two 50 mg. tablets 3 times daily with food. Decrease dosage when positive reaction occurs.)

Glandulars (adrenal gland concentrates) 1–3 times daily, but not at night, because they might cause insomnia.
(CAUTION: Glandulars should not be taken by anyone who is allergic to beef or pork.)

Beta carotene (water soluble) 10,000–25,000 IU daily
Vitamin B2 (riboflavin) 100 mg., 3–4 times daily
Vitamin B5 (pantothenic acid) 1,000–2,000 mg. daily
Vitamin B6 (pyridoxine) 200 mg. 1–4 times daily
Vitamin E (dry form) 400–1,200 IU daily

215. Blood Pressure—High and Low

HIGH

Over sixty million Americans have high blood pressure, which has been intimately linked to heart attacks and strokes. The importance of keeping your blood pressure down cannot be overestimated, and there are a number of natural ways that can help.

• Talk slower (fast talkers often don't breath properly and this can result in elevated blood pressure)
• Reduce, if you are overweight (controlled, sensible dieting can significantly lower blood pressure in overweight individuals)

• Decrease sodium and increase potassium in your diet (see section 270 on hidden salt in foods)
• Decrease your sugar intake (see section 267)
• Eliminate caffeine (see section 242)
• Eat more onions and garlic
• Stop smoking
• Avoid stress or anxiety-provoking situations (jangling everyday noises, even loud televisions, can cause stress and elevate blood pressure).
• Exercise regularly (brisk walking) and get adequate rest.

Regimen

Lecithin granules, 3 tbsp. daily, or 3 caps 3 times daily
Potassium may be necessary if you are taking an antihyper-
    tensive, but check with your doctor to be sure it's not
    contraindicated for your particular medication.
MVP (see section 136)
Calcium 1,000 mg. daily
Magnesium 500 mg. daily
Vitamin E (dry form), 100 IU daily and work up to higher
    strengths (check with your doctor)
Garlic pills (deodorized) 1–3 daily

LOW

Low blood pressure, unless extreme, is a far better condition to have than its alternative. Nonetheless, hypotensives
often suffer from dizziness and occasional fainting spells and
blackouts.

Regimen
1–3 kelp tablets daily
(If you're taking thyroid medication, check with your doctor,
    as kelp might decrease the need for the amount you're
    currently taking.)
MVP (see section 136)

216. Bronchitis

This inflammation of the bronchial tube lining is quite common and extremely enervating. The stress it puts on the body is high, and even antibiotics are the bad guys as far as nutrients are concerned (see section 250).

Beta carotene 25,000 IU daily
Rose hips vitamin C, 1,000 mg. A.M. and P.M.
MVP (see section 136)
Vitamin E (dry form) 400 IU 1–3 times daily
Water, 6–8 glasses daily
3 acidophilus caps 3 times daily, or 1–2 tbsp. liquid 3 times
  daily

217. Candida Albicans

This yeast infection takes advantage of circumstances in the body that are conducive to its growth, and there are many. For example: antibiotics, birth control pills, cortisone, diabetes mellitus, nutritional deficiencies, chronic constipation or diarrhea, and physical or emotional stress.

Symptoms can range from all those associated with vaginitis (discharge, itching, bladder infection, menstrual irregularities and cramps) to severe depression, acne, anxiety, fatigue, nervousness, and mental confusion.

The first step in treating candida albicans is to deprive the body of all yeast-containing foods. For example: cheese, leavened breads, sour cream, buttermilk, beer, wine, cider, mushrooms, soy sauce, tofu, vinegar, dried fruits, melons, and frozen or canned juices.

If your doctor has not yet put you on a yeast fungus-killing drug, such as Nystatin, there are many natural and surprisingly effective dietary combatants. Among them are garlic, broccoli, cabbage, onions, plain yogurt, turnips and other vegetables.

And an effective supplement regimen would be:

MVP (see section 136) twice daily

Propolis, 500 mg. 3 times daily
Vitamin E (dry form) 200–400 IU daily
Free-form amino acids (balanced formula) daily
Caprylic acid supplement, 1–3 times daily
Acidophilus (yeast free) 1 capsule 3 times daily

218. Chicken Pox

This childhood staple is caused by a virus closely related to that of shingles. The fever and itching deplete a good amount of nutrients. Many mothers have found their children up and about faster by adding the following supplements to their diets.

Rose hips vitamin C, 500 mg. 3 times daily
Vitamin E (dry form), 100–200 IU 1–3 times daily
Beta carotene, 10,000 IU daily (check pediatrician for proper
    dosage according to age and weight).
Multivitamin and mineral A.M. and P.M.

219. Chronic Fatigue Syndrome

It's known by different names in different countries, but the common symptoms are: sudden onset, extreme fatigue, chills or low-grade fever, sore throat, tender lymph nodes, muscle pain, headaches, joint pain (without swelling), confusion, memory loss, visual disturbances, and sleep disorders, among others.

Two to five million Americans have been stricken with this illness—now being called "the disease of the nineties." The British and Canadians know it as "ME" (myalgic encephalomyelitis) and the Japanese refer to it as "low natural killer cell syndrome." In this country it's referred to as chronic fatigue immune dysfunction syndrome (CFIDS) or chronic fatigue syndrome (CFS).

Originally thought to be caused by the Epstein-Barr virus (the herpes virus that causes infectious mononucleosis), it is now known that CFS victims develop high amounts of antibodies to numerous other bugs.

According to a report in *Newsweek* magazine, Dr. Jay

Goldstein, a southern California physician, has theorized that the illness begins "when an unknown chemical or contagion damages the immune system . . . enabling viruses ordinarily held in check to start running amok. The immune system's helper T cells then start churning out tougher chemicals called 'cytokines,' which can themselves cause CFS symptoms." And the normal killer T cells that should attack anything foreign become mysteriously underactive (or, in some cases, unhealthily overactive).

There's no "silver bullet" treatment for CFS, but the body's immune system can use all the nutritional help it can get.

MVP (see section 136) A.M. and P.M.
Beta carotene, 10,000–25,000 IU daily, 5 days a week (stop for 2 days)
Vitamin C, 1,000 mg. 1–3 times daily
Vitamin E (dry form), 200–400 IU, 1–3 times daily
Ornithine, 2,000 mg. daily (taken with water, no protein, and on an empty stomach)
Cysteine, 1 daily with vitamin C (3 times as much vitamin C as cysteine)
Selenium, 50–100 mcg. daily
Zinc, chelated, 15–50 mg., 1–3 times daily
Propolis, 500 mg., 1–3 times daily
Evening Primrose Oil, 500 mg., 1–3 times daily

MY ADVICE:

Because the herpes virus is implicated, I'd suggest avoiding arginine-rich foods (see section 80). I'd also advise steering clear of refined carbohydrates, caffeine, alcohol, highly allergenic foods and foods containing artificial flavors, colors, and other additives that can stress the immune system.

220. Colds

No one pays too much attention to a cold, except the body —it pays plenty.

MPV (see section 136)
Rose hips vitamin C, 1,000 mg. 3 times daily

Beta carotene, 10,000 IU 1–3 times daily (take for 5 days
and stop for 2)
Vitamin E (dry form) 200–400 IU daily
Water, 6–8 glasses daily
3 acidophilus capsules 3 times daily, or 1–2 tbsp. liquid 3
times daily

221. Colitis

As a rule this illness is more common in women than men
and often is triggered by emotional upset. Alternating diarrhea
and constipation, as well as abdominal pain, are its distressing
hallmarks. Diet is of prime importance and vitamins are recommended.

MVP (see section 136)
Potassium, 99 mg. (elemental) 1–3 times daily
Raw cabbage juice (vitamin U), 1 glass 3 times daily
Water, 6–8 glasses daily
Aloe vera gel (for internal use), 1 tbsp. 3 times daily or 1–
3 capsules 3 times daily
3–6 acidophilus caps 3 times daily or 2 tbsp. liquid 3 times
daily
1 tbsp. bran flakes 3 times daily or 3–6 bran tablets

222. Diabetes

What happens in diabetes, primarily, is that the pancreas fails
to produce adequate insulin and the blood sugar rises uncon-
trollably. In mild cases diet alone can control the condition.
(Beware of hidden sugars. See section 268.) In severe cases,
replacement insulin is necessary. In all cases, the care of a
physician is essential.

Supplements that have aided diabetics are:

MVP (see section 136)
Glucose Tolerance Factor (GTF) chromium 200 mcg. Potas-
sium, 99 mg. 3 times daily
Chelated zinc, 50 mg. 1–3 times daily
Water, 6–8 glasses daily

223. Eye Problems

From simple inflammations to refraction difficulties to serious diseases, eye problems should never be ignored, nor should visits to the ophthalmologist be postponed. There are, however, generally beneficial supplements you can take.

Beta carotene, 25,000 IU 1–3 times daily
B complex, 100 mg. (time release) A.M. and P.M.
Rose hips vitamin C complex, 500 mg. A.M. and P.M.
Vitamin E (dry form) 400 IU A.M. and P.M.

224. Heart Conditions

With any heart condition, you should be under a doctor's care. Though the following supplements have been found to be quite safe and helpful, you should check with your physician to make sure they are not contraindicated in your particular case. (Vitamin E can increase the imbalance between the two sides of the heart for some people with rheumatic hearts.)

Vitamin B, 100 mg. (time release) A.M. and P.M.
Extra niacin, 100 mg. 1–3 times daily
Vitamin E (dry form) 400 IU, 1 daily
MVP (see section 136)
3 lecithin capsules or 3 tbsp. granules 3 times daily
Chrondroitin Sulphate A (CSA) daily
EPA and DHA, 1–3 capsules daily

HEART ATTACK *PREVENTION* TACTICS

• Decrease sugar and salt consumption.
• Stop smoking.
• Exercise regularly.
• Watch your weight.
• Practice relaxation techniques such as meditation and biofeedback to reduce stress.
• Decrease intake of saturated fats, hydrogenated oils and cholesterol.
• Eat more garlic, fresh fruit, and fish.

- Increase your soy protein intake (use in place of animal protein whenever possible).
- Get enough calcium and magnesium in your diet (supplements of 1,000 mg. calcium and 500 mg. magnesium daily are recommended).
- Be sure you're getting enough vitamins C, B6, and E.
- Supplement lecithin in your diet.
- Laughter is great medicine (not only does it release pent-up emotions and stress . . . it's fun and feels good, too).

225. Hypoglycemia

Though an estimated 20 to 40 million Americans have it, this disease is one of the most often undiagnosed. It is a condition of low blood sugar, and, like diabetes, presents a situation where the body is unable to metabolize carbohydrates normally. Since a hypoglycemic's system overreacts to sugar, producing too much insulin, the key to raising blood sugar levels is not by eating rapidly metabolized refined carbohydrates but by eating more complex carbohydrates and protein.

Recommended supplements:

Beta carotene and vitamin D capsules (10,000 and 400 IU) daily
Vitamin C, 500 mg. with or after each meal
Vitamin E, 100–200 IU 3 times daily
B complex, 50 mg. 3 times daily
Vitamin F, 1 capsule 3 times daily
Multiple mineral tab A.M. and P.M. (niacin as needed and tolerated; see section 44)
Pantothenic acid, 500 mg. twice daily
2 lecithin capsules (19 grains = 1,200 mg.) 3 times daily
Digestive enzymes if necessary
1 kelp tablet 3 times daily
3 acidophilus capsules or 1–2 tbsp. liquid 3 times daily
GTF chromium, 200 mcg. 3 times daily

226. Impetigo

Caused by germs similar to those that cause boils—staphylococcus or streptococcus—it occurs more in children than adults, but no one is immune. It often results from scratching and infecting insect bites, allowing the germs to get into broken skin.

Vitamin A and D capsules (10,000 and 400 IU) daily
    (reduce dose for child) for 5 days, then stop for 2
Vitamin E (dry form), 100–400 IU once a day
Rose hips vitamin C, 500 mg. A.M. and P.M.

227. Measles

You can get measles at any age, though it's more common among children. It is the most contagious of the communicable diseases. There is now a preventive vaccine for it, but the virus still manages to get a large number of the unprotected each year. The disease and rash can be mild, or severe with a heavy cough. Your body needs vitamins to help fight and recover from it.

Beta carotene, 10,000 IU (reduce dose for child) 1–3 times
    daily
Rose hips vitamin C, 500–1,000 mg. A.M. and P.M.
Vitamin E (dry form), 200–400 IU A.M. or P.M.

228. Mononucleosis

Commonly contracted by adolescents and young adults, mono (glandular fever) or "the kissing disease" as it is often called, can happen to anyone and can deplete the body of massive amounts of nutrients.

Diet is important and supplements are generally considered essential during the long convalescence.

MVP (see section 136) A.M. and P.M. with food
Extra vitamin C, 1,000 mg. A.M. and P.M. for 3 months
Potassium, 99 mg. 3 times daily
B complex, 100 mg. (time release) A.M. and P.M.
Zinc, chelated, 15–50 mg. daily
Propolis, 500 mg. A.M. and P.M.

229. Mumps

A vaccine for mumps exists, but the disease is still quite common and just as nutritionally debilitating. The virus can spread through the patient's entire system, involving not only the salivary glands but the testicles or ovaries, the pancreas, the nervous system, and sometimes even the heart.

Beta carotene, 10,000 IU (reduce dose for children) 1–3 times daily for 5 days, then stop for 2
Rose hips vitamin C, 500–1,000 mg. twice daily
Vitamin E, 200–400 IU (dry form) daily

230. P. M. S. (Premenstrual Syndrome)

For two to ten days before the onset of menstruation, millions of women are affected by a wide range of physical discomforts and mood disorders—from bloating, depression, and insomnia to severe pains, uncontrolled rages, crying spells, and even suicidal depression. This is known as P. M. S., premenstrual syndrome.

FOODS AND BEVERAGES TO AVOID

- Salt and salty foods (see section 271)
- Licorice (it stimulates the production of aldosterone which causes further retention of sodium and water)
- Cold foods and beverages (these adversely affect abdominal circulation and worsen cramping)
- Caffeine in all forms (see section 241) Caffeine increases the craving for sugar, wastes B vitamins, washes out potassium and zinc, and increases hydrochloric acid (HC1) secretions which can cause abdominal irritation.
- Astringent dark teas (tannin binds important minerals and prevents absorption in the digestive tract)
- Alcohol (adversely affects blood sugar, depletes magnesium levels, and can interfere with proper liver function, which can aggravate P. M. S.)
- Spinach, beet greens, and other oxalate-containing vegetables (oxalates make minerals nonassimilable, difficult to be properly absorbed)

FOODS AND BEVERAGES TO INCREASE

• Strawberries, watermelon (eat seeds), artichokes, asparagus, parsley, and watercress (these are natural diuretics)
• Raw sunflower seeds, dates, figs, peaches, bananas, potatoes, peanuts, and tomatoes (rich in potassium)
• Try Don Quai, it's an herb known as the female ginseng and can improve circulation, regulate liver function, and help remove excess water from the system.

Suggested supplements
Vitamin B6, 50–300 mg. daily (work up from 50 mg. gradually)
MVP (see section 136)
Magnesium, 500 mg. and calcium 250 mg. daily
(Yes, with P.M.S. it is twice as much magnesium as calcium, because a magnesium deficiency causes many of the P.M.S. symptoms.)
Vitamin E (dry form), 100–400 IU daily
Pantothenic acid (vitamin B5), 1,000 mg. (1 g.) daily
Evening Primrose Oil, 500 mg., 1–3 times daily
And exercise! Aside from the fact that this will improve abdominal circulation, perspiration helps remove excess fluids.
Brisk walking for 30 minutes twice daily and/or swimming are highly recommended.

231. Shingles

Shingles (herpes zoster) is caused by a virus much like the one that causes chicken pox. But where chicken pox causes a general skin eruption, shingles usually erupts along a nerve path. Differences aside, the nutritional deficit caused by both diseases is high.

Beta carotene, 25,000
Vitamin B complex, 100 mg. (time release) A.M. and P.M.
Rose hips vitamin C with bioflavonoids, 1,000–2,000 mg. A.M. and P.M.
Vitamin D, 1,000 IU daily for 5 days, then stop for 2

232. Tonsillitis

An inflammation of the tonsils that can afflict any age group, though it is more common in children. Good nutrition and supplements have been effective in preventing it as well as recovering from it.

MVP (see section 136) A.M. and P.M. with food
Beta carotene, 10,000 IU (reduce dose for children) 1–3 times daily
Extra vitamin C complex, 1,000 mg. A.M. and P.M.
Vitamin E (dry form) 200–400 IU daily
3 acidophilus caps or 1–2 tbsp. 3 times daily
Water, 6–8 glasses daily

233. Ulcers

There are two types of peptic ulcer, one in the stomach and the other in the duodenum, usually associated with excessive acidity in the stomach juices (see section 9). For both of these conditions, supplements have been found helpful.

Beta carotene, 25,000
Vitamin B complex, 100 mg. (time release) A.M. and P.M.
Rose hips vitamin C with bioflavonoids, 1,000 mg. (time release) A.M. and P.M.
High-potency multiple mineral A.M. and P.M.
Aloe vera gel, 1–3 capsules or 1–3 tbsp. liquid daily

234. Venereal Disease

Syphilis and gonorrhea are still among the most widespread venereal diseases, and though sulfa drugs, penicillin, tetracycline, erythromycin, and newer antibiotics are the most effective treatments for them, these remedies cause almost as much need for supplements as the diseases themselves.

MVP (see section 136)
3 acidophilus capsules or 1–2 tbsp. liquid 3 times daily
Extra vitamin C 1,000 mg. A.M. and P.M.
Vitamin K, 100 mcg. daily if on extended antibiotic program

Genital herpes, America's #1 venereal disease of the '80s, has, unfortunately, made it to the '90s. Like herpes simplex type I, which causes cold sores (see section 180), type II herpes, which causes genital infection, also seems to respond well to lysine-rich foods. As a preventative, it wouldn't be a bad idea to increase your intake of cottage cheese, flounder, tuna fish, peanuts, raw chick peas (garbanzos), and soybeans. *Acyclovir* (ZOVIRAX) is a drug that—at this writing—seems to be effective in blocking herpes replication, but the final results are not yet in. Meanwhile, I'd suggest a preventative supplement of lysine, 500 mg. daily (with water or juice— no protein) and vitamin C, 1,000 mg. A.M. and P.M. If you already have the virus: Lysine, 3 g. (3,000 mg.) 3 times daily—in divided doses—between meals.

CAUTION: If you have symptoms of herpes virus simplex I or II, avoid supplementation of arginine and argine-rich foods (see section 80).

235. Any Questions About Chapter XIV?

When you talk about blood pressure, what's normal and what's "high"?

You are considered within the normal range if your higher (systolic) pressure is between 100 and 140, and your lower (diastolic) pressure is in the range of 60 to 90. For a healthy young adult, a reading of 120/80 is considered normal.

XV

It's Not All in Your Mind

236. How Vitamins and Minerals Affect Your Moods

The first scientifically documented discovery to relate mental illness to diet occurred when it was found that pellagra (with its depression, diarrhea, and dementia) could be cured with niacin. After that, it was shown that supplementation with the whole B complex produced greater benefits than niacin alone.

Evidence of biochemical causes for mental disturbances continues to mount. Experiments have shown that symptoms of mental illness can be switched off and on by altering vitamin levels in the body.

Even normal, happy people can become depressed when made deficient in niacin or folic acid.

Dr. R. Shulman, reporting in the *British Journal of Psychiatry*, found that forty-eight out of fifty-nine psychiatric patients had folic-acid deficiencies. Other research has shown that the majority of the mentally and emotionally ill are deficient in one or more of the B-complex vitamins or vitamin C. And even normal, happy people have been found to become depressed and experience other symptoms of emotional disturbance when made niacin or folic-acid deficient.

237. Nutrients That Combat Depression, Anxiety and Stress

Vitamin B1 (thiamine)	Above-average amounts can help alleviate depression and anxiety attacks.
Vitamin B6 (pyridoxine)	Aids in the proper production of natural antidepressants such as dopamine and norepinephrine.
Pantothenic acid	A natural tension-reliever.
Vitamin C (ascorbic acid)	Essential for combatting stress.
Vitamin B12 (cobalamin)	Helps relieve irritability, improve concentration, increase energy, and maintain a healthy nervous system.
Choline	Sends nerve impulses to brain and produces a soothing effect.
Vitamin E (dry form) (alpha-tocopherol)	Aids brain cells in getting needed oxygen.
Folic acid (folacin)	Deficiencies have been found to be contributing factors in mental illness.

Zinc	Promotes mental alertness and aids in proper brain function.
Magnesium	The antistress mineral, necessary for proper nerve functioning.
Manganese	Helps reduce nervous irritability.
Niacin	Vital to the proper function of the nervous system.
Calcium	Alleviates tension, irritability, and promotes relaxation.
Tyrosine	Helps increase the rate at which brain neurons produce the antidepressants dopamine and norepinephrine.
Tryptophan	Works with vitamin B6, niacin, and magnesium to synthesize the brain chemical serotonin, a natural tranquilizer.
Phenylalanine	Necessary for the brain's release of the antidepressants dopamine and norepinephrine.

238. Other Drugs Can Add to Your Problem

Alcohol is a nerve depressant. If you take tranquilizers and a drink, the combination of the two can cause a severe depression—or even death.

> If you're on the pill and depressed,
> it's not surprising.

If you take a sedative with an antihistamine (such as any found in over-the-counter cold preparations) you might find yourself experiencing tremors and mental confusion.

Oral contraceptives deplete the body of B6, B12, folic acid, and vitamin C. If you're on the pill and depressed, it is not surprising. Your need for B6, necessary for normal tryptophan metabolism, is fifty to a hundred times a non-pill-user's requirement.

DRUGS AND MEDICATIONS THAT YOU MIGHT NOT THINK WOULD CAUSE DEPRESSION—BUT CAN

The following list is not all-inclusive, but all mentioned deplete the body—in varying degrees—of important mood-regulating nutrients. (See section 250.) So if you're taking medication to get well and feeling down, there's a good chance that it's not all in your mind!

- Adrenocorticoids
- Ammonium chloride
- Arthritis medicines
- Antihistamines
- Antihypertensives
- Baclofen
- Barbiturates
- Beta-blockers (INDERAL)
- Chloramphenicol
- Diuretics

- Estrogens
- Fluorides
- Glutethimide (DORIDEN)
- Indomethacin (INDOCIN)
- Isoniazid (INH, NYDRAZID)
- Laxatives, lubricant
- Meprednisone (BETAPAR)
- Methotrexate (MEXATE)
- Nitrofurantoin (FURADANTIN, MACRODANTIN)
- Oral contraceptives
- Penicillamine (CUPRIMINE)
- Penicillin (all forms)
- Phenylbutazone (AZOLID, BUTAZOLIDIN)
- Phenytoin (DILANTIN)
- Potassium supplements
- Prednisone
- Procainamide
- Propoxyphene (DARVON)
- Pyrimethamine (DARAPRIM)
- Sulfonamides, systemic
- Tetracyclines
- Triamterene (DYRNIUM)
- Trimethobenzamide (TIGAN)

239. Any Questions About Chapter XV?

As the producer of a daily television show, I live in Stress City. I eat sporadically, so I'd like to know if there are some foods that would be better for me than others.

There are. Whether it's a power breakfast or an on-the-set lunch, go for the complex carbohydrates instead of the protein. In other words, take the pasta, rice or cereal instead of the steak and eggs. Complex carbohydrates help boost your brain levels of the chemical *serotonin*, making you calmer and less stressed—but no less alert.

Every once in a while I find myself depressed when there's really nothing in my life to be depressed about. I'm a 29-

year-old male, happily married, and I don't know why I got into these depressions. Could there be a dietary reason?

Absolutely! Especially if you're consoling yourself with sugar-rich foods. Sugar, be it in refined carbohydrates, alcohol, or whatever, can deplete your body of B vitamins, especially vitamin B1, which can bring on depression. Amino acids (see section 75–77) such as tyrosine, tryptophan and phenylalanine can all be used as anti-depressants. Check with your doctor, but I'd recommend 500–2,000 mg. (2 g.) of a combination of these amino acids, taken at bedtime or in the morning, with water or juice (no protein).

XVI

Drugs and You

240. Let's Start With Caffeine

There are no doubts about it, caffeine is a powerful drug.
That's right, *drug*. Chances are you're not just enjoying your
daily coffees or colas, you're addicted to them.

> Caffeine is the most psychoactive
> drug in the world.

Caffeine acts directly upon the central nervous system. It
brings about an almost immediate sense of clearer thought
and lessens fatigue. It also stimulates the release of stored
sugar from the liver, which accounts for the "lift" coffee,
cola, and chocolate (the caffeine big three) give. But these
benefits may be far outweighed by the side effects:

• The release of stored sugar places heavy stress on the endocrine system. (Eventually, adrenal exhaustion can occur,
resulting in hypoglycemia.)
• Heavy coffee drinkers often develop nervousness or become jittery.
• Daily intake adds up over a year, and a lot of caffeine
accumulates in the body's fat tissue—and is not easily eliminated.
• Coffee-drinking housewives demonstrated symptoms typ-

ical of drug withdrawal when switched to a decaffeinated beverage.

• Dr. John Minton, professor of surgery at Ohio State University and specialist in cancer oncology, has found that excessive intake of methylxanthines (active chemicals in caffeine) can cause benign breast disease and prostate problems.

• Caffeine can rob the body of B vitamins, especially inositol, as well as vitamin C, zinc, potassium, and other minerals.

• Coffee increases the acidity in your gastrointestinal tract and can cause rectal itching.

• Many doctors consider caffeine a culprit in hypertensive heart disease.

• The British medical journal *Lancet* reported a strong relationship between coffee consumption and cancer of the bladder and the lower urinary tract.

• People who drink five cups of coffee daily have a 50 percent greater chance of having heart attacks than non-coffee drinkers.

• The *Journal of the American Medical Association* reports a disease called caffeinism, with symptoms of appetite loss, weight loss, irritability, insomnia, feelings of flushing, chills, and sometimes a low fever.

• Caffeine has been shown to interfere with DNA replication.

• The Center for Science in the Public Interest advises pregnant women to stay away from caffeine, since studies have shown that the amount contained in about four cups of coffee per day causes birth defects in test animals.

• High doses of caffeine will cause laboratory animals to go into convulsions and then die.

• Can dangerously increase heart rate and blood pressure when taken with decongestants or pulmonary bronchodilators such as the inhalers Proventil, Ventolin, Bronkaid, and Primatine.

Caffeine can be highly toxic (the lethal dose estimated to be around 10 g.). New research shows that one quart of coffee consumed in three hours can destroy much of the body's thiamine.

241. You're Getting More Than You Think

The following table shows the amount of caffeine (in milligrams) consumed in specific beverages and drugs:

BEVERAGE	12-OUNCE CAN OR BOTTLE
Coca-Cola	64.7 mg.
Dr. Pepper	60.9 mg.
Mountain Dew	54.7 mg.
Diet Dr. Pepper	54.2 mg.
Tab	49.4 mg.
Pepsi-Cola	43.1 mg.
R.C. Cola	33.7 mg.
Diet R.C.	33.0 mg.
Diet-Rite	31.7 mg.

Coffee	Per Serving
Instant	66.0 mg.
Percolated	110.0 mg.
Dripolated	146.0 mg.

Tea Bags	
Black 5-minute brew	46.0 mg.
Black 1-minute brew	28.0 mg.

Loose Tea	
Black 5-minute brew	40.0 mg.
Green 5-minute brew	35.0 mg.
Cocoa	13.0 mg.

DRUGS	PER PILL
Anacin (also available without caffeine)	32.0 mg.
Bio Slim T capsules	140.0 mg.
Cafergot	100.0 mg.
Dexatrim (also available without caffeine)	200.0 mg.
Empirin	32.0 mg.
Emprazil	30.0 mg.

Excedrin	65.0 mg.
(Excedrin PM has no caffeine, but does have an antihistamine.)	
Florinal	130.0 mg.
Midol	32.4 mg.
NoDoz	100.0 mg.
Soma Compound	32.0 mg.
Triminicin	30.0 mg.
Vanquish	33.0 mg.
Vivarin	200.0 mg.

242. Caffeine Alternatives

Decaffeinated coffee is *not* the best solution to the caffeine problem. Trichlorethylene, which was first used to remove caffeine, was found to cause a high incidence of cancer in test animals. Though the manufacturers have switched to methylene chloride, which is safer, it, too, introduces the same carbon-to-chloride bond into the body that is characteristic of so many toxic insecticides.

> Ginseng can give you a
> real lift.

Regular tea is not the answer either, since that has nearly as much caffeine. But herb teas can be quite invigorating, and most natural-food stores have a wide variety to choose from. Then, too, ginseng can give you a real lift, much like the one you get from caffeine, without the side effects.

Colas, diet or regular, have become as popular as coffee for those who enjoy the caffeine boost. Try substituting club soda or mineral water, or even a flavored soda if you must. You won't get the caffeine lift, but you'll be doing your body a big favor.

243. What Alcohol Does to Your Body

Alcohol is the most widely used drug in our society, and because it is so available, most people don't think of it as a drug. But it is; and if misused, it can cause a lot of damage to your body.

- Alcohol is not a stimulant, but actually a sedative-depressant of the central nervous system.
- It is capable of rupturing veins.
- It does not warm you up, but causes you to feel colder by increasing perspiration and body heat loss.
- It destroys brain cells by causing the withdrawal of necessary water from them.
- It can deplete the body of vitamins B1, B2, B6, B12, folic acid, vitamin C, vitamin K, zinc, magnesium, and potassium.
- Four drinks a day are capable of causing organ damage.
- It can hamper the liver's ability to process fat.

244. What You Drink and When You Drink It

Just because the alcohol content varies in different beverages, don't be fooled. It is true that beer has only about 4 percent alcohol, wine about 12 percent, and whiskey up to 50 percent; but a can of beer, a glass of wine, and a shot of whiskey all have virtually the identical inebriation potential. In other words, four cans of beer can get you just as tipsy as four shots of tequila.

> A Bloody Mary at breakfast is
> more harmful than a whiskey
> sour at dinner.

Surprisingly, what you drink doesn't matter nearly as much as *when* you drink it. Dr. John D. Palmer, of the University of Massachusetts, reports that the length of time alcohol remains in circulation in your blood varies throughout the day. Which means, of course, the more time the alcohol spends in your blood, the more time it has to act on your brain cells. Between 2 A.M. and noon are the most vulnerable hours, while late afternoon to early evening are the least. A cocktail at dinner will be burned away 25 percent faster than a Bloody Mary at breakfast, and the last drink of a party, consumed after midnight, is metabolized relatively more slowly than the ones that preceded it, producing a more lasting rise in blood alcohol.

245. Vitamins To Decrease Your Taste For Alcohol

> Heavy drinkers can break
> the habit.

Research at the University of Texas has shown that if alcoholic mice are fed nutritious, vitamin-enriched diets, they quickly lose their interest in alcohol. This seems to hold true for people, since heavy drinkers have been able to break the habit—and even lose interest—with the right diet and proper nutritional supplements. Vitamins A, D, E, C, and all the B vitamins—especially B12, B6, and B1—along with calcium and magnesium, choline, inositol, niacin, and a very high-protein diet have brought about the best results. Dr. H. L. Newbold, of New York, who has worked with alcoholics, recommends building up to 5 glutamine capsules (200 mg.) —not glutamic acid—three times a day to control drinking, and working with a good nutritionally oriented doctor for the best all-around regimen. (See section 293.)

In experiments done by the Veterans' Administration, a supplement of tryptophan, given in larger concentrations than occur in a normal diet, has helped alcoholics achieve normal sleeping patterns by reducing or normalizing the fragmentation of dreaming (REM). Because serotonin, a natural tranquilizer substance in the brain, has been shown to be reduced in alcoholism, tryptophan (500 mg. to 3 g. at bedtime) can help alcoholics stay dry by relieving some of the symptoms of alcohol-related body chemistry disorders. (NOTE: At the time of this writing, tryptophan was not available as an over-the-counter supplement in the United States or Canada.)

246. The Lowdown on Marijuana and Hashish

Marijuana and hashish come from the hemp plant *cannabis sativa*. The marijuana consists of the chopped leaves and stems of the plan, while the hashish is formed from the resin scraped from the flowering tops.

Both of these drugs can be either smoked or eaten. If smoked, the effects usually last from 1 to 3 hours. If eaten, they can last from 4 to 10 hours, though it takes longer for the user to feel them.

Unlike other illicit drugs, marijuana and hashish have the unusual property of "reverse tolerance," meaning that seasoned users need less of the drug to get high than first-timers. Essentially, these drugs act as intoxicants, relaxants, tranquilizers, appetite stimulants, and mild hallucinogens, though effects very with the individual.

The smoking of one joint can cause a rise in blood pressure, an increased heartbeat, a lowering of body temperature and vitamin C levels in the blood. It has been found, too, that smoking marijuana during pregnancy can cause low birth weight in newborns and increase the risk of lung cancer.

CAUTION: Toxic psychosis can occur if *cannabis* is eaten and the user hasn't been able to judge the amount ingested.

Supplements and foods that can help users

Increase your intake of citrus fruits and green leafy vegetables. (Those "munchies" usually give you more than your share of refined sugars and carbohydrates, meaning that you've deprived yourself of necessary B vitamins.)

Vitamin C (time release), 1,000 mg. A.M. and P.M.

Vitamin E, 100–400 IU 1 to 3 times daily to protect your lungs

247. Cocaine Costs a Lot More Than You Think—In More Ways Than One

Cocaine is a vasoconstrictor, a stimulant of the central nervous system, and potentiates the effects of nerve stimulation.

Applied externally, it blocks nerve impulses and produces a numbing sensation.

> The wrong "cut" can kill.

What users get—no matter how much they pay—is rarely more than 60 percent pure cocaine. The rest is the "cut," which is used by dealers to dilute or enhance the drug for more profit. Some cuts are relatively harmless: lactose, dextrose, inositol (a B vitamin), and mannitol. Other nondrug cuts such as cornstarch, talcum powder, and flour can be dangerous because they are basically insoluble in blood and can clot up in the body. *Benzocaine*, which is pharmacologically active, can also cause blood clots and serious complications when used as a cut for cocaine.

Because the drug is absorbed rapidly through the mucous membranes, nasal inhalation is the most popular form of taking cocaine, though it is also often applied locally under the tongue and eyelids, and on the genital region. It can also be injected intravenously or smoked in a process called "freebasing," or as crack, which is cocaine, baking soda, and water distilled into an instantly smokable "rock."

The short-lived effects of coke (about ½ hour) are usually euphoria, feelings of psychic energy and self-confidence, but then more of the drug is necessary to recapture the high. Dependence is intense.

Aside from causing nosebleeds, rapid heartbeat, cold sweats, appetite loss, and in some cases the feeling that gnats or bugs are crawling on you, cocaine can cause convulsions, vomiting, anaphylactic shock, and death. Its toxicity is unpredictable. Even small doses with the wrong cut or taken by susceptible individuals can be lethal.

Supplements and foods to help users
High-potency multiple vitamin and mineral A.M. and P.M.
High-potency multiple mineral A.M. and P.M.
Vitamin C, 1,000 mg., vitamin E, 200–400 IU, and vitamin
B complex, 100 mg., all 1–3 times daily

248. Help for Coming Down or Kicking the Cocaine Habit

Tyrosine, an amino acid that's usually found in meat and wheat (see section 82), has been found to alleviate the depression, fatigue, and irritability that make quitting cocaine so difficult. At Fair Oaks Hospital in Summit, NJ, addicts took the amino acid in their orange juice for 12 days. They also took vitamin C, the B vitamins (thiamine, niacin, and riboflavin), and tyrosine hydroxylase, the enzyme that helps the body use tyrosine. The results were remarkably effective.

249. Whether Rx or Over-the-Counter, There Are Alternatives to Drugs

Americans consume over 1.5 million pounds of tranquilizers, more than 800,000 pounds of barbiturates, and well over 4 million pounds of antibiotics a year. Are all these drugs necessary? Probably not; but when people pay for a visit to their doctor, they expect to walk away with a prescription.

But there are alternatives, which orthomolecular physicians and nutritionally minded individuals are trying before resorting to drugs.

> Inositol and pantothenic acid
> instead of sleeping pills

Dr. Robert C. Atkins, author of *Dr. Atkins' Diet Revolution*, has his patients try pantothenic acid and about 2,000 mg. of inositol as sleep-inducers, instead of Seconal, Nembutal, Butisol, or other barbiturate sleeping pills. He has also had success using B15 to control blood sugar, and B13 (oratic acid) to lower high blood pressure.

So before you pop that next pill, you might want to consider some natural alternatives.

> Inositol and pantothenic acid
> instead of sleeping pills

DRUG	NATURAL ALTERNATIVES
Antacids	Papaya and multiple digestive enzymes
Antibiotics and antihistamines	Garlic, vitamin C, and (yep, it's true) chicken soup have amazing antibiotic and antihistamine properties. Other fine infection-fighters are vitamin A, pantothenic acid, and folic acid.
Antidepressants	Choline, calcium, and magnesium; vitamins B1, B6, and B12, L-tryptophan and L-phenylalanine
Antidiarrhesis	Carrots, niacin, and *lactobacillus acidophilus* yogurt for diarrhea caused by antibiotics
Antinauseants	Vitamins B1 and B6 can help alleviate nausea due to motion or morning sickness. Niacin and vitamin P can help in the treatment of dizziness and queasiness due to diseases of the inner ear.
Decongestants	Vitamin A, C, P, garlic, and potassium
Diuretics (water pills)	Alfalfa and vitamin B6 can work as natural diuretics
Laxatives	Vitamin C, vitamins B1, B2, B6, and B12, potassium, acidophilus, alfalfa, bran, and water
Tranquilizers (sedatives, relaxants, etc.)	Choline, vitamins B1, B6, B12, niacin, calcium, and magnesium; manganese, zinc, pantothenic acid and inositol, and L-tryptophan

Aspirin can *triple* the excretion
rate of vitamin C.

250. The Great Medicine Rip-Off

More than ever before, Americans are gulping down drugs. What most people don't realize is that a lot of these medications—prescription as well as over-the-counter—are taking as much as they're giving, at least nutritionally. All too often the drugs either stop the absorption of nutrients or interfere with the cells' ability to use them.

A recent study showed that ingredients found in common over-the-counter cold, pain, and allergy remedies actually lowered the blood level of vitamin A. Since vitamin A protects and strengthens the mucous membranes lining the nose, throat, and lungs, a deficiency could give bacteria a cozy home to multiply in, prolonging the illness the drug was meant to alleviate.

> Aspirin can *triple* the excretion
> rate of vitamin C.

Aspirin, the household wonder drug, the most common ingredient in pain-relievers, cold and sinus remedies, is a vitamin-C thief. Even a small amount can *triple* the excretion rate of vitamin C from the body. It can also lead to a deficiency of folic acid and vitamin B, which could cause anemia as well as digestive disturbances.

Corticosteroids (cortisone, prednisone), used for easing arthritis pain, skin problems, blood and eye disorders, and asthma, have been found to be related to lowered zinc levels.

According to a study that appeared in the *Postgraduate Medical Journal*, a significant number of people who take barbiturates have low calcium levels.

Laxatives and antacids, taken by millions, have been found to disturb the body's calcium and phosphorus metabolism. And any laxative taken to excess can deplete large amounts of potassium as well as vitamins A, D, E, and K.

Diuretics, commonly prescribed for high blood pressure, and antibiotics are also potassium thieves.

The following is a list of drugs that induce vitamin defi-

ciencies and the vitamins they deplete. Look it over before
you take your next medicine.

THIEVING DRUG	NUTRIENTS DEPLETED
Alcohol (including alcohol-containing cough syrups, elixirs, and OTC medications such as NYQUIL	Vitamins A, B1, B2, biotin, choline, niacin, vitamin B15, folic acid, & magnesium
Ammonium Chloride (e.g., AMBENYL, EXPECTORANT, TRIAMINICOL, DECONGESTANT COUGH SYRUP, P.V. TUSSIN SYRUP)	Vitamin C
Antacids (e.g., MAALOX, MYLANTA, GELUSIL, TUMS, ROLAIDS	B complex & Vitamin A
Anticoagulants (e.g., COUMADIN, DICUMAROL, PANWARFIN)	Vitamins A & K
Antihistamines (e.g., CHLORTRIMETON, PYRIBENZAMINE)	Vitamin C
Aspirin (and remember, APC drugs contain *aspirin*)	Vitamins A, B complex, C; calcium, potassium
Barbiturates (e.g., PHENOBARBITAL, SECONAL, NEMBUTAL, BUTISOL, TUINAL)	Vitamins A, D, folic acid, & C
Caffeine (present in all APC medicines)	B1, inositol & biotin; potassium, zinc, can also

	inhibit calcium & iron assimilation Vitamin K & niacin
Chloramphenicol (CHLOMYCETIN)	
Cholestyramine (QUESTRAN)	Vitamins A, D, E, and K, and potassium
Cimetidine (TAGAMET)	Vitamin B1
Clofibrate (ATROMID-S)	Vitamin K
Colchicine (COLBENEMID)	B12, A, and potassium
Diethylstilbestrol (DES)	Vitamin B6
Diuretics (e.g., DIURIL, HYDRODIURIL, SER-AP-ES, LASIX)	B complex, potassium, magnesium, & zinc
Fluorides	Vitamin C
Glutethimide (DORIDEN)	Folic acid
Indomethacin (INDOCIN)	Vitamins B1 & C
Isoniazid (INH, NYDRAZID)	B6
Kanamycin (KANTREX)	Vitamins K & B12
Laxatives, lubricant (e.g., castor oil, mineral oil)	Vitamins A, D, E, K, calcium, & phosphorus
Meprednisone (BETAPAR)	Vitamins B6, C, zinc, & potassium
Methotrexate (MEXATE)	Folic acid
Nitrofurantoin (e.g., FURADANTIN, MACRODANTIN)	Folic acid

Oral contraceptives (e.g., BREVICON, DEMULEN, ENOVID, LO/OVRAL, NORINYL, OVRAL)	Folic acid, vitamins C, B2, B6, B12, & E
Penicillamine (CUPRIMINE)	Vitamin B6
Penicillin (in all its forms)	Vitamins B6, niacin, & K
Phenylbutazone (e.g., AZOLID, BUTAZOLIDIN)	Folic acid
Phenytoin (DILANTIN)	Folic acid & vitamin D
Prednisone (e.g., METICORTEN, PREDNISOLONE, ORASONE)	Vitamins B6, D, C, zinc, & potassium
Propantheline (PRO-BANTHINE)	Vitamin K
Pyrimethamine (DARAPRIM)	Folic acid
Sulfonamides, systemic (e.g., BACTRIM, GANTANOL, TANTRISIN, SEPTRA)	Folic acid, vitamins K & B2
Sulfonamides and topical steroids (e.g., AEROSPORIN, CORTISPORIN, NEOSPORIN, POLYSPORIN)	Vitamins K, B12, & folic acid
Tetracyclines (e.g., ACHROMYCIN-V, SUMYCIN, TETRACYN)	Vitamin K, calcium, magnesium, & iron
Tobacco	Vitamins C, B1, and folic acid; calcium
Trifluoperazine (STELASINE)	Vitamin B12
Triamterene (DYRENIUM)	Folic acid

251. Any Questions About Chapter XVI?

I know that coffee can give you the jitters, but I've switched to drinking decaffeinated, and still find myself getting moody and uptight. Can such a small amount of caffeine do this?

Caffeine isn't the only substance in coffee that has an effect on behavior. There is, though not yet identified, another substance in both regular and decaffeinated coffee (but not in tea) which blocks the normal activity of brain opiates (endorphins), which act as pain-killers and mood elevators.

Some prescription medications that I take are specifically labeled: "Do not drink alcoholic beverages while taking this medication." If there is no label, does that mean it's safe to have a drink while on them?

Only if you think that Russian roulette is safe. Alcohol can interact adversely with almost all drugs. In fact, any drug that's available in time-release or spansule form can become dangerous if taken in conjunction with alcohol. The coating that's supposed to allow the drug to be released slowly over an extended time period (usually 8–12 hours) can dissolve rapidly in alcohol and give you an uncomfortable and potentially toxic dose of the medication. My advice is get well first, then celebrate afterwards.

XVII
Losing It—Diets by the Pound

252. The Atkins' Diet

This diet (*Dr. Atkins' Diet Revolution, Dr. Atkins' Super-energy Diet*), ignores calorie content and focuses on carbohydrate restriction; but unlike other low-carbohydrate programs, Dr. Atkins' calls for *no* carbohydrates (at least for the first week). By doing this, the body begins to throw off ketones (tiny carbon fragments that are by-products of incompletely burned fat) in amounts sufficient to account for substantial weight loss. According to Dr. Atkins, because carbohydrates are the first fuel your body burns for energy, if none are taken in then the body will draw upon stored fat for fuel, and as ketones are excreted, hunger as well as weight will disappear.

The pros and cons are many (especially since the diet also encourages high-fat consumption despite its inherent health hazard), but if you are on this diet, Dr. Atkins does recommend a high-potency vitamin supplement. I would suggest following the MVP program outlined in section 136, and taking an additional 1,000 mg. vitamin C with bioflavonoids if you've cut out all citrus fruit. Also at least 50 mg. B complex with morning and evening meal, 1 g. potassium divided over three meals, and 400 to 800 mcg. folic acid daily.

253. The Stillman Diet

Dr. Irwin Stillman's Quick Weight Loss Diet, often called "The Water Diet" because it requires drinking eight glasses of water daily (in addition to all other beverages), is essentially an all-protein program—no fats or carbohydrates. It permits no vegetables or fruits, no dairy products or grains, and is said to burn up about 275 more calories daily than a diet that contains the same number of calories but includes other elements, such as carbohydrates and fats. You don't count calories, but you're not supposed to stuff yourself either, and the average weight loss is said to be between five and fifteen pounds per week.

Even Dr. Stillman recognized the need for supplementation while on his diet. He recommended a multivitamin-mineral tablet for anyone following his regimen, and a high-potency multivitamin-mineral tablet for anyone on it who is over forty or eating very small amounts of food.

My own feeling is that anyone on Dr. Stillman's all-protein regimen should be taking a high-potency vitamin and chelated mineral tablet twice daily, along with 1,000 mg. vitamin C complex (time release) and a high-potency multiple chelated mineral tablet. Also, because the heavy water intake tends to flush the B vitamins as well as C from the body more quickly, a time-release vitamin B complex would be advisable, as would 400 to 800 mcg. folic acid and 1 g. potassium divided over three meals.

254. The Scarsdale Diet

This fourteen-day crash diet, on which you can lose up to twenty pounds, was created by the late Dr. Herman Tarnower and made famous in his book *The Complete Scarsdale Medical Diet* (Rawson, Wade Publishers, Inc.). It is basically a variation on the low-calorie, low-fat, low-carbohydrate, high-protein regimen. The difference between the Scarsdale diet and the Stillman and Atkins diets is that Dr. Tarnower added a no-decision factor to his plan. In other words, you eat exactly what's on the menu for each meal every day. And no switching, at least not for two weeks.

Taking all responsibility from the dieter—except that of following instructions—made the Scarsdale a popular and effective regimen.

As with any diet, because of the sudden cut in food intake, supplements are advised. A basic MVP (see section 136) should be taken if you're on the Scarsdale. Also recommended are vitamin E (dry form), 200 to 400 IU daily, and a good B complex.

255. Weight Watchers

This is a long-term regimen that advocates three meals a day with measured portions of protein, carbohydrates, and fat.

Though the program is nutritionally well rounded, most Weight Watchers that I've met agree that supplements have helped them keep up their energy levels while their calorie intake goes down. A multivitamin-mineral tablet, a multiple chelated mineral, and a vitamin C complex, 500 to 1,000 mg. taken one to two times daily should fill the bill.

256. The Drinking Man's Diet

This is another low-carbohydrate, high-fat and high-protein diet, but with the added appeal of allowing alcohol to be part of the regimen. Allegedly based on the Air Force diet (the Air Force denies it), this one advocates keeping your carbohydrate count to no more than 60 g. a day.

The diet states specifically that it is for healthy people, and cautions adherents to get at least 30 g. of carbohydrates daily and enough vitamin C.

Anyone on this diet would be well advised to take a vitamin-C supplement, along with a general MVP (see section 136) regimen, and B complex three times a day because of the alcohol.

257. Liquid Protein and Cambridge Diets

These diets are dangerous and potentially lethal. In fact, the Food and Drug Administration has issued a new ruling that all protein supplements (liquid or powder) used in reducing diets must carry the following label:

Warning—Very low-calorie protein diets (below 800 calories per day) may cause serious illness or death. Do not use for weight reduction without medical supervision. Use with particular care if you are taking medication. Not for use by infants, children, or pregnant or nursing women.

The Cambridge Diet offers three liquid *allegedly* "nutritionally balanced" meals a day totaling 330 calories, which is an intake that can be aligned to semistarvation. Dr. Sami Hashim, a world-renowned expert in the treatment of obesity, has stated that "anyone who is on a diet of 600 calories or less should be in the hospital."

Radical diets, such as these, can cause disastrous effects on the body, not the least of which being abnormal heart function and severe deficiencies in vital minerals due to extremely rapid weight loss. I couldn't in good conscience offer supplement suggestions, since I firmly believe that these diets should not be undertaken without strict medical supervision.

258. Zen Macrobiotic Diet

Contrary to popular belief, this diet is not connected with the Zen Buddhists, but is the creation of a Japanese man named George Ohsawa. Though it has gained many adherents, it is nutritionally dangerous when strictly followed.

There are ten stages to the diet, and milk is prohibited. You start by giving up dessert and work backwards until you're in the highest stage and eating nothing but grains, preferably brown rice. The diet, based on the oriental yin/ yang philosophy, restricts fluid intake, which is dangerous, as is the lack of nutrients provided in meals consisting of nothing but brown rice. Followers believe that if your thoughts are right you can produce vitamins, minerals, and proteins within your own body, and actually change one element to another.

Just in case your thoughts aren't always right, it would be advisable if you are on this diet, or just a strict vegetarian one, to take supplements. A high-potency vegetarian multiple-vitamin and mineral tablet twice daily along with a good B complex with folic acid is recommended. Also vitamin B12, 100 mcg. one to three times a day.

259. Fructose Diet

This fourteen-day diet is for people who crave sweets. The secret is a supplement of fructose, a natural sugar, that not only satisfies your hunger and keeps up your energy, but allows you to lose a pound a day.

Developed by Dr. J. T. Cooper, the fructose diet is basically a low-calorie program, but by taking 36 to 42 g. of fructose a day you are supposed not to crave food. Unlike other dietary sugars, fructose doesn't require insulin to enter the body's cells. It is absorbed directly, eliminating the hypoglycemic (low blood sugar) reaction brought on by excess insulin, which is what makes dieters feel hungry.

Fructose is obtained from vegetables such as artichokes and corn. It is available in powder, flavored 2-g. chewable tablets, and syrup.

Ten glasses of water daily are recommended along with supplements. An MVP (see section 136) is important, as is potassium, 99 mg. (elemental) taken three times a day—one tablet with each meal.

260. Kelp, Lecithin, Vinegar, B6 Diet

This low-profile but effective diet has been around for more than a decade and is still popular. The basic components of the diet can be obtained in 1 tablet that contains kelp, lecithin, apple cider vinegar, and vitamin B6. There are two potencies available: single and double strength. (With the single strength you take two tablets with each meal and with the double strength you take one.)

As with any diet that cuts down caloric intake, a good multiple-vitamin and mineral tablet taken with breakfast and dinner is recommended. Also a B complex and 1,000 mg. vitamin C (time release) twice daily.

261. Mindell Dieting Tips

• Before starting any diet, check with your physician. If you don't feel that your family doctor understands your dieting needs, contact a bariatrician, who specializes in the field. For the name of one in your area, write to the American Society of Bariatric Physicians, Suite 300, 5200 South Quebec, Englewood, Colorado 80111. (Enclose a stamped self-addressed envelope.)

• If you're on a low- or no-carbohydrate diet, beware of artificially sweetened "sugarless" or "dietetic" gum or candy that has sorbitols, mannitols, or hexitols. These ingredients are metabolized in the system as carbohydrates, *only more slowly*!

• If you're on a diet that allows alcohol, a glass of wine before dinner stimulates the gastric juices and aids in proper digestion.

• If you do have wine, remember that dry white has less calories than red.

• If you're eating popcorn as a low-calorie snack, be aware that movie theater popcorn has twice the calories per cup as "light" microwave—and two-and-a-half times that of air-popped.

• When a recipe calls for a cup of sour cream, substitute low-fat yogurt and you'll save over 300 calories.

• Remember that the body's natural response to a decreased food intake is to burn *fewer* calories—which is why diets without exercise don't work in the long run.

• Watch out for such diet fallacies as:

Gelatin dessert is nonfattening.
Grapefruit causes you to lose weight.
Fruits have no calories.
High-protein foods have no calories.
A pound of steak is not as fattening as a potato.
Toast has much fewer calories than bread.

• Whatever you're eating, sit down to eat it, and eat it slowly. (You might expend more calories standing than sitting, but

you tend to eat more that way, too.) Also, don't read or watch TV until you finish your meal.
• When selecting fruit, remember that all fruits are not equal, that an apple, a banana, or a pear has more calories and carbohydrates than a half cantaloupe, a cup of raw strawberries, or a fresh tangerine.
• When choosing your vegetable, take green beans instead of peas (you save 40 calories on a half-cup serving), spinach instead of mixed vegetables (you save 35 calories), and mashed potatoes—if you must—instead of hashed browns (you save 139 calories).
• Carbohydrate watchers, don't underestimate onions; one cup of cooked onions has 18 g.
• If you're counting every calorie, realize that 1 tablespoon of lecithin granules contains 50 calories and a lecithin capsule about 8.
• Try a one-day-a-week water fast (the ancient Greeks did it). Limit yourself to cold tap or bottled water (not iced) or herb tea with lemon or lime juice. Nothing else. This should pep you up, too.

DIET NEWS FLASH: And one of the best to come along in a while. Dr. William Fry, clinical professor emeritus at Stanford University Medical School, says hearty laughter may help you shape up. Laughter, according to Dr. Fry, is a form of "internal jogging." In fact, a good laugh can be the equivalent of three minutes of aerobic exercise (it doubles the heart rate for three to five minutes, increases oxygen consumption, and gives abdomen and diaphragm muscles a workout). In addition, when the laughter stops, the heart rate drops below normal, creating a relaxed feeling that can last for more than half an hour. This gives new meaning to "laughing off weighty problems." Forget about Fonda. Heard any good jokes lately?

262. Mindell Vitamin-balanced Diet To Lose and Live By

I know your mother told it to you, but it is true anyway—breakfast *is* the most important meal of the day. It comes after the longest period of time that you've been without food, and you cannot catch up nutritionally by eating a good lunch or dinner later.

If you're dieting, it is especially important to perk up your energy level at the start of the day.

BREAKFAST

8 oz. nonfat or low-fat milk (or juice)

A flavored low-calorie protein powder that contains nutritional yeast, lecithin, and fructose

4 ice cubes

Mix well in blender for 60 seconds. Calories, approximately: 150

This mixture can be frozen and used as a dessert for dinner or a pick-me-up snack if your calories quotient allows.

Lunch is a tricky meal. Fast-food restaurants are seductively convenient, and nothing blows a diet faster than "a few french fries" and a "tiny milkshake." If you really want to lose weight, think more along these lines:

LUNCH

A modest portion (3–5 ounces) of water-packed canned or fresh fish, skinless chicken or white meat turkey, a raw vegetable salad (with lemon or vinegar dressing), and a piece of fruit.

OR

2 eggs (prepared without fat) or cottage or pot cheese (no more than ¾ cup), raw vegetables, 1 slice of whole wheat bread with a light coating of margarine, and a fruit for dessert. (The American Heart Association suggests only 3 whole eggs per week, though many doctors allow more. Check with your own physician.)

OR

A low-cal turkey sandwich (3 oz. turkey, 1 tsp. mayo, 2 slices whole wheat bread, lettuce, thin-slice tomato), small carrot, ½ cup unsweetened applesauce, mixed with ½ cup nonfat yogurt.

OR

A diet pizza (2 oz. sliced low-fat mozzarella cheese, ½ whole wheat muffin, small sliced tomato, 1 tsp. olive oil with oregano sprinkled on top), ¼ cantaloupe or 1 cup frozen melon balls.

(Vary lunches from day to day.)

Dinner is usually a dieter's downfall, but it doesn't have to be that way:

DINNER

Five nights a week you should have fish (sole, trout, salmon, halibut, etc.) or poultry broiled, boiled, or roasted (remove skin before eating—but leave on for cooking—poultry); and two nights a week you can have meat, once again broiled, boiled, or roasted; a cooked vegetable; a large salad (no more than 1 teaspoon oil in the dressing); a small boiled or baked potato once or twice a week; and a fresh fruit for dessert.

BEVERAGES

For best results (and improved health) stay away from alcohol—try sparkling mineral water with lime instead. Also be sure to drink at least six 8-ounce glasses of water daily. Herb teas, hot or iced, are recommended alternatives to diet sodas—especially those that contain caffeine. (See section 241.)

SUPPLEMENTS

[Take supplements six days a week and rest on the seventh. By doing this, you'll never have to worry about a buildup of fat-soluble vitamins in the system.]

Time-release multiple vitamin with chelated minerals (at least 50 mg. B1, B2, and B6 per tablet) taken A.M. and P.M.

Time-release vitamin C, 1,000 mg. with rose hips bioflavonoids, 2 tablets taken A.M. and P.M.

A multiple chelated mineral tablet with at least 500 mg. calcium and 250 mg. magnesium per tablet (must also have manganese, zinc, iron, selenium, chromium, copper, iodine, and potassium) taken A.M. and P.M.

Dry vitamin E, 500 IU-D-alpha-tocopherol with selenium, chromium, vitamin C, and ascorbates taken A.M. and P.M.

RNA 100 mg.—DNA 100 mg., 3 tablets daily, 6 days a week SOD 125 mcg. daily, 6 days a week
Lecithin, 1,200 mg. (6 capsules) daily. (If you use lecithin granules in breakfast drink, this supplement is not necessary.)
Vitamin B15, 50 mg. in the A.M.

263. Supplements For Eating More and Gaining Less

The amino acids arginine and ornithine (see section 80) have been found to stimulate the pituitary gland to continue to produce growth hormone, which can rejuvenate your metabolism. While some hormones encourage the body to store fat, growth hormone acts as a mobilizer of fat, helping you to look trimmer and have more energy as well.

> You can rejuvenate your metabolism
> while you sleep.

Best of all, you can rejuvenate your metabolism while you sleep because that's when growth hormone is secreted!
Supplements are available in tablets or powder and work best when taken on an empty stomach with water or juice (no protein). For reducing benefits, take 2 grams (2,000 mg.) immediately before retiring.

CAUTION: Arginine is contraindicated for growing children, persons with schizophrenic conditions, and anyone who has a herpes virus infection. Doses exceeding 20 grams can be dangerous.

264. Any Questions About Chapter XVII?

I know that no more than 20–30 percent of my daily calories should come from fat. But I'm not good at figuring out percentages. I read labels, but I'm still confused. Is there an easy way to determine how much I'm getting?

As a matter of fact, a newsletter called *Alternatives* has come up with one. Always keep in mind that 1 gram of fat equals about 9 calories. Therefore, to keep your fat intake below 30 percent daily, when you check food labels be sure that for every 100 calories there are no more than 3 grams of fat.

What is a "setpoint"? And what does it have to do with losing weight?

The "setpoint" theory is one of the most widely accepted on weight gain and loss. It holds that fatness is caused by the setting of an area in the hypothalamus (part of the brain), sometimes called an "appestat," which controls your appetite for food. Needless to say, everyone's appestat is not on the same setting.

Glycerol, which is bound and released according to the fat content of a cell, along with the blood level of insulin, informs the brain of the body's fat reserves and sets your appestat accordingly. Unfortunately, external influences—such as the aroma and taste of delectable food—can *raise* your appestat.

But you can reset your setpoint by exercising regularly. In other words, you'll reduce your appetite by lowering the point at which you feel full.

To reset for weight loss, the minimum requirement is half an hour of aerobic exercise three times a week. A simple and effective way to do this is by walking two miles in half an hour three times a week (or one mile in fifteen minutes six times a week).

Does grapefruit really help you lose weight?

If you eat it instead of chocolate cake it does. Grapefruit, which has been touted as a miracle diet food, is little more than a fine source of vitamin C, and other nutrients in lesser amounts. Despite its being sold in pill form, it's still just grapefruit. On the bright side, half a grapefruit only has 58 calories.

What's your feeling about the Nutri/System weight loss program?

In theory it's fine, based as it is on varied low-fat, low-sodium and low-calorie foods with high nutritional content and a variety of tastes and textures. The Nutri/System belief is that overweight people have a craving for an overabundance of taste, smell and texture sensations (an exaggerated "set point").

Therefore, providing foods with texture, taste and aroma —even if low calorie—will enable these people to lose weight.

What I worry about, though, are those dieters who rely solely on the pre-packaged Nutri/System foods. These tend to become dieting "crutches" and don't help change poor eating and cooking habits. Even with the best of diets, there is no "quick fix."

I've heard that you're likely to be more successful dieting in warm weather. Is this true?

If this were completely true, dieters would be moving to Florida and southern California in droves. What has been purported by Susan Perry and Jim Dawson in *The Secrets Our Body Clocks Reveal* (Rawson Associates) is that we are genetically disposed to have extra fat layers in fall and winter. Therefore, when days start getting longer, in spring, it's allegedly easier for us to lose weight. The question is, easier than what?

What real dangers are there in liquid dieting, the kind that Oprah did—aside from running the risk of gaining the weight back?

Extremely real dangers. Many people who go on very-low-calorie diets (VLCD) do so without proper medical supervision. They are unaware that a VLCD is designed for people who are at least 30 percent over their ideal weight (as determined by a physician—not a fashion model.) Once on a VLCD, a dieter must be medically monitored (receiving regular blood tests, electrocardiograms and blood pressure checks).

If you are less than 30 percent over your ideal weight, and you go on one of the over-the-counter (OTC) liquid diets, substituting it for all meals (instead of the recommended one or two for a limited period), you risk losing too much muscle, bone, and lean body mass in proportion to fat—causing possible heart arrhythmia, permanently slowed metabolism, fatigue, and, in extreme cases, even death.

XVIII

So You Think You Don't Eat Much Sugar and Salt

265. Kinds of Sugars

More than a hundred substances that qualify as sweet can be called sugars. The ones we come in contact with most often are *fructose*, a natural sugar found in fruit and honey; *glucose*, the body's blood sugar and the simplest form of sugar in which a carbohydrate is assimilated; *dextrose*, made from cornstarch and chemically identical to glucose; *lactose*, milk sugar; *maltose*, the sugar formed from the starch by the action of yeast; and *sucrose*, the sugar that is obtained from sugar cane or beets and refined to the product that reaches us as granules.

> Brown sugar is merely sugar crystals
> coated with molasses syrup.

Brown sugar, which many people assume to be healthier than white sugar, is merely sugar crystals coated with molasses syrup. (In the United States most brown sugar is made by simply spraying refined white sugar with the molasses syrup.) Raw sugar is banned in the United States because it contains contaminants. When it's partially refined and cleaned up, it can be sold as turbinado sugar. *Honey* is a blend of fructose and glucose.

266. Other Sweeteners

Sorbitol, mannitol and *xylitol* are natural occurring sugar alcohols that are absorbed more slowly into the blood than glucose or sucrose. The biggest misconception about these sweeteners is that they have no calories. The fact is, they have as many calories as sugar—and in some instances, products using them as sweeteners contain *more* calories than they would if made with regular sugar. In other words, these are not low–or no-calorie sugar substitutes, even though products containing them are often sold in the dietetic section of food markets. Always check labels. Products using these sweeteners must reveal that they are "not a reduced calorie food" or be marked "not for weight control."

> Just because a product is marked "sugarless"
> doesn't mean it's low-calorie!

Aspartame (EQUAL, NUTRASWEET) is a combination of amino acids phenylalanine and aspartic acid (see sections 77 and 82) and has no calories. *Acesulfame K* (SUNETTE, SWEETONE) looks like sugar, but is derived from acetoacetic acid and has no calories. And *saccharin* (SWEET 'N LOW, SWEET 10), a noncaloric petroleum derivative estimated to be 300 to 500 times sweeter than sugar, and chemically similar to acesulfame K, is absorbed but not modified by the body, and is excreted unchanged in the urine.

CAUTION: If you have diabetes or hypoglycemia, be sure to check with your doctor or a nutritionally oriented dietician before adding any products containing alternative sweeteners to your diet.

267. Dangers of Too Much Sugar

> Ketchup has 8 percent more sugar
> than ice cream.

The big problem with sugar is that we eat too much of it (over 154 pounds) and often don't even know it. All carbohydrate sweeteners qualify as sugar, even though they may be called by other names; and when sucrose is the number-three ingredient on a box of cereal, corn syrup number five, and honey number seven, you don't realize it but you're eating something that is 50 percent sugar!

The consumer today is hooked on sugar right from the start. Baby formulas are often sweetened with sugar, as are many baby foods (check labels). Because sugar also acts as a preservative, retains and absorbs moisture, it's often in products we never think of as containing it, products such as salt, peanut butter, canned vegetables, bouillon cubes, and more. Would you believe that the ketchup you put on your hamburger has just less than 8 percent more sugar than ice cream? That cream substitute for coffee is 65 percent sugar compared to 51 percent for a chocolate bar?

The fact is, we're eating too much sugar for our health. It is beyond argument that sugar is a prime factor in tooth decay. Also, one-third of our population is overweight, and obesity increases the possibility of heart disease, diabetes, hypertension, gallstones, back problems, and arthritis. Not that sugar alone is the cause, but its presence in foods induces you to eat more, and if you cut your calorie count without cutting your sugar intake, you'll lose nutrients faster than pounds. Sugar is also the villain where hypoglycemia is concerned, and, though there have been arguments pro and con, directly or indirectly a factor in diabetes and heart disease.

268. How Sweet It Is

Hidden sugars are where you least expect them. (Would you believe that Canada Dry tonic water has approximately 18¼ teaspoons of sugar in a 12 oz. serving?) If you want to be a sugar detective, my advice is to check labels. Look for sucrose substitutes such as corn syrup or corn sugar, and watch out for words ending in "-ose," which indicates the presence of sugar. A sugar by any name is still a sugar. And remember that not even medicines are immune from added sweeteners!

MEDICINES	SUGAR PER TABLESPOON
Alternagel Liquid	2,000 mg.
Basaljel Extra-Strength Liquid	375 mg.
Gaviscon Liquid	1,500 mg.
Gaviscon-2 tablets	2,400 mg.
Maalox plus tablets	575 mg.
Mylanta Liquid	2,000 mg.
Riopan Plus Chew Tablets	610 mg.

(When in doubt about sugar or saccharin content of any medication—ask your pharmacist.)

269. Dangers of Too Much Salt

Taking things with a grain of salt is all well and good, but eating things with it might be a different story. The normal intake of sodium chloride (table salt) is 6 to 18 g. daily, but the American Heart Association recommends an intake of no more than 3 g. (3,000 mg.) daily. An intake over 14 g. is considered excessive. And too many of us are being excessive. The average American consumes about 15 pounds (a bowling ball) of salt each year!

Too much salt can cause hypertension (high blood pressure), which increases the chances of heart disease, and has recently been cited as one of the causes for migraine headaches. It causes abnormal fluid retention, which can result in dizziness and swelling of the legs. Also it may cause potassium to be lost in the urine and interfere with the proper utilization of protein foods. In addition, recent studies have linked excess sodium in the diet and low potassium to sodium ratios as high risk factors for colorectal cancer—particularly in men.

270. High-Salt Traps

Just because you stay away from pretzels and snack foods and don't pour on the table salt doesn't mean you're not getting more salt than you should. Salt traps are as hidden from view as sugar ones.

If you want to keep your salt intake down:

● Hold back on beer. (There's 25 mg. sodium in every 12 ounces.)
● Avoid the use of baking soda, monosodium glutamate (MSG, Accent), and baking powder in food preparation.
● Stay away from laxatives, most of which contain sodium.
● Do not drink or cook with water treated by a home water softener; it adds sodium to the water.
● Look for the words SALT, SODIUM, or the chemical symbol *Na* when reading food labels.
● Watch out for tomato juice. It's low in calories, but very high in sodium.
● Don't eat cured meat such as ham, bacon, corned beef, or frankfurters, sausage, shellfish, any canned or frozen meat, poultry, or fish to which sodium has been added.
● When dining out, ask for an inside cut of meat, or chops or steaks without added salt.
● Watch out for diet sodas—the calories might be low, but in many the sodium content is still *high*!
● Be aware that 2 slices of most processed breads (even if "lite" or whole wheat) contain approximately 230 mg. of salt.

271. How Salty Is It?

APPROXIMATE SODIUM CONTENTS OF COMMON FOODS

Item	Amount	Salt (mg.)
Pickle, dill	1 large	1,928
Frozen turkey three-course dinner (Swanson)	1 (17 oz.)	1,735
Soy sauce	1 tbsp.	1,320
Pancakes (Hungry Jack Complete)	3 pancakes 4 in. each	1,150

Chicken noodle soup (Campbell's)	10 oz.	1,050
Tomato soup (Campbell's)	10 oz.	950
Green beans, canned (Del Monte)	1 cup	925
Cheese, pasteurized, processed American (Kraft)	2 oz.	890
Baked red kidney beans (B and M)	1 cup	810
Pizza, frozen (Celeste)	4 oz.	656
V8 vegetable juice	6 oz.	654
Danish cinnamon rolls w/raisins (Pillsbury)	1 serving	630
Pudding, instant chocolate (Jell-O)	½ cup	486
Bologna (Oscar Mayer)	2 slices	450
Tuna, in oil (Del Monte)	3 oz.	430
Frankfurter, beef (Oscar Mayer)	1	425

272. Any Questions About Chapter XVIII?

Isn't it true that in very hot weather you need salt supplements, especially if you do exercise and perspire heavily?

No! This is not only a myth, but one that could result in dangerous consequences. The truth is that salt tablets have a dehydrating effect, and are never indicated. When you exercise, your body uses mechanisms to conserve salt—and since the average American eats somewhere around 60 or more times the salt than is needed by the body, salt depletion is highly unlikely. In fact, too much salt under those conditions can contribute to heat exhaustion and heat stroke. (In the very, *very* rare case where a salt deficiency might occur, replacement should be administered with a 0.1% solution of salt administered in drinking water—and a doctor should be consulted.)

I know that some diet sodas are high in salt, but I've heard that plain club soda is also. How much could it really have?

It could really have a lot—and it does! An 8-oz. glass of Canada Dry club soda has 75.0 mg.! You can get the same fizz from salt-free seltzer.

I've been told that eating a candy bar before running is not good for you. I don't understand why a quick energy fix would be bad. Can you explain?

Eating sugar or drinking a sugar drink within half an hour before exercise has been shown to stimulate the release of insulin, causing a drop in blood sugar (and, therefore, needed energy). Research done at the Human Performance Lab at Ball State University in Muncie, Indiana, found that once exercise starts, the insulin response is inhibited, which is why athletes can then drink beverages, such as Gatorade, that contain sugar in a glucose form that won't cause bloating.

Does sugarless chewing gum really help prevent cavities?

The claim for sugarless gum is that it doesn't *promote* cavities. There is no claim that it actually has a prophylactic effect. In fact, sugarless gum, or candy, that contains sorbitol or mannitol can increase your chances of tooth decay!

No, sorbitol and mannitol don't actually promote cavities, but both of them nourish and increase the type of bacteria in your mouth—namely, *Streptococcus mutans*—that do. According to Dr. Paul Keyes, founder of the International Dental Health Foundation, *Streptococcus mutans* have the mechanism to stick to teeth but will remain harmless until you eat something containing sugar or sucrose, with which they then quickly combine to cause decay. Because the sorbitol and mannitol have swelled the ranks of these bacteria, there are more of them available to use passing sugars to attack your teeth.

Rinsing your mouth with water within 15 minutes after eating or drinking anything containing sucrose is the best preventive.

XIX

Staying Beautiful—Staying Handsome

273. Vitamins for Healthy Skin

What you look like on the outside depends a lot on what you do for yourself on the inside. And as far as your skin is concerned, vitamins and proper nutrition are essential.

To look your best, make sure you're getting 55 to 65 g. of protein a day. Drink eight glasses of water daily (herbal teas can count for a few of them), and keep your milk and yogurt consumption restricted to the nonfat variety. Keep away from chocolates, nuts, dried fruits, fried foods, cola drinks, coffee, alcohol, cigarettes, and excessive salt. Also, do not use sugar. Small amounts of honey or blackstrap molasses will sweeten just as well and you'll look better for it.

A good start toward healthy, glowing skin is a daily protein drink. It can be taken in place of any meal, but it makes an especially good breakfast.

PROTEIN DRINK

6 oz. raw nonfat milk
1 tbsp. nutritional yeast powder (lots of B vitamins)
3 tbsp. acidophilus (promotes friendly bacteria)
1 tbsp. granulated lecithin (breaks down bumps or cholesterol under the skin)
1 tbsp. protein powder
½ tbsp. blackstrap molasses or honey

Carob powder, bananas, strawberries, or any fresh fruit for
flavoring
Mix in blender. (Add 3–4 ice cubes, if desired.)

SUPPLEMENTS

Multiple-vitamin and mineral-complex—1 daily
Take after any meal. Important for skin tone and nerve
health.
B complex, 100 mg. (time release)—1 daily
Take after any meal. B2 (riboflavin) and B6 (pyridoxine)
reduce facial oiliness and blackhead formation.
Beta carotene, 25,000 IU daily
Take 1 after breakfast and 1 after dinner. Maintains soft,
smooth, disease-free skin. Builds resistance to infections.
Rose hips vitamin C, 1,000 mg. with bioflavonoids—3 daily
Take 1 after each meal and at bedtime. Aids in preventing
the spread of acne. Promotes healing of wounds, bruising,
and scar tissue. Helps to prevent breakage of capillaries
on face.
Vitamin E (dry form), 400 IU—1–3 daily
Take 1 after each meal. Improves circulation in tiny face
capillaries. Aids in healing by replacing cells on the skin's
outer layer. Works with vitamin C in making skin less
susceptible to acne. Use vitamin-E oil (28,000 IU per oz.)
externally on skin for healing burns, abrasions, and scar
tissue.
Multiple chelated minerals—6 daily
Take 2 tablets after each meal (or 3 in A.M. and P.M.).
Helps maintain the acid-alkaline balance of the blood necessary for a clear complexion. Calcium is for soft, smooth
skin tissue; copper for skin color; iron to improve pale skin;
potassium for dry skin and acne; zinc for external and
internal wound-healing.
Choline and inositol, 1,000 mg. daily, after a large meal
(Lecithin granules, 2 tbsp. daily, can be substituted for
choline and inositol tabs.) Helps emulsify cholesterol (fatty
deposits or bumps under the skin). Purifies the kidneys
which aids the skin.

Acidophilus—6 tbsp. daily
    Take 2 tbsp. or 6 capsules after each meal. Helps fight skin eruptions caused by unfriendly bacteria in the system.
Chlorophyll—3 tsp. or 9 tablets daily
    Take 1 tsp. or 3 tablets after each meal. Reduces hazard of bacterial contamination. Possesses antibiotic action. An excellent aid to wound-healing, after washing thoroughly with a soap substitute made from the comfrey plant.
Cysteine, 1 g. daily
    Take between meals with juice. Helps maintain supple, young-looking skin.

If face is badly blemished, extra zinc (chelated) is advised, 15–50 mg. daily. Aids in growth and repair of injured tissues.

274. Vitamins for Healthy Hair

Shampoos and conditioners are not enough. To make sure that you're giving your crowning glory its due, you have to be aware that nutrition plays a very important role in having terrific, shiny hair. Unlike the skin, hair cannot repair itself; but you *can* get new, healthier hair to grow.

    The first thing to do is examine your diet. Does it include fish, wheat germ, yeast, and liver? It should. The vitamins and minerals that these foods supply are what your hair needs, along with frequent scalp massage, a good pH-balanced, protein-enriched shampoo, and supplements.

SUPPLEMENTS

Multiple-vitamin and mineral complex—1 daily
    Take after any meal. Important for general health of hair.
B complex, 100 mg. (time release)—1 daily
    Taken after any meal, B vitamins are essential for hair growth. Pantothenic acid, folic acid, and PABA help restore gray hair to its natural color.
Beta carotene, 10,000 IU—1–2 daily 5 days a week
Take A.M. and P.M. Works with vitamin B to keep hair shiny.
    Cysteine, 1 g. daily

Take between meals with juice. Hair is 10–145: cysteine, and this supplement can keep tresses looking lustrous.
Multiple chelated minerals—1 daily
Take with breakfast. Minerals such as silicon, sulfur, iodine, and iron help prevent falling hair.

Keep in mind that you need some fatty acids, vitamin B, and choline in your body for vitamin A to survive.

275. Vitamins for Hands and Feet

Your hands take lots of abuse. Detergents strip away natural oils, and water and weather alone can cause chapping. Rubber gloves are a good idea, but if you already have splits in your skin or some sort of dermatitis, they could *not* be put directly on your hands. (A pair of cotton gloves beneath the rubber ones will absorb perspiration and prevent reinfection.) Also, do not use cornstarch in the gloves; it can promote the growth of microorganisms. If you want to use something to absorb the moisture, try plain unscented talcum powder.

As for toenails and fingernails, the best remedy for problems is diet. Gelatin is commonly accepted as the cure for weak nails, but this is a misconception. The nails do need protein, but gelatin is a poor supplier. Not only are two essential amino acids missing, but another amino acid, glycine, is supplied in amounts you do not need. Foods rich in sulfur, such as egg yolks, should be part of your diet, and desiccated, defatted liver (tablets) should be taken as a supplement.

SUPPLEMENTS

Multiple-vitamin and mineral complex—1 daily
Take after any meal. Promotes general skin health and growth of nails.
B complex, 100 mg. (time release)—1 daily
Take after any meal. Helps build resistance to fungus infections and vital to nail growth.
Beta carotene 10,000 IU daily
Take after any meal. Helps to prevent splitting nails.

Vitamin E, 100–400 IU—1–2 daily
    Take in A.M. and P.M. Necessary for proper utilization of
    vitamin A.
Multiple chelated minerals—1 daily
    Take after any meal. Iron helps strengthen brittle nails,
    zinc gets rid of white spots.

276. Natural Cosmetics—What's in Them?

Many cosmetics nowadays are advertised as "natural," but
looking at the ingredients can cause you to wonder. To be
sure of what you're getting, read the label carefully. The
following explanations of cosmetic ingredients should make
things clearer.

Amyl Dimethyl PABA—a sunscreening agent from PABA,
    a B-complex factor
Annatto—a vegetable color obtained from the seeds of a
    tropical plant
Avocado oil—a vegetable oil obtained from avocados
Caprylic/Capric triglyceride—an emollient obtained from co-
    conut oil
Carrageenan—a natural thickening agent from dried Irish
    moss
Castor oil—an emollient oil collected from the pressing of
    castor bean seeds
Cetyl alcohol—a component of vegetable oils
Cetyl palmitate—a component of palm and coconut oils
Citric acid—a natural organic acid found widely in citrus
    plants
Cocamide DEA—a thickener obtained from coconut oil
Coconut oil—obtained by pressing the kernels of the seeds
    of the coconut palm
Decyl oleate—obtained from tallow or coconut oil
Disodium monolaneth-5-sulfosuccinate—obtained from lan-
    olin and used to improve the texture of hair
Fragrance—oils obtained from flowers, grasses, roots, and
    stems that give off a pleasant or agreeable odor
Goat milk whey—protein-rich whey obtained from goat's
    milk

Glyceryl stearate—an organic emulsifier obtained from glycerin

Hydrogenated castor oil—a waxy material obtained from castor oil

Imidzaolidinyl urea—a preservative derived naturally as a product of protein metabolism (hydrolysis)

Lanolin alcohol—a constituent of lanolin that performs as an emollient and emulsifier

Laureth-3—an organic material obtained from coconut and palm oils

Methyl glucoside sesquistearate—an organic emulsifier obtained from a natural simple sugar

Mineral oil—an organic emollient and lubricant

Olive oil—a natural oil obtained from olives

Peanut oil—a vegetable oil obtained from peanuts

Pectin—derived from citrus fruits and apple peel

PEG lanolin—an emollient and emulsifier obtained from lanolin

Petrolatum—petroleum jelly

P.O.E. (20) methyl glucoside sesquistearate—an organic emulsifier from a simple natural sugar

Potassium sorbate—obtained from sorbic acid found in the berries of mountain ash

Safflower oil-hybrid—a natural emollient obtained from a strain of specially cultivated plants

Sesame oil—oil of pressed sesame seeds

Sodium cetyl sulfate—a detergent and emulsifier obtained from coconut oil

Sodium laureth sulfate—a detergent obtained from coconut oil

Sodium lauryl sulfate—a detergent obtained from coconut oil

Sodium PCA—a natural-occurring humectant found in the skin where it acts as the natural moisturizer

Sorbic acid—a natural preservative derived from berries of mountain ash

Tocopherol—a natural vitamin E

Undecylenamide DEA—a natural preservative derived from castor oil

Water—the universal solvent, and the major constituent of all living material

277. Not So Pretty Drugs

Medications are necessary for certain conditions, but doctors often fail to mention their possible side effects. It is a rare physician who puts his patient on the pill and tells her that her face might break out, or that she might suffer hair loss; but many women on oral contraceptives find this out soon enough. In fact, many drugs can be the cause of skin and other cosmetic problems. The following is a list of just a few:

Amytal	Skin rash, swollen eyelids, itchy skin
Butisol	Acne, pimples
Coumadin	Skin rash, itching, hives
Dalmane	Rash, flushes
Dexamyl	Swollen patches, itchy skin
Dexedrine	Swollen patches, itchy skin
Equanil	Rash, welts, dermatitis
Librium	Pimples
Miltown	Welts, flaking skin, itching
Nembutal	Skin rash
Phenobarbital	Rash, itchy skin, swollen eyelids
Placidyl	Itchy skin, swollen patches
Quaalude	Pimples, welts
Talwin	Rash, facial swelling, skin peeling
Tetracycline	Taken during pregnancy and in infancy may cause permanent discoloration of child's teeth
Thorazine	Peeling skin, jaundice, welts, swelling
Tofranil	Rash, itchy skin, jaundice
Tuinal	Can aggravate existing skin condition
Valium	Jaundice, rash, swollen patches

278. Any Questions About Chapter XIX?

What do you think of jojoba oil as a beauty aid?

Personally, I think it's one of the best. It's available in a variety of forms—an oil, a cream, a soap, a shampoo—and it works wonders naturally!

For example: As a moisturizer, use a few drops under your makeup. Massage gently into your skin, particularly around the eyes where lines occur. (Be careful to avoid direct contact with the eyes and if any irritation results, discontinue use.) At night, use the oil to soften your skin as you sleep. Just apply a light layer over your face and neck—after they've had a good cleansing, of course.

The oil can also be used to soften skin after showers (all you need is a few drops) and as a luxuriant bath oil (again, just a few drops). For dry, chapped, or recently shaved skin, it should be applied directly.

After shampooing your hair, try rubbing a few drops of the oil into your hair and scalp. (Don't rinse.) Daily use will help even the driest hair return to its natural luster.

My nails just won't grow. I've tried all sorts of vitamins, but they don't work. Where do I go from here?

It's possible that you might have a thyroid problem, so you might want to check with a nutritionally oriented physician (see section 293).

In the meanwhile, you could try silica, an organic herb that's also known as horsetail and *Equisetum arvense*, which is changed by the body into readily available calcium—which nourishes nails, skin, hair, bones, and the body's connective tissue.

XX

Staying Young, Energetic, and Sexy

279. Retarding the Aging Process

Aging is caused by the degeneration of cells. Our bodies are made up of millions of these cells, each with a life of somewhere around two years or less. But before a cell dies, it reproduces itself. Why, then, you might wonder, shouldn't we look the same now as we did ten years ago? The reason for this is that with each successive reproduction, the cell goes through some alteration—basically, deterioration. So as our cells change, deteriorate, we grow old.

> You can look and feel six
> to twelve years younger.

Dr. Benjamin S. Frank, author of *Nucleic Acid Therapy in Aging and Degenerative Disease*, found that deteriorating cells can be rejuvenated if provided with substances that directly nourish them—substances such as nucleic acids.

DNA (deoxyribonucleic acid) and RNA (ribonucleic acid) are our nucleic acids. DNA is essentially a chemical boilerplate for new cells. It sends out RNA molecules like a team of well-trained workers to form them. When DNA stops giving the orders to RNA, new cell construction ceases—as does life. But by helping the body stay well-supplied with nucleic acids, Dr. Frank has found that you can look and feel six to twelve years younger than you actually are.

According to Dr. Frank, we need 1 to 1½ g. of nucleic acid daily. Though the body can produce its own nucleic acids, he feels they are broken down too quickly into less useful compounds and should be supplied from external sources if the aging process is to be regarded, even reversed.

Foods rich in nucleic acids are wheat germ, bran, spinach, asparagus, mushrooms, fish (especially sardines, salmon, and anchovies), chicken liver, oatmeal, and onions. He recommends a diet where seafood is eaten seven times a week, along with two glasses of skimmed milk, a glass of fruit or vegetable juice, and four glasses of water daily.

After only two months of RNA-DNA supplementation and diet, Dr. Frank found that his patients had more energy and that there was a substantial diminution of lines and wrinkles, with healthier, rosier, and younger-looking skin in evidence.

One of the most recent arrivals in the battle to combat aging is SOD (superoxide dismutase). This enzyme fortifies the body against the ravages of free radicals, destructive molecules which speed the aging process by destroying healthy cells as well as attacking collagen (''cement'' that holds cells together).

As we age, our bodies produce less SOD, so supplementation—along with a natural diet that restricts free radical formation—can help increase our energetic and productive years. It's important to note, though, that SOD can become inactive very quickly if essential minerals, such as zinc, copper, and manganese, are not supplied.

A new product called PYCNOGENOL, made from a patented blend of nutrients found in fruits and vegetables and other plants, is now available and being touted as a potent free-radical fighter and anti-aging supplement. It improves circulation, helping each cell get the food it needs. And, unlike most other antioxidants, it crosses the blood-brain barrier to help protect brain and nerve tissue from oxidation. It has also been found to bond to collagen fibers and help reverse some of the damage caused over the years by free-radicals.

Coenzyme Q-10, a substance that can be synthesized by the body (although it is also obtained from food) is used by our cells during the process of respiration, and deficiencies are common in the course of normal aging. In fact, studies have shown that reduced levels of Coenzyme Q-10 may directly contribute to aging and that increasing levels retard the process as well as:

• reduces the risk of heart attack (aids respiration of the heart muscle; appears to provide a protective effect against viral-caused heart inflammations; helps prevent cardiac arrhythmias)
• stimulates the immune system
• aids in the treatment of periodontal disease
• lowers blood pressure
• shares many of vitamin E's antioxidant properties
• aids in the prevention of toxicity from drugs used to treat many diseases associated with aging.

As a supplement, the recommended dosage is 10 mg. three times daily.

DHEA (dehydroepiandrosterone), a natural hormone that is produced by the adrenal glands, and has been used in anti-aging regimens, since one of its properties is that it can "de-excite" the body's processes and thereby slow down the production of fats, hormones, and acids that contribute to aging, is no longer available as a supplement. It has been found to also contain anti-cancer and weight loss properties and is currently being formulated as a prescription drug.

280. Basic Keep Yourself Young Program

Along with proper diet, a good supplement regimen is important to the success of looking, feeling, and keeping yourself young.

High-potency multiple vitamin with chelated minerals (time release preferred) A.M. and P.M.
Vitamin C, 1,000 mg. with bioflavonoids A.M. and P.M.

Vitamin E (dry form), 400 IU with antioxidants A.M. and
 P.M.
Pychogenol, 100 mg. for 7–10 days then cut back to 50 mg.
 daily
RNA-DNA, 100-mg. tablets, 1 daily for one month, then 2
 daily for the next month, then 3 daily thereafter, 6 days a
 week
Stress B complex, A.M. and P.M.
SOD, 125 mcg. daily, 6 days a week

281. High-Pep Energy Regimen

Whether you want to feel good, or just look good, exercise,
diet, and the right supplements are the tickets to high energy.

If you're not into jogging, can't afford the sneakers, don't
play tennis, find yourself reluctant to swim in twenty-below
weather, and hate calisthenics, I have the perfect exercise for
you—jumping rope.

A jump rope is inexpensive, convenient (you can take it
everywhere), and lots of fun to use. And it works! In terms
of calories burned, jumping rope can outdo bicycling, tennis,
and swimming. An average person of about 150 pounds uses
up 720 calories an hour jumping rope (120 to 140 turns per
minute). When you realize that an hour of tennis uses up only
420 calories, you have a better idea of just how good jumping
rope can be for you.

For keeping energy high, remember to eat a combination
of two protein foods (or a protein drink) at each meal; drink
at least six glasses of water daily (a half-hour before or after
meals); avoid refined sugar, flour, tobacco, alcohol, tea, coffee, soft drinks, processed and fried foods.

A good pep-up protein drink:

1 tbsp. protein powder
1 tbsp. lecithin granules
2 tbsp. acidophilus liquid
1 tbsp. nutritional yeast
1 tbsp. safflower oil (optional)

Blend with milk, water, or juice in blender for 1 minute. (Add fresh fruit if desired.)

282. High-Pep Supplements

With breakfast:

High-potency multiple vitamins with chelated minerals (time release preferred)
Vitamin E (dry form), 400 IU
High-potency multiple chelated mineral
Acidophilus, 3 capsules or 2 tbsp. liquid
Lecithin granules, 1 tbsp. or 3 1,200 mg. capsules
3 calcium and magnesium tablets
Vitamin B15, 50 mg.
Coenzyme Q-10, 50 mg.

With lunch:

Acidophilus, 3 capsules or 2 tbsp. liquid
Lecithin granules, 1 tbsp. or 3 1,200 mg. capsules
Coenzyme Q-10, 50 mg.
Optional: Vitamin B12, liver tablets, digestive enzymes

With dinner:

Vitamin E (dry form), 400 IU
Acidophilus, 3 capsules or 2 tbsp. liquid
Lecithin granules, 1 tbsp. or 3 1,200 mg. capsules
Coenzyme Q-10, 50 mg.
Optional: digestive enzymes

283. Vitamins and Sex

The important thing to remember is that if you're not feeling up to par, your sex drive is going to suffer along with the rest of you.

There have been many claims for vitamin E in relation to sex. Studies have indeed shown that it increases the fertility in males and females and helps restore male potency. That it strongly influences the sex drive in men and women has yet to be proven, thought I have met many vitamin-E takers who are happily convinced that it does.

The largest percentage of zinc
in a man's body is found in
the prostate.

Another noteworthy sex nutrient is zinc. The largest percentage of zinc in a man's body is found in the prostate, and a lack of the mineral can produce testicular atrophy and prostate trouble.

Remember, vitamins that keep up your energy levels (see section 282) will also do a lot for your sexual performance.

284. Food and Supplements for Better Sex

Oysters (yes, they're high in zinc), shellfish of all kinds, brewer's yeast, wheat bran, wheat germ, whole grains, barley, brown rice, and sunflower seeds. Incorporating these foods in a program that includes a high-protein and low-refined carbohydrate diet, exercise, and supplements is as good as an aphrodisiac for lovers.

Supplements
MVP (see section 136)
Vitamin B complex, 50 mg., 1–3 times daily
Vitamin E, 400 IU, 1–3 times daily
Zinc, 50 mg. (chelated) daily
Ginseng, 500 mg., 3 times daily 1 hour before meals

285. Any Questions About Chapter XX?

I understand that octacosanol can improve a male's sexual performance enormously. What do you feel about this?

I feel that a lot is still going to depend on the male involved. It is true, though, that octacosanol (which is a natural food substance present in very small amounts in many vegetable oils, the levels of alfalfa and wheat, wheat germ, and other foods) has an energy-releasing function, increasing strength and stamina, and in laboratory experiments it seems to improve reproductive disturbances.

If you try it, don't be impatient, it often takes 4 to 6 weeks for beneficial effects from octacosanol to be noticed.

Always keep in mind, too, that an energizing diet of raw or lightly cooked foods, rich in B vitamins and amino acids, will contribute to a good sex life.

I've heard athletes talk about the energizing properties of propolis. But I still don't know exactly what it is, or if it's something I should be taking at the age of 72?

If you start now, there's a good chance you'll still be taking it at 102! Propolis is a resinlike material, found in leaf buds and the bark of many common trees, that is collected by bees, who use their enzymes to convert it into pollen. Aside from being a rich source of minerals, B vitamins, and natural antibiotics, propolis has been shown to give athletes increased staying power. It can also stimulate the thymus gland, enhance the body's immune system, and be used externally to heal bruises and blemishes.

As a supplement, it's available in tablet, granule, and tincture form. (There are also creams for external use.) It works best when taken in conjunction with vitamin C and zinc.)

I'm a 45-year-old woman who works out daily. What natural energy enhancers would you recommend?

Along with vitamins A, B complex, C, E, iron and zinc, I'd recommend *Cytochrome C*. This simple compound of amino acids increases muscle performance, acts as a carrier of oxygen to the mitochondria (the cell powerhouse of skeletal muscle), and is an essential part of the metabolic process that makes prolonged exercise possible. In actively working muscles, the aerobic process of energy production is dependent on cytochromes. If this system becomes ineffective, the muscle cell metabolism switches to an alternate aerobic pathway that produces lactic acid. As the lactic acid builds, muscle fatigue ensues and thus reduces working endurance.

I would also recommend *inosine*. Known as an anti-fatigue

nutrient, inosine is found in meat, meat extracts, and sugar beets. A naturally occurring metabolic product that's readily utilized by the body, inosine increases the oxygen-carrying capacity of the blood, allowing more oxygen to be delivered to muscles and thereby reducing fatigue.

Other natural fatigue reducers are *propolis, octocosanol, ginseng* and *amino acids*. In order for the body to effectively use and synthesize protein, *all* the essential amino acids (see section 70) must be present and in the proper proportions. For general energy enhancement, they're best taken in balanced formula supplements. And for optimal potency, remember your diet must include ample vitamins B6, B12, and niacin.

What is "Spanish Fly" and is it really a natural aphrodisiac?

Far from it! "Spanish Fly" is actually "cantharides" made from the outer skeletons of beetles. It causes itching, but not necessarily for sex. In fact, it's a poisonous substance that can be anything *but* a turn-on. It has been linked to convulsions and kidney disorders, and has been reported to make urination virtually impossible, to say nothing of causing men to experience extremely painful erections.

What's legally marketed in this country as "Spanish Fly" is generally nothing more than dried herbs that are no more potent than parsley. I'd advise saving your money for a romantic dinner. As old-fashioned as it sounds, I feel that a candlelight dinner will beat a beetle skeleton as an aphrodisiac every time.

I've been told that there's something called "DMG" that is an aphrodisiac. Have you heard of it and does it work?

I've heard of it, but I can't vouch for its effectiveness. DMG is dimethyglycine, a nutrient found in grains. It aids in increasing the supply of oxygen to the bloodstream and body tissues. Those touting it as an aphrodisiac say that the increased oxygen in the tissues enhances your sexual response. (Maybe eating those Wheaties does work.) Anyway, it is available as a supplement, so you might want to give it a try. It might not be your ticket to ecstasy—but it won't hurt.

My grandmother used to say that sweet potatoes and carrots were women's fertility foods. She ate them frequently and had nine children. Was this just coincidence?

Maybe yes and maybe no. Carrots and sweet potatoes (yams) have been found to have chemical structures similar to estrogen—a necessary female fertility hormone.

XXI

Pets Need Good Nutrition Too

286. Vitamins for Your Dog

Dogs need vitamins as much as people do. Their requirements, of course, are not the same as ours, but they too need all the nutrients. (If you want to know exactly what they need for basic nutrition, write for the National Research Council's *Nutrient Requirements of Dogs*, National Academy of Sciences, Washington, D.C.)

An adult dog needs 4.4 g. protein daily, along with 1.3 g. fat, 0.4 g. linoleic or arachidonic acid, and 15.4 g. carbohydrate. Puppies need twice that amount.

Proteins are essential for a dog's growth and body repair. Those with a high biological value, such as eggs, muscle meat, fish meat, soybeans, milk, and yeast, are the best. If you want to give your dog eggs, be sure that they're cooked. Raw egg white contains avidin, which prevents biotin from being absorbed. Milk, though good for dogs, often causes diarrhea, so yogurt and cottage cheese are recommended.

Carbohydrates are used by dogs for energy, but it is suggested that no more than 50 to 60 percent of their food include them.

Fats, the most concentrated energy source, supply the essential fatty acid for healthy skin and hair. A deficiency can retard puppies' growth and lead to coarse hair and flaking skin. One teaspoon of safflower or corn oil added to the dog's dry food can help.

> Imbalanced supplements can
> harm your dog.

Calcium and phosphorus, in a ratio of 1.2 to 1, should be included in the dog's diet. If the ratio is incorrect, abnormal mineralization can occur in the bones of growing puppies as well as adult dogs. There must also be sufficient vitamin D for proper absorption of these two minerals. Because the balance is so important, *be certain that the vitamin supplements you give are balanced.* Too much bonemeal or cod liver oil can result in problems as severe as those you're trying to combat.

Cod liver oil is not advised as a routine supplement; it can lead to vitamin-D overload.

All-meat diets are not good for your pet because the calcium-phosphorus ratio is wrong and there are inadequate amounts of vitamins A, D, and E.

> Stop fleas with brewer's
> yeast.

Brewer's yeast, mixed in with your dog's food, will help prevent fleas. (It works for cats too.) Fleas despise the odor it gives off after your dog ingests it.

Do not give your dog supplemental vitamins A, D, or niacin. They can have an adverse effect on the animal. (See section 290 for "Cautions.")

287. Arthritis and Dysplasia Regimen for Dogs

Dogs, unlike humans, manufacture their own vitamin C, but recent research has shown that supplemental C can be effective in the treatment of arthritis and dysplasia. I recommend, though, that you consult your vet before starting any vitamin program. Ask him or her about this regimen:

Vitamin C, 300 mg.
4–5 alfalfa tablets
Vitamin E, 100 IU
Mix with food daily.

288. Vitamins for Your Cat

Cats need vitamins, just as people and dogs do, but nutritional requirements for them have not been as well established. (For the most recent available information, you can write for the National Research Council's *Nutrient Requirements of Laboratory Animals*, National Academy of Sciences, Washington, DC.)

> Cow's milk is insufficient
> for a growing kitten.

Protein requirements for cats are high, considerably higher than those of dogs or people. And kittens need one-third more protein than adult cats. Muscle meats, organ meat, poultry, fish, cheese, eggs, and milk are all good sources. (Eggs should be cooked or, if given raw, only the yolk should be used.) If you are giving a kitten milk, use a dry powdered milk at double the concentration given a human baby; cow's milk isn't nutritious enough for an infant cat.

Carbohydrates are not actually required in a cat's diet, but they are used as energy. If there are adequate levels of fats and protein, 33 percent of the diet can be made up of carbohydrates.

> Give your cat the fats
> you shouldn't eat.

Fats are a cat's most concentrated source of energy. Unlike people, cats can have diets of up to 64 percent fat and show no signs of vascular problems. Only because fats are more costly than carbohydrates do most cat foods have low percentages. In fact, you can give your cat the fats you need to cut down on—butter, animal fat, vegetable. Where cats are concerned, polyunsaturates are not the good guys. Too much polyunsaturated fatty acid is antagonistic to vitamin E, and fat deposits in the cat's body can be seriously affected.

Although levels of all the essential vitamins haven't been established for cats, the importance of certain vitamins in a cat's diet should be noted. For example, cats are dependent on their diet for fully formed vitamin A. (Their requirement is much higher than that of dogs because unlike dogs they cannot manufacture vitamin A in the body from carotene.) On the other hand, too much vitamin A can result in bone deformities. Liver as a supplement (not a total diet) is recommended, as is a *balanced* vitamin-mineral preparation. Fish, butter, milk, and cheese are also high in vitamin A.

The B vitamins are also important for a cat's nerve stability, outer coat, and inner tissues. B6 (pyridoxine) helps prevent urinary calculi, a serious problem for altered male cats. (A diet low in ash is recommended.) In general, cats require twice the amount of B vitamins needed by dogs, and feeding dog food to a cat for an extended period of time can result in a B-complex deficiency. It should also be noted that B1 (thiamine) can be destroyed by an antagonist in raw fish. (For foods high in B vitamins, see sections 27, 28, and 29.)

All-fish diets are not
healthy for cats.

Vitamin-E deficiency can occur from feeding excessive amounts of red meat tuna. (It can also occur because of any all-fish diet.) Lack of appetite, fever, pain, and a reluctance to move are characteristic symptoms of pansteatitis, which results from vitamin E deficiency. If this occurs, see your vet, don't feed tuna unless it is supplemented with vitamin E, and don't use fish oils as supplements.

The calcium-phosphorus ratio in a cat's diet should be about one to one, with adequate amounts of vitamin D. Since manufacturers of canned cat foods usually add irradiated yeast, a source of vitamin D, supplements of D are unnecessary—and can be dangerous. (See section 290 for "Cautions.")

A multiple vitamin with iron—prepared especially for cats— is often given for feline anemia. The disease is rare in cats on a balanced diet that includes cooked and raw muscle meat, organ meats, cooked meats, cooked or canned chicken, and fish, vitamin-rich cereals, and vegetables.

Keep in mind that pregnant or lactating cats, who often eat 10 to 15 ounces of food a day, have double or triple the vitamin requirements of an average five- to seven-pound cat.

289. Any Questions About Chapter XXI?

If selenium is an important antioxidant for humans, shouldn't it be given to dogs who live in cities, too?

I would not recommend selenium supplementation for dogs or cats unless such supplementation is prescribed by a vet and carefully monitored. Casual supplementation can be hazardous, particularly if your dog is old or sick.

XXII

Vitamin "Yeses" and "Nos" You Should Know

290. Cautions

Though we all know that vitamins are good for us, there are times, situations, and metabolic conditions where caution and special adjustments are advised. I recommend you look over the following list carefully for your own well-being and in order to get the most from your vitamins.

- Chronic hypervitaminosis A can occur in patients receiving megadoses as treatment for dermatological conditions.
- A deficiency of vitamin A can lead to loss of vitamin C.
- Large doses of vitamin A may cause birth defects, particularly if taken in the first trimester, and should be avoided by pregnant women.
- An oversupply of vitamin B1 (thiamine) can affect thyroid and insulin production and might cause B6 deficiency, as well as loss of other B vitamins.
- Prolonged ingestion of any B vitamin can result in significant depletion of the others.
- Pregnant women should check with their doctors before taking sustained doses of over 50 mg. of vitamin B6 (pyridoxine).
- B6 should not be taken by anyone under L-dopa treatment for Parkinson's disease.
- Large doses of vitamin B2 (riboflavin), especially if taken

without antioxidant supplements, may cause a sensitivity to sunlight.

• Because vitamin D promotes absorption of calcium, a large excess of stored vitamin D can cause too much calcium in the blood (hypercalcemia).

• Don't eat raw egg whites. They deactivate the body's biotin.

• It is possible that large amounts of vitamin C might reverse the anticoagulant activity of the blood thinner warfarin, commonly prescribed as the drug Coumadin.

• Diabetes and heart patients should check with their doctors, because vitamin C might necessitate a lower dosage of pills.

• Megadoses of vitamin C wash out B12 and folic acid, so be sure you are taking at least the daily requirement of both.

• Excessive doses of choline, taken over a long period of time, may produce a deficiency of vitamin B6.

• If you have a heart disorder, check with your physician for the proper vitamin-D dosage to take.

• Vitamin E should be used cautiously by anyone with an overactive thyroid, diabetes, high blood pressure, or rheumatic heart disease. (If you have any of these conditions, start at a very low dosage and build up gradually by 100 IU daily each month to between 400 and 800 IU.)

• Rheumatic heart fever sufferers should know that they have an imbalance between the two sides of their hearts and large vitamin-E doses can increase the imbalance and worsen the condition. (Before using supplements, consult your physician.)

• Vitamin E can elevate blood pressure in hypertensives, but if supplementation is started with a low dosage and increased slowly, the end result will be an eventual lowering of the pressure through the vitamin's diuretic properties.

• Diabetics have been able to reduce their insulin levels with E. Check with your physician.

• Decreases in vitamin E should be gradual, too.

• An excessive intake of folic acid can mask symptoms of pernicious anemia.

• High doses of folic acid for extended periods of time are not recommended for anyone with a medical history of convulsive disorders or hormone-related cancer.

- Folic acid and PABA might inhibit the effectiveness of sulfonamides, such as Gantrisin.
- Megadoses of vitamin K can build up and cause a red cell breakdown and anemia.
- Folic acid supplements are contraindicated for anyone taking the anticonvulsant phenotoin.
- Patients on the blood thinner Dicumarol should be aware that synthetic K could counteract the effectiveness of the drug. Conversely, the drug inhibits the absorption of natural vitamin K.
- Sweats and flushes can occur from too much vitamin K.
- Niacin should be used cautiously by anyone with severe diabetes, glaucoma, peptic ulcers, impaired liver function, or gout.
- Do not give niacin to your dog or cat; it causes flushing and sweating and greatly discomforts the animal. Do not supplement a pet's diet with vitamins A or D unless your vet specifically advises it.
- Excessive amounts of PABA (Para-aminobenzoic acid) in certain individuals can have a negative effect on the liver, kidneys, and heart.
- Iron should not be taken by anyone with sickle-cell anemia, hemochromatosis, or thalassemia.
- If your iron supplement is ferrous sulfate, you're losing vitamin E.
- Large quantities of caffeine can inhibit iron absorption.
- Anyone with kidney malfunction should not take more than 3,000 mg. of magnesium on a daily basis.
- Too much manganese will reduce utilization of the body's iron.
- High doses of manganese can cause motor difficulties and weakness in certain individuals.
- Diets high in fat increase phosphorus absorption and lower your calcium levels.
- If you take cortisone and aldosterone drugs, such as Aldactone and prednisone, you lose potassium and retain sodium. Check with your physician for proper supplements.
- Excessive perspiration can cause a depletion of sodium.
- Too much sodium can cause a potassium loss.

- Excessive zinc intakes can result in iron and copper losses.
- If you add zinc to your diet, be sure you're getting enough vitamin A.
- Anyone suffering from Wilson's disease is susceptible to copper toxicity.
- Too much cobalt may cause an unwanted enlargement of the thyroid gland.
- Anyone taking thyroid medication should be aware that kelp also affects that gland. If you have been using both, a consultation with your doctor and retesting are advised. You might need *less* prescription medicine than you think.
- Large amounts of raw cabbage can cause an iodine deficiency and throw off thyroid production in individuals with existing low-iodine intakes.
- Oyster shells, dolomite and bonemeal, although good sources of calcium, may contain lead or other toxic substances.
- Milk that contains synthetic vitamin D can deplete the body of magnesium.
- Heavy coffee and tea drinkers—cola drinkers, too—should be aware that large caffeine ingestion creates an inositol shortage.
- Inform your doctor if you're taking large amounts of vitamin C. C can change results of lab tests for sugar in the blood and urine and give false negative results in tests for blood in stool specimens.
- Don't engage in strenuous physical activity within four hours after taking vitamin A if you want optimum absorption.
- Copper has a tendency to accumulate in the blood and deplete the brain's zinc supplies.
- RNA-DNA supplements increase serum uric acid levels and should *not* be taken by anyone with gout.
- Tyrosine and phenylalanine may increase blood pressure and should *not* be taken with MAO inhibitors or other antidepressant drugs. These amino acids are also contraindicated for anyone with pigmented malignant melanomas.
- PABA is contraindicated with *methotrexate* (MEXATE), a cancer-fighting drug.

• People taking MAO inhibitors should avoid aged foods high in tyramine (cheese, wine, etc.) and be aware that the tyramine content of foods generally *increases* with age.

• Folacin (folic acid) decreases the anticonvulsant action of *phenytoin* (DILANTIN).

• Antibiotics are reduced in their effectiveness when taken with supplements. (Take supplements at least an hour before or two hours after prescription antibiotics.)

• Calcium can interfere with the effectiveness of tetracycline.

• High doses of vitamin D or calcium ascorbate are contraindicated if you are taking the heart medication *digoxin* (LANOXIN).

• Broad spectrum antibiotics should not be taken with high doses of vitamin A.

• Vitamin A should not be taken in conjunction with the acne drug ACCUTANE (*isotretinoin*).

• Choline is not recommended during the depressive phase of manic-depressive conditions, since it can deepen this particular sort of depression.

• Papaya, as well as raw pineapple, is not recommended for anyone with an ulcer.

291. Quick Reference Cancer Defense Guide

Along with antioxidant vitamins and minerals (see section 49), there are many naturally occurring substances in foods that appear to have even more powerful anti-cancer properties. Among them: beta-carotene, quercetin, indoles and isothiocyanatos (in cruciferous vegetables) and omega-3 fatty acids.

Since your best defense against cancer is a strong nutritional offense—be sure you put the following winning foods in your diet.

CANCER-FIGHTING FOODS TO INCREASE IN DIET

Food	Comments
Carrots	Highest in beta-carotene; more easily absorbed when cooked.
Cantaloupe	Great vitamin A, beta-carotene, and vitamin C source; low calorie and high fiber; aids in combatting excess sodium.
Cabbage	A cruciferous vegetable; can lower risk of colorectal cancer; just 2 tablespoons cooked daily has been found to help prevent stomach cancer.
Squash	Same as carrots above.
Sweet Potatoes	Same as carrots above.
Papaya	Same as cantaloupe.
Spinach	Same as cantaloupe. (See Cautions in section 290.)
Broccoli	A cruciferous vegetable that contains indoles and isothiocyanates (substances that help reduce and prevent certain cancerous tumors); rich in carotenoids.
Brussel sprouts	Same as broccoli and other crucifers.
Bok choy	Same as broccoli and other crucifers.
Cauliflower	Same as broccoli and other crucifers.
Kale	Same as broccoli and other crucifers.
Radish	Same as broccoli and other crucifers.
Horseradish	Same as broccoli and other crucifers.

Rutabaga	Same as broccoli and other crucifers.
Kohlrabi	Same as broccoli and other crucifers.
Celery	Same as broccoli and other crucifers.
Onions	High in quercertin (not destroyed by cooking): can suppress malignant cells before they become tumors.
Tuna	Rich in omega-3 fatty acids; helps immune system to prevent and inhibit spreading of cancers. (May help halt metastasis once tumor occurs.)
Salmon	Same as tuna.
Sardines	Same as tuna.
Mackerel	Same as tuna.
Bluefish	Same as tuna.
Wheat bran	Dietary fiber content helps prevent colon cancer. (The National Cancer Institute suggests 35 grams of fiber daily.)
Corn bran	Provides protection against carcinogens.
Rice bran	Same as corn and wheat bran.
Oat bran	Same as corn and wheat bran.
Fruits and vegetables high in vitamins A, C, E, and selenium	(See sections 26, 35, 39 and 63.)

HIGH-RISK CANCER FOODS TO DECREASE IN DIET

Bacon	Contains nitrite, an additive that can interact with natural chemicals in our foods and

	bodies to form nitrosamines, potent cancer-causing substances.
Luncheon meats	Same as bacon above.
Frankfurters	Same as bacon above.
Knockwurst	Same as bacon above.
Smoked fish	Same as bacon above.
Butter, margarine, mayonnaise, oils	It's recommended that no more than 20–30 percent of the calories in your diet come from fat. (Individuals whose diets contain over 40 percent fat, saturated as well as unsaturated, are more likely to develop colon, breast, and prostate cancers.) In these foods, 100 percent of the calories are fat.
Coffee (regular or decaffeinated)	Implicated in bladder and pancreatic cancers.
Liver and high-fat meat	Contaminants accumulate in an animal's liver and fat cells.
Tobacco	Cigarettes, cigars, pipes, chewing tobacco and snuff have been implicated in the development of cancer of the mouth, throat, esophagus, pancreas and bladder as well as the lung. (Smoking—as well as side-stream smoke—also increases the risk of cervical cancer for women.
Alcohol	Found to cause liver cancer and to contribute to cancers of the mouth, layrnx and esophagus, particularly among smokers.
Food additives, particularly BHA, BHT, Food Dyes Red	Highly-suspect carcinogens.

No. 3, Blue No. 2.
Green No. 3, and
Citrus Red No. 2;
propyl gallate and
sodium nitrite.

> Cancer is more common among people
> who are obese than people who are at or
> below their ideal body weight.

292. Any Questions About Chapter XXII?

*Is it true that licorice candy can be dangerous to people
taking antihypertensive medication?*

Surprisingly, yes. In fact, just two or more candy twists
made with "natural" licorice can interfere with many antihypertensive (and diuretic) medicines by increasing sodium
reabsorption, potassium excretion and water retention.

*I've been told to stay away from foods containing MSG, so
I read labels carefully and generally avoid Chinese food. But
are all foods that contain MSG labeled?*

The FDA requires products containing MSG to list it on
their labels. But recent studies have shown that there are
foods—tomatoes and cheese, for instance—that contain
monosodium glutamate (MSG) naturally! In other words, an
Italian meal may contain as much MSG as an Asian one.
(You might be interested to know that Asian foods frequently
contain natural chemicals such as salicylates and amines that
can also cause allergic reactions.)

XXIII

Locating a Nutritionally Oriented Doctor

293. How To Go About It

If you want to consult a nutritionally oriented physician but don't know any in your area, the following organizations can help you find one. If you're seeking a Board-certified physician, you should specify that, as not all nutritional health professionals are M.D.s.

It should be understood that no endorsement or other opinion of any practitioner contacted through these services (or such practitioner's diagnoses, treatments, or credentials) is implied or should be inferred.

As a courtesy, please be sure to enclose a self-addressed, stamped envelope with all queries.

ADDRESS

American Academy of Environmental Medicine
P.O. Box 16106
Denver, CO 80216
(303) 622-9755

American Association of Naturopathic Physicians
P.O. Box 20386
Seattle, WA 98102
(206) 323-7610

American College of Advancement in Medicine (ACAM)
23121 Verdugo Drive, Suite 204
Laguna Hills, CA 92653
(714) 583-7666

American Holistic Medical Association
4101 Lake Boone Trail
Raleigh, NC 27607
(919) 787-5146

American Holistic Nurses' Association
Box 116
Telluride, CO 81435

Arizona Homeopathic Medical Association
333 W. Cypress St.
Phoenix, AZ 85003
(602) 252-0443

Association for the Promotion of Herbal Healing
2000 Center St., Suite 1475
Berkeley, CA 94704

Coalition for Alternatives in Nutrition and Health Care
(CANAH)
P.O. Box B-12
Richlandtown, PA 18955
(215) 346-8461

Council for Responsible Nutrition
1300 19th St. NW
Washington, D.C. 20036
(202) 872-1609

Consulting Nutritionists
3150 E. 41st Street
Tulsa, OK 74135

Consulting Nutritionists in Private Practice
P.O. Box 345
Cold Springs, NY 10515

HEAL (Human Ecology Action League)
P.O. Box 1369
Evanston, IL 60204

Health Associates
1990 Broadway, Suite 1206
New York, NY 10023
(212) 307-1399

Hippocrates Health Institute
25 Exeter Street
Boston, MA 02116

The Huxley Institute
210 East 31st Street
New York, NY 10016

Huxley Institute for Biosocial Research
900 N. Federal Highway, Suite 330
Boca Raton, FL 33432
(800) 847-3802

International Academy of Holistic Health & Medicine
218 Avenue B
Redondo Beach, CA 90277
(213) 540-0564

International Academy of Nutrition and
Preventive Medicine
P.O. Box 5832
Lincoln, NE 68505
(402) 467-2716

International Academy of Preventive Medicine
34 Corporate Woods, Suite 469
Overland Park, KS 66210

International Foundation for Homeopathy
2366 Eastlake Ave. East, Suite 301
Seattle, WA 98102
(206) 324-8230

National Association of Naturopathic Physicians
2613 N. Stevens
Tacoma, WA 98407
(206) 789-7237

National Center for Homeopathy
1500 Massachusetts Ave. NW
Washington, D.C. 20005
(202) 223-6182

National Health Federation
P.O. Box 688
Monrovia, CA 91017
(818) 357-2181

Northwest Academy of Preventive Medicine
15615 Bellevue-Redmont Road, Suite E
Bellevue, WA 98008

Nutrition for Optimal Health Association
P.O. Box 380
Winnetka, IL 60093

Society for Clinical Ecology
2005 Franklin St., Suite 490
Denver, CO 80205

294. Finding Specialized Nutritional Help

(Enclose a self-addressed, stamped envelope with all queries.)

For alcoholism

Alcoholics Anonymous
P.O. Box 459
Grand Central Station
New York, NY 10163

For allergies

National Institute of Allergy and
    Infectious Diseases
NIH, Dept. of Health and
    Human Services
Bldg. 31, Room 7A32
Bethesda, MD 20205

For Alzheimer illnesses

Alzheimer's Disease and Related
    Disorders
P.O. Box 5675
Chicago, IL 60601
(800) 621-0379

ALS Society of America
15300 Ventura Blvd., Suite 315
Sherman Oaks, CA 91403

For arthritis

Arthritis Information
    Clearinghouse
Box 34427
Bethesda, MD 20817

For breast-feeding

La Leche League, Int., Inc.
9616 Minneapolis Ave.
P.O. Box 1209
Franklin Park, IL 60131-8209
(312) 455-7730

For cancer

Cancer Control Society
2043 N. Berendo St.
Los Angeles, CA 90027
(213) 663-7801

International Association of
   Cancer Victors and Friends,
   Inc.
7740 West Manchester Ave.,
   Suite 110
Playa del Rey, CA 90293
(213) 822-5032

National Cancer Institute
NIH, Bldg. 31, Rm 10A18
Bethesda, MD 20205

For cardiovascular
disorders

Association for Cardiovascular
   Therapy
P.O. Box 706
Bloomfield, CT 06002

Association of Heart Patients
P.O. Box 54305
Atlanta, GA 30308

For chronic fatigue
syndrome

Chronic Fatigue and Immune
   Dysfunction Syndrome
   Association
1-800-44-CFIDS or 1-800-442-
   3437

Chronic Fatigue Immune
   Dysfunction Syndrome Society
   International
P.O. Box 320108
Portland, OR 97223

For cardiovascular
disorders

Association for Cardiovascular
   Therapy
P.O. Box 706
Bloomfield, CT 06002

Association of Heart Patients
P.O. Box 54305
Atlanta, GA 30308

The Stroke Foundation
898 Park Avenue
New York, NY 10021

For communicative
disorders

American Tinnitus Association
P.O. Box 5
Portland, OR 97207
(503) 248-9985

National Council of Stutterers
P.O. Box 8171
Grand Rapids, MI 49508

For depression

Academy of Orthomolecular
   Psychiatry
P.O. Box 372
Manhasset, NY 11030

For diabetes

National Diabetic Information
   Clearinghouse
805 15th St. NW, Rm. 500
Washington, D.C. 20005

For eating disorders

American Anorexia and Bulimia
   Association, Inc.
418 E. 76th Street
New York, NY 10021
(212) 734-1114

ANAD (National Association of
   Anorexia Nervosa and
   Associated Disorders)
Box 271
Highland Park, IL 60035
(708) 831-3438

Anorexia Nervosa and Related
   Eating Disorders, Inc.
P.O. Box 5102
Eugene, OR 97405
(503) 344-1144

Bulimia Anorexia Self-Help
P.O. Box 39903
St. Louis, MO 63139
(800) 762-3334

For epilepsy

Epilepsy Foundation of America
4351 Garden City Drive
Landover, MD 20785
(301) 459-3700

For hypoglycemia

National Hypoglycemia
    Association
P.O. Box 885
Ithaca, NY 14850

For pets

The American Veterinary
    Holistic Medical Association
2214 Old Emmerton Road
Bel Air, MD 21014

For sleep disorders

Association for Sleep Disorders
    Center (ASDC)
Box 2604
Del Mar, CA 92014

For women

Coalition for the Medical Rights
    of Women
2845 24th Street
San Francisco, CA 94110

National Women's Health
    Network
1325 G St. NW
Washington, D.C. 20005
(202) 347-1140

295. Free Calls for Fast Answers

The National Health Information Clearinghouse, sponsored by the Department of Health and Human Services, can direct you to numerous free health information services. Just call: 1-800-336-4797.

Among the toll-free hotlines are:

- Acne Help Line: 1-800-222-SKIN; in California, 1-800-221-SKIN
- Alzheimer's Disease and Related Disorders Association: 1-800-621-0379; in Illinois, 1-800-572-6037
- American Council for the Blind: 1-800-424-8666
- American Society for Dermatologic Surgery: 1-800-441-ASDS
- Arthritis Medical Center: 1-800-327-3027
- Bulimia and Anorexia Self-Help: 1-800-762-3334
- Cancer Information Service: 1-800-4-CANCER
- Dial-a-Hearing Screening Test: 1-800-222-EARS
- Epilepsy Foundation of America: 1-800-EFA-1000
- Heartlife: 1-800-241-6993
- Herbs: Penn Herb 1-800--523-9971; Herbal Pathways, 1-800-631-3575; Green Mountain Herbs, 1-800-525-2696; Foodscience Corporation, 1-800-451-5190
- Juvenile Diabetes Foundation International: 1-800-JDF-CURE
- National AIDS Hotline: 1-800-342-AIDS
- National Center for Stuttering: 1-80-221-2483
- National Drug Abuse Treatment Referral and Information Service: 1-800-COCAINE
- National Institute on Drug Abuse: 1-800-662-4357
- Second Surgical Opinion Hotline: 1-800-638-6833
- Sexually Transmitted Disease Hotline: 1-800-227-8922
- Sudden Infant Death Syndrome Hotline: 1-800-221-7437
- Vegetarian Information Service (Morningstar Farms—A division of Miles Laboratories): 1-800-243-4143
- Y-Me Breast Cancer Support Program: 1-800-221-2141

Afterword

As more and more people have become aware of the importance of vitamins in their daily lives, the need for clear, uncomplicated information has become evident. And with more and more research showing that the right vitamins at the right time are much more important to us than anyone ever realized, the need has become a necessity. It is my hope that this newly revised book has fulfilled that need, that it has debunked the myths surrounding food and nutrition, and erased any uncertainties about the nature, function, and safety of vitamins.

Whether you have read the book cover to cover or simply thumbed through to personally relevant points, I believe you'll find its reference value will increase as new life situations arise. My intention was to provide an omnibus guide that could answer not only your present vitamin questions, but future ones as well. As times goes by, the sections on staying young, energetic and sexy, and retarding the aging process will bear rereading, as will those offering regimens for whatever your new particular circumstance happens to be. In other words, the information I have set down is meant to be pursued, and is intended not just for today, but for many, many happy and healthy tomorrows.

DR. EARL MINDELL, R.PH., PH.D.
Beverly Hills, California
May 16, 1991

Glossary

Absorption: the process by which nutrients are passed into the bloodstream.

Acetate: a derivative of acetic acid.

Acetic acid: used as a synthetic flavoring agent, one of the first food additives (vinegar is approximately 4 to 6 percent acetic acid); it is found naturally in cheese, coffee, grapes, peaches, raspberries, and strawberries; Generally Recognized As Safe (GRAS) when used only in packaging.

Acetone: a colorless solvent for fat, oils, and waxes, which is obtained by fermentation (inhalation can irritate lungs, and large amounts have a narcotic effect).

Acid: a water-soluble substance with sour taste.

Adrenals: the glands, located above each kidney, that manufacture adrenaline.

Alkali: an acid-neutralizing substance (sodium bicarbonate is an alkali used for excess acidity in foods).

Allergen: a substance that causes an allergy.

Alzheimer's disease: a progressively degenerative disease, involved with loss of memory, which new research indicates might be helped with extra choline.

Amino acid chelates: chelated minerals that have been produced by many of the same processes nature uses to chelate minerals in the body; in the digestive tract, nature surrounds the elemental minerals with amino acid, permitting them to be absorbed into the bloodstream.

Amino acids: the organic compounds from which proteins are constructed; there are twenty-two known amino acids, but only nine are indispensable nutrients for man—histidine, isoleucine, leucine, lysine, total S-containing amino acids, total aromatic amino acids, threonine, tryptophan, and valine.

Anorexia: loss of appetite.

Antibiotic: any of various substances that are effective in inhibiting or destroying bacteria.

Anticoagulant: something that delays or prevents blood-clotting.

Antigen: any substance not normally present in the body that stimulates the body to produce antibodies.

Antihistamine: a drug used to reduce effects associated with histamine production in allergies and colds.

Antioxidant: a substance that can protect another substance from oxidation; added to foods to keep oxygen from changing the food's color.

Antitoxin: an antibody formed in response to, and capable of neutralizing, a poison of biologic origin.

Assimilation: the process whereby nutrients are used by the body and changed into living tissue.

Ataxia: loss of coordinated movement caused by disease of nervous system.

ATP: a molecule called adenozine triphosphate, the fuel of life, a nucleotide—building block of nucleic acid—that produces biological energy with B1, B2, B3, and pantothenic acid.

Avidin: a protein in egg white capable of inactivating biotin.

Bacteriophage: a virus that infects bacteria.

Bariatrician: a weight-control doctor.

B-Cells: white blood cells, made in the bone marrow, which produce antibodies upon instructions from T-cells, white blood cells manufactured in the thymus.

BHA: butylated hydroxyanisole; a preservative and antioxidant used in many products; insoluble in water; can be toxic to the kidneys.

BHT: butylated hydroxytoluene; a solid, white crystalline antioxidant used to retard spoilage of many foods; can be more toxic to the kidney than its nearly identical chemical cousin BHA.

Bioflavonoids: usually from orange and lemon rinds, these citrus-flavored compounds needed to maintain healthy bloodvessel walls are widely available in plants, citrus fruits, and rose hips; known as vitamin P complex.

Calciferol: a colorless, odorless crystalline material, insoluble in water; soluble in fats; a synthetic form of vitamin D made by irradiating ergosterol with ultraviolet light.

Calcium gluconate: an organic form of calcium.

Capillary: a minute blood vessel, one of many that connect the arteries and veins.

Carcinogen: a cancer-causing substance.

Carotene: an orange-yellow pigment occurring in many plants and capable of being converted into vitamin A in the body.

Casein: the protein in milk that has become the standard by which protein quality is measured.

Catabolism: the metabolic change of nutrients or complex substances into simpler compounds, accompanied by a release of energy.

Catalyst: a substance that modifies, especially increases, the rate of chemical reaction without being consumed or changed in the process.

Chelation: a process by which mineral substances are changed into easily digestible form.

Chronic: of long duration; continuing; constant.

CNS: central nervous system.

Coenzyme: the major portion, though nonprotein, part of an enzyme; usually a B vitamin.

Collagen: the primary organic constituent of bone, cartilage, and connective tissue (becomes gelatin through boiling).

Congenital: condition existing at birth, not hereditary.

Dehydration: a condition resulting from an excessive loss of water from the body.

Dermatitis: an inflammation of the skin; a rash.

Desiccated: dried; preserved by removing moisture.

Dicalcium phosphate: a filler used in pills, which is derived from purified mineral rocks and is an excellent source of calcium and phosphorus.

Diluents: fillers; inert material added to tablets to increase their bulk in order to make them a practical size for compression.

Diuretic: tending to increase the flow of urine from the body.

DNA: deoxyribonucleic acid; the nucleic acid in chromosomes that is part of the chemical basis for hereditary characteristics.

Endogenous: being produced from within the body.

Enteric coated: a tablet coated so that it dissolves in the intestine, not in the stomach (which is acid).

Enuresis: bed-wetting.

Enzyme: a protein substance found in living cells that brings about chemical changes; necessary for digestion of food.

Excipient: any inert substance used as a dilutant or vehicle for a drug.

Exogenous: being derived or developed from external causes.

FDA: Food and Drug Administration.

Fibrin: an insoluble protein that forms the necessary fibrous network in the coagulation of blood.

Free-radicals: highly reactive chemical fragments that can produce an irritation of artery walls, start the arteriosclerotic process if vitamin E is not present; generally harmful.

Fructose: a natural sugar occurring in fruits and honey; called fruit sugar; often used as a preservative for foodstuffs and an intravenous nutrient.

Galactosemia: a hereditary disorder in which milk becomes toxic as food.

Glucose: blood sugar; a product of the body's assimilation of carbohydrates and a major source of energy.

Glutamic Acid: an amino acid present in all complete proteins; usually manufactured from vegetable protein; used as a salt substitute and a flavor-intensifying agent.

Glutamine: an amino acid that constitutes, with glucose, the major nourishment used by the nervous system.

Gluten: a mixture of two proteins—gliadin and glutenin—present in wheat, rye, oats, and barley.

Glycogen: the body's chief storage carbohydrate, primarily in the liver.

GRAS: Generally Recognized As Safe; a list established by Congress to cover substances added to food.

Hesperidin: part of the C complex.

Holistic treatment: treatment of the whole person.

Homeostasis: the body's physiological equilibrium.

Hormone: a substance formed in endocrine organs and transported by body fluids to activate other specifically receptive organs.

Humectant: a substance that is used to preserve the moisture content of materials.

Hydrochloric acid: a normally acidic part of the body's gastric juice.

Hydrolyzed: put into water-soluble form.

Hydrolyzed protein chelate: water-soluble and chelated for easy assimilation.

Hypervitaminosis: a condition caused by an excessive ingestion of vitamins.

Hypoglycemia: a condition caused by abnormally low blood sugar.

Hypovitaminosis: a deficiency disease owing to an absence of vitamins in the diet.

Ichthyosis: a condition characterized by a scaliness on the outer layer of skin.

Idiopathic: a condition whose causes are not yet known.

Immune: protected against disease.

Insulin: the hormone, secreted by the pancreas, concerned with the metabolism of sugar in the body.

IU: International Units.

Lactating: producing milk.

Laxative: a substance that stimulates evacuation of the bowels.

Linoleic acid: one of the polyunsaturated fats, a constituent of lecithin; known as vitamin F; indispensable for life, and must be obtained from foods.

Lipid: a fat or fatty substance.

Lipofuscin: age pigment in cells.

Lipotropic: preventing abnormal or excessive accumulation of fat in the liver.

Megavitamin therapy: treatment of illness with massive amounts of vitamins.

Metabolize: to undergo change by physical and chemical processes.

Mucopolysaccharide: thick gelatinous material that is found many places in the body; it glues cells together and lubricates joints.

Nitrites: used as fixatives in cured meats; can combine with natural stomach and food chemicals to cause dangerous cancer-causing agents called nitrosamines.

Orthomolecular: the right molecule used for the right treatment; doctors who practice preventive medicine and use vitamin therapies are known as orthomolecular physicians.

OSHA: Occupational Safety and Health Administration.

Oxalates: organic chemicals found in certain foods, especially spinach, which can combine with calcium to form calcium oxalate, an insoluble chemical the body cannot use.

PABA: para-aminobenzoic acid; a member of the B complex.

Palmitate: water-solubilized vitamin A.

PKU (phenylketonuria): a hereditary disease caused by the lack of an enzyme needed to convert an essential amino acid (phenylalanine) into a form usable by the body; can cause mental retardation unless detected early.

Polyunsaturated fats: highly nonsaturated fats from vegetable sources; tend to lower blood cholesterol.

Predigested protein: protein that has been processed for fast assimilation and can go directly to the bloodstream.

Prostaglandins: hormone-like substances that aid in regulation of the immune system.

Provitamin: a vitamin precursor; a chemical substance necessary to produce a vitamin.

PUFA: polyunsaturated fatty acid.

RDA: Recommended Dietary Allowances as established by the Food and Nutrition Board, National Academy of Sciences, National Research Council.

RNA: the abbreviation used for ribonucleic acid.

Rose hips: a rich source of vitamin C; the nodule underneath the bud of a rose called a hip, in which the plant produces the vitamin C we extract.

Rutin: a substance extracted from buckwheat; part of the C complex.

Saturated fatty acids: usually solid at room temperature; higher proportions found in foods from animal sources; tend to raise blood cholesterol levels.

Sequestrant: a substance that absorbs ions and prevents changes that would affect flavor, texture, and color of food; used for water softening.

Syncope: brief loss of consciousness; fainting.

Synergistic: the action of two or more substances to produce an effect that neither alone could accomplish.

Synthetic: produced artificially.

Systemic: capable of spreading through the entire body.

T-Cells: white blood cells, manufactured in the thymus, which protect the body from bacteria, viruses, and cancer-causing agents, while controlling the production of B-cells, which produce antibodies, and unwanted production of potentially harmful T-cells.

Teratological: monstrous or abnormal formations in animals or plants.

Tocopherols: the group of compounds (alpha, beta, delta, episilon, eta, gamma, and zeta) that make vitamin E; obtained through vacuum distillation of edible vegetable oils.

Toxicity: the quality or condition of being poisonous, harmful, or destructive.

Toxin: an organic poison produced in living or dead organisms.

Triglycerides: fatty substances in the blood.

Unsaturated fatty acids: most often liquid at room temperature; primarily found in vegetable fats.

USAN: United States Adopted Names Council; cosponsored by the American Pharmaceutical Association (APhA), the American Medical Association (AMA), and the United States Pharmacopeia (USP) for the specific purpose of coining suitable, acceptable, nonproprietary names in the drug field.

USRDA: United States Recommended Daily Allowances.

Xerosis: a condition of dryness.

Zein: protein from corn.

Zyme: a fermenting substance.

Bibliography and Recommended Reading

I owe a great debt of thanks to the many scientists, doctors, nutritionists, professors, and researchers whose painstaking and all too often unrewarding work in the field of vitamins and nutrition has made this book possible.

The following list is given to show my sincere appreciation and make known the foundation upon which I have built my knowledge. Many of the books are highly technical and confusing for the layman, meant as they are for professionals in the field. But others, which I have marked with an asterisk, I heartily commend to you for further reading and a healthier future.

*Abrahamson, E.M., and Pezet, A.W. *Body, Mind and Sugar*. New York: Avon Books, 1977.

*Abravanel, Elliot D., M.D., and King, Elizabeth A. *Anti-Craving Weight Loss Diet*. New York: Bantam Books, 1990.

*Adams, Ruth. *The Complete Home Guide to All the Vitamins*. New York: Larchmont Books, 1972.

*Adams, Ruth, and Murray, Frank. *Minerals: Kill or Cure*. New York: Larchmont Books, 1976.

*Aguilar, Nona. *Totally Natural Beauty*. New York: Rawson Associates Publishers, 1977.

*Airola, Paavo. *Are You Confused?* Phoenix, AZ: Health Plus, 1972.

*————. *How To Get Well*. Phoenix, AZ: Health Plus, 1975.

*————. *Hypoglycemia, A Better Approach*. Phoenix, AZ: Health Plus, 1977.

Amberson, Rosanne. *Raising Your Cat*. New York: Bonanza Books, 1969.

*Atkins, Robert C. *Dr. Atkins' Diet Revolution*. New York: David McKay, 1972.

*Atkins, Robert C. *Dr. Atkins' Nutrition Breakthrough*. New York: William Morrow and Company, Inc., 1981.

*Bailey, Hubert. *Vitamin E: Your Key to a Healthy Heart*. New York: ARC Books, 1964, 1966.

Bieri, John G. "Fat-soluble vitamins in the eighth revision of the Recommended Dietary Allowances." *Journal of the American Dietetic Association* 64 (February 1974).

Blood: The River of Life. American National Red Cross, 1976.

*Bolles, Edmund Blair. *Learning to Live with Chronic Fatigue Syndrome*. New York: Dell Medical Library, 1990.

*Borsaak, Henry. *Vitamins: What They Are and How They Can Benefit You*. New York: Pyramid Books, 1971.

"Bread: You Can't Judge a Loaf by Its Color." *Consumer Reports* 41 (May 1976).

*Bricklin, Mark. *Practical Encyclopedia of Natural Healing*. Emmaus, PA: Rodale Press, 1976.

Brody, Jane E. "Cancer-blocking Agents Found in Foods." *New York Times*, 6 March 1979.

*————. *The New York Times Guide to Personal Health*. New York: Times Books, 1982.

*Burack, Richard, with Fox, Fred J. *New Handbook of Prescription Drugs*. New York: Pantheon Books, 1967.

Burton, Benjamin. *Human Nutrition*. 3rd ed. New York: McGraw-Hill, 1976.

"Buying Beef." *Consumer Reports* 39 (September 1974).

*Carr, William H.A. *The Basic Book of the Cat*. New York: Gramercy Publishing Co., 1963.

*Chapman, Esther. *How To Use the 12 Tissue Salts*. New York: Pyramid Books, 1977.

*"Chronic Fatigue Syndrome: A Modern Medical Mystery." *Newsweek* (November 12, 1990).

*Clark, Linda. *The Best of Linda Clark*. New Canaan, CT: Keats Publishing Co., 1976.

*————. *Know Your Nutrition*. New Canaan, CT: Keats Publishing Co., 1973.

*————. *Secrets of Health and Beauty*. New York: Jove Publication, 1977.

*Consumer Reports, Editors of. *The Medicine Show*. Mount Vernon, NY: Consumers Union, 1981.

Cooper, Barber, Mitchell, Rynberge, Green. *Nutrition in Health and Disease*. New York: Lippincott, 1963.

Cooper, Kenneth H., M.D. *Overcoming Hypertension*. New York: Bantam Books, 1990.

Cumulative Index for Journal of Applied Nutrition. La Habra, CA: International College of Applied Nutrition, 1947–76, 1976.

*Davis, Adelle. *Let's Eat Right To Keep Fit*. New York: Harcourt, Brace and World, 1954.

*————. *Let's Get Well*. New York: Harcourt, Brace and World, 1965.

*————. *Let's Have Healthy Children*. 2nd ed. New York: Harcourt, Brace and World, 1959.

*Dufty, William. *Sugar Blues*. Pennsylvania: Chilton Book Co., 1975.

*Ebon, Martin. *Which Vitamins Do You Need?* New York: Bantam Books, 1974.

Farrar, Jill. "Health & Fitness." *Vogue Australia* (December 1990).

Flynn, Margaret A. "The Cholesterol Controversy." *Journal of the American Pharmacy* NS18 (May 1978).

"Food Facts Talk Back." *Journal of the American Dietetic Association*, 1977.

*Frank, Benjamin S. *No-Aging Diet*. New York: Dial, 1976.

*Fredericks, Carlton. *Eating Right for You*. New York: Grosset and Dunlap, 1972.

*————. *Look Younger/Feel Healthier*. New York: Grosset and Dunlap, 1977.

*————. *Psycho Nutrients*. New York: Grosset and Dunlap, 1975.

*Gomez, Joan, and Gerch, Marvin J. *Dictionary of Symptoms*. New York: Stein and Day, 1963.

Goodhart, Robert S., and Shills, Maurice E. *Modern Nutrition in Health and Disease*. 5th ed. Philadelphia: Lea and Febiger, 1973.

*Graedon, Joe. *The People's Pharmacy*. New York: St. Martin's Press, 1976.

Guidelines for the Eradication of Iron Deficiency Anemia. New York: International Nutritional Anemia Consultative Group (INACG), 1976.

Guidelines for the Eradication of Vitamin-A Deficiency and Xerophthalmia. International Vitamin-A Consultative Group (IVACG).

Harper, Alfred E. "Recommended Dietary Allowances: Are They What We Think They Are?" *Journal of the American Dietetic Association* 64 (February 1974).

Holvey, David, ed. *The Merck Manual*. 12th ed. Rahway, NJ: Merck and Co., 1972.

Howe, Phyllis S. *Basic Nutrition in Health and Disease*. 6th ed. Philadelphia: W.B. Saunders Co., 1976.

"How Nutritious Are Fast-Food Meals?" *Consumer Reports* (May 1975).

*Hunter, B.T. *The Natural Foods Primer*. New York: Simon and Schuster, 1972.

Index of Nutrition Education Materials. Washington, DC: Nutrition Foundation, 1977.

Journal of Applied Nutrition. International College of Applied Nutrition, La Habra, CA, 1974–76.

*Karelitz, Samuel. *When Your Child Is Ill*. New York: Random House, 1969.

Katz, Marcella. *Vitamins, Food, and Your Health*. Public Affairs Committee, 1971, 1975.

*Kordel, L. *Health Through Nutrition*. New York: MacFadden-Bartell, 1971.

*Kowalsi, Robert E. *The 8-Week Cholesterol Cure*. New York: Harper and Row, 1987.

Lewin, Renate. "Chronic Fatigue Syndrome: It's Not All in Your Head." *Let's Live* (February 1991).

*Linde, Shirley. *The Whole Health Catalog*. New York: Rawson Associates Publishers, 1977.

"The Losing Formula." *Newsweek* (April 30, 1990).

*Lucas, Richard. *Nature's Medicines*. New York: Prentice-Hall, 1965.

*McGinnis, Terri. *The Well Cat Book*. New York: Random House-Bookworks, 1975.

*————. *The Well Dog Book*. New York: Random House-Bookworks, 1974.

"Marijuana: The Health Questions." *Consumer Reports* 40 (March 1975).

*Martin, Clement G. *Low Blood Sugar: The Hidden Menace of Hypoglycemia*. New York: Arco Publishing Co., 1976.

Martin, Marvin. *Great Vitamin Mystery*. Rosemont, IL: National Dairy Council, 1978.

*Mayer, Jean. *A Diet for Living*. New York: David McKay, 1975.

Mitchell, Helen S. "Recommended Dietary Allowances Up to Date." *Journal of the American Dietetic Association* 64 (February 1974).

National Health Federation Bulletin. November 1973. National Research Council. *Recommended Dietary Allowances*. 8th ed., revised. Washington, DC: National Academy of Sciences, 1974.

National Research Council. *Recommended Dietary Allowances*. 10th ed. Washington, DC: National Academy Press, 1989.

*Newbold, H.L. *Dr. Newbold's Revolutionary New Discovery About Weight Loss*. New York: Rawson Associates Publishers, 1977.

*————. *Mega-Nutrients for Your Nerves*. New York: Peter H. Wyden, Publisher, 1973.

*Null, Gary. *The Natural Organic Beauty Book*. New York: Dell, 1972.

*Null, Gary and Steve. *The Complete Book of Nutrition*. New York: Dell, 1972.

Nutrition Almanac. New York: McGraw-Hill, 1973.

Nutrition—Applied Personally. La Habra, CA: International College of Applied Nutrition, 1978.

Nutrition Information Resources for the Whole Family. National Nutrition Education Clearing House, 1978.

Nutrition Labeling: How It Can Work for You. National Nutrition Consortium, American Dietetic Association, 1975.

Nutrition Source Book. Rosemont, IL: National Dairy Council, 1978.

"Organic Chemical in Water: A Major Health Concern." *Consumer Reports* (February 1983):69.

*Passwater, Richard A. *Super Nutrition*. New York: Dial, 1975.

*Passwater, Richard A. *The New Supernutrition*. New York: Pocket Books, 1991.

*Pauling, Linus. *Vitamin C and the Common Cold*. New York: Bantam Books, 1971.

*Pearson, Durk, and Shaw, Sandy. *Life Extension*. New York: Warner Books, 1983.

Piltz, Albert. *How Your Body Uses Food*. Rosemont, IL: National Dairy Council, 1960.

*Pommery, Jean. *What To Do till the Veterinarian Comes*. Radnor, PA: Chilton Book Company, 1976.

"Present Knowledge in Nutrition." *Nutrition Reviews*. Nutrition Foundation, Inc., 1976.

*Pritikin, Nathan. *The Pritikin Permanent Weight-Loss Manual*. New York: Grosset & Dunlap, 1981.

*Rodale, J. I. *The Complete Book of Minerals for Health*. 4th ed. Emmaus, PA: Rodale Books, 1976.

*———. The Encyclopedia of Common Diseases. Emmaus, PA: Rodale Press, 1976.

*Rosenberg, Harold, and Feldzaman, A.N. *Doctor's Book of Vitamin Therapy: Megavitamins for Health*. New York: Putnam's, 1974.

*Schiffman, Susan S., and Scobey, Joan. *The Nutri/System Flavor Set-Point Weight-Loss Cookbook*. Boston: Little Brown and Company, 1990.

*Seaman, Barbara, Gideon. *Women and the Crisis in Sex Hormones*. New York: Rawson Associates Publishers, 1977.

*Shute, Wilfrid E., and Taub, Harold J. *Vitamin E for Ailing and Healthy Hearts*. New York: Pyramid Books, 1969.

*Smith, Lendon, M.D. *Feed Yourself Right*. New York: McGraw Hill, 1983.

*Spock, Benjamin. *Baby and Child Care*. New York: Simon and Schuster, 1976.

*Steinman, David. *Diet For A Poisoned Planet*. New York: Harmony Brooks, Crown Publishers, 1990.

*Stoff, Jesse A., M.D. *Chronic Fatigue Syndrome: The Hidden Epidemic*. New York: Harper and Row, 1988.

Thompson, Trisha. "Eat Your Heart Out?" *Fame* (February 1990).

"Too Much Sugar." *Consumer Reports* 43 (March 1973).

Underwood, Eric J. *Trace Elements in Human and Animal Nutrition*. 4th ed. New York: Academic Press, 1977.

United Nations, Food and Agriculture Organization. *Calorie Requirements*, 1957, 1972.

U.S. Department of Agriculture. *Amino Acid Content of Food* by M.L. Orr and B.K. Watt, 1957; rev. 1968.

U.S. Department of Agriculture. Consumer and Food Economics Institute, Agricultural Research Service. *Composition of Foods: Raw, Processed, Prepared* by Bernice K. Watt and Annabel L. Merrill, 1975.

U.S. Department of Agriculture. *Energy Value of Foods: Basis and Derivation* by Annabel L. Merrill and Bernice K. Watt, 1973.

U.S. Department of Agriculture. *Nutritive Value of American Foods* by Catherine F. Adams, 1975.

U.S. Department of Health, Education and Welfare. *Consumer Health Education: A Directory*, 1975.

U.S. Department of Health, Education and Welfare. *Ten-State Nutrition Survey*. Washington, DC: U.S. Government Printing Office, 1968–70.

"The U.S. Food and Drug Administration: On Food and Drugs." *Consumer Reports* 38 (March 1973).

U.S. President's Council on Physical Fitness and Sports. *Exercise and Weight Control* by Robert E. Johnson. Urbana, IL: University of Illinois Press, 1967.

U.S. Senate. Select Committee on Nutrition and Human Needs. *Diet and Killer Diseases with Press Reaction and Additional Information*. Washington, DC: U.S. Government Printing Office, 1977.

U.S. Senate. Select Committee on Nutrition and Human Needs. *National Nutrition Policy: Nutrition and the Consumer II*. Washington, DC: U.S. Government Printing Office, 1974.

"Vitamin-Mineral Safety, Toxicity and Misuse." *Journal of the American Dietetic Association*, 1978.

*Wade, Carlson. *Magic Minerals*. West Nyack, NY: Parker Publishing Co., 1967.

*————. *Miracle Protein*. West Nyack, NY: Parker Publishing Co., 1975.

*————. *Vitamin E: The Rejuvenation Vitamin*. New York: Award Books, 1970.

*Whelan, Elizabeth M., Ph.D. and Stare, Fredrick J., M.D. *The 100% Natural, Purely Organic, Cholesterol-Free, Megavitamin, Low-Carbohydrate Nutrition Hoax*. New York: Atheneum, 1983.

"Which Cereals Are Most Nutritious?" *Consumer Reports* 40 (February 1975).

Williams, Roger J. *Nutrition Against Disease*. New York: Pitman Publishers, 1971.

*Winter, Ruth. *A Consumer's Dictionary of Food Additives*. New York: Crown, 1973.

*Young, Klein, Beyer. *Recreational Drugs*. New York: Macmillan, 1977.

*Yudkin, John. *Sweet and Dangerous*. New York: Peter H. Wyden, 1972.

Index

Acacia (gum arabic), 20
Acesulfame K, 273
Acidophilus, 137, 138, 281
Acne, 27, 28, 54, 137, 152,
    178, 210–211, 280, 318
Aconite, 149
Actors, splmt for, 204
Adaptogens, 138, 158–59
Age reversing/retarding, 2, 89,
    27, 33, 37, 43, 51, 65–67,
    118, 287–88
Aging, 37, 43, 68, 73, 82, 86,
    95, 110, 111, 133, 200,
    208, 289–90
AIDS, 118–19, 144; hotline,
    318
Alcohol, 7, 38, 39, 104, 113,
    114, 118, 121, 141, 214,
    234, 241, 247–49, 258,
    260, 308, 314; depletion of
    vit./min., 12, 34, 35, 42,
    47, 48, 58, 61, 65, 68, 81,
    82, 88, 214, 248, 255;
    splmt for drinkers, 30, 32,

37, 49, 56, 95, 114, 206–
    07, 249
Alfalfa, 59, 138–39
Algin, warning, 20–21
Allergy, 118, 133, 160, 182,
    189, 194, 223–24, 254,
    255, 309, 314; splmt for,
    43, 47, 67, 87, 212, 223–
    24
Aloe vera, 149–50, 212
Alzheimer's, 48, 68, 314, 319
Amino acids, 14, 75, 91, 100,
    103–21, 243, 294
Anemia: iron deficiency, 71, 79,
    187; nutri. macrocytic, 55;
    pernicious, 36, 133, 302;
    splmts, 34, 35, 36, 52, 55,
    66, 74, 75, 84, 110, 138
Anise, 150
Antacids, 30, 115, 133, 135,
    255; natural, 135, 253
Antibiotics, 42, 46, 59, 61, 257,
    305; natural, 253
Anticoagulants, 51, 59, 255, 303

Anticonvulsants, 50, 116–17

Antidepressants, 33, 104, 106, 108, 121, 239–40, 242, 253

Antihistamine, 24, 252, 255; vitamin C, 214, 216, 219

Antioxidants, 28, 51, 66–67, 88, 89, 118, 198, 289

Anxiety, 104, 116, 121, 133, 151, 239–42

Appetite, 55, 96, 106, 116, 117–18, 120, 121, 139, 144, 150, 269; loss, 164–65

Aphrodisiacs, 292, 294–95

Apples, 13; craving, 182

Arginine, 101, 110–13, 119, 120, 121, 268

Arteriosclerosis, 48, 73, 94, 122, 123

Arthritis, 35, 75, 118, 119, 120, 129, 140, 145, 314, 318; herbal rem., 149, 151, 152, 157; pain, 86, 108; splmts, 47, 67, 224

Aspartame, 106, 273

Aspartic acid, 101, 114, 117, 120, 273

Aspirin, 12, 56, 59, 81, 253, 254, 255

Asthma, 39, 224–25

Astragalus, 150

Atherosclerosis, 115, 129

Athletes, 40, 114, 118, 200–01, 293

Athlete's foot, remedy, 211

Atkins diet, 252, 259

Backaches, 71, 108

Bacon, 90, 91, 183, 307

Bad breath, 61, 115, 137, 157, 165, 211

Baking soda/powder, 91, 186, 276

Balanced diet, 161–62

Bananas, 82, 87, 104, 182

Barbiturates, 215, 252, 254, 255

Basil, 149

B-complex vitamins, 16, 17, 22, 23, 28, 30, 46, 47, 56, 57, 60, 79, 91, 94, 105, 133, 280; deficiency, 166, 169, 172, 174, 178, 179, 238–39

Bee stings, splmt, 211–12

Beriberi, 29

Beta-carotene, 14, 26, 66, 67, 68, 280

Bile, 9–10, 91, 141

Bioflavonoids, 11, 18, 45, 53, 62–64, 166, 177, 280

Biotin, 11, 41–42, 83, 164, 172, 174, 176, 179

Bleeding, 58; gums, 63, 64, 212

Blessed Thistle, 150–51

Blood, 46, 52, 55, 74, 75, 79; clots, 43, 52, 58; coagulation, 66, 129; PH, 72, 93, 115; testing, 45, 304

Blood pressure, 52, 60, 73, 87, 90, 91, 107, 108, 129, 138, 139, 152, 172–73, 237, 250, 275; lowering, 225–26, 289; regimens, 226; splmt, 173

Body odor, 115, 165–66

Bonemeal, 70, 86, 304

Bones, 13, 69, 70, 75, 76, 83, 180, 212

Boron, 13, 15, 71

Brain, 104, 113, 115, 116, 120

Bran/fiber, 146–47, 288

Branched Chain Amino Acids (BCAAs), 119–20, 201–02

Breakfast, 198, 265–66, 291

Breast: cancer, 308; cancer help line, 318; disease, 245

Brewer's yeast, 292, 297

Bronchitis, 227
Bruising, 64, 166, 212, 293
Burning sensation, 187
Burns, 52, 64, 212
Butter, 129, 308; craving, 182

Cabbage, 66, 78, 139, 227, 304, 306
Caffeine, 30, 47, 126, 184, 234, 244–46, 255, 303, 304; alternatives, 247; beverages/drugs containing, 246–47
Calcium, 11, 12, 14, 15, 28, 45, 49, 51, 54, 69–71, 81, 82, 83, 84, 85, 86, 95, 97–98, 99, 240, 305; deficiency, 70, 86, 174, 180
Calcium pantothenate, 10, 35, 46–47, 55, 64, 139, 252
Calories, 102, 131, 162, 194, 269
Cambridge Diet, 261–62
Cancer, 32, 45, 98, 118, 127–28, 133, 245, 247, 258, 275, 304, 308–09, 314–15, 318; high-risk foods, 307–08
Cancer-fighting: DHEA, 289; food, 12, 13, 67–68, 144, 305–07; splmts, 12, 40–41, 43, 67, 89, 222
Canker sores, 55, 61
Capillary health, 63
Carbohydrates, 131, 137, 169, 242; high consumption, 53, 54; metabolism, 84, 90, 123; need for, 131–32
Cardiovascular health, 69, 81; help for, 315
Cats, 298–99, 303, 317; vits., 28, 51, 298–300
Celiac disease, 58
Cells, 38, 55, 93, 119, 223

Cellulose, 20, 33, 140
Chamomile, 151
Cheese, craving for, 182
Chelation, 19, 193
Children, 12, 27, 36, 77, 80, 81, 100, 101, 111, 184, 268; hyperactive, 152; junk food, 186–87; splmts, 50, 197
Chinese food, craving for, 184
Chlorella, 145–46
Chlorine, 71, 72, 97, 170, 172, 173, 176
Chlorophyll, 139–40, 281
Chocolate, 71, 110, 215, 244; craving, 184
Cholesterol, 29, 57, 115, 120, 122, 166, 187–88; HDL, 123, 124, 127; LDL, 122–23, 124, 127; levels, raising/lowering, 124–27, 129, 139, 141, 143, 157; "low" label, 127; splmts to lower, 39, 43, 47, 48, 53, 54, 57, 60, 62, 92, 94, 166; VLDL, 124
Choline, 11, 46–49, 51, 52, 57, 58, 68, 115, 122, 239, 305
Chromium, 62, 73–74, 125
Chronic fatigue, 228–29, 315
Cobalt, 14, 74, 79, 177, 304
Cocaine, 116, 250–51, 252, 318; splmts/foods to help, 251
Coenzyme Q-10, 289
Coffee, 13, 58, 81, 88, 215, 221, 244, 246; decaf, 247, 258
Cola, 215, 221, 244, 246, 247; craving, 182
Cold, common, 43, 49, 150–53, 254, 255; regimen, 229–30
Colitis, 58, 230

Collagen, 43, 288
Colon, 9; cancer, 141, 275, 308
Comfrey, 151
Conjunctivitis, 49, 152
Connective tissue, 63, 112
Constipation, 71, 96, 137, 141, 166–67, 214
Construction workers, 203
Convulsions, 83, 116, 302, 303
Cooking, 76, 77, 185–86
Copper, 14, 15, 75–76, 79, 114, 179, 185, 304
Corticosteroids, 123, 254, 303
Cosmetics, natural, 283–85
Cramps: legs, 33, 52, 108, 200, 216–17; menstrual, 71, 217
Cravings, 182–84, 187
Cuts, splmt to heal, 213
Cysteine/Cystine, 101, 114–15, 119, 120, 281
Cystitis, 149
Cytochrome C, 146, 293

Dancers, splmt for, 202
Dandruff, 89, 170–71
Decongestant, natural, 253
Deficiencies, 162–64, 182–84; symptoms, 164–81
Dental: caries, 50, 76, 274, 277; pain, 29
Deodorant, natural, 140, 153
Depression, 42, 76, 106, 113, 116, 117, 238–41, 243, 305, 316; drugs/med. and, 241–42
Dermatitis, 34, 41, 61, 178–79
Dexatrim, 117
DHA, 126, 128, 129
DHEA, 289
Diabetes, 32, 35, 45, 62, 73, 95, 114–15, 118, 141, 200, 230, 273, 274, 302, 316, 318

Diarrhea, 59, 60, 151, 153, 167; natural remedy, 253
Diets, 259–71; anti-aging, 288–90; better sex, 292; carbohydrate vs. protein, 136; fad, 54; laughter and, 265; liquid, 262, 270–71; low/no-carbohydrate, 88, 259–62, 264; Mindell tips, 264–65; Mindell Vitamin-Balanced Diet, 265–68; splmts, 259–63, 267–68; very low calorie, 262, 270–71; warnings, 261–62, 270–71
Digestion, 7–10, 29, 60, 72, 95, 142, 145, 170, 264
Dilantin, 56, 116–17, 305
Dill, 157
Dinner, diet, 267, 291
Diuretics, 82, 88, 139, 150, 151, 152, 157, 235, 254, 256; vitamins as, 29, 33, 52, 253
Dizziness, 63, 84, 110, 152, 167, 226
DL-Phenylalanine, 107–09
DMG (dimethyglycine), 294–95
DNA, 93, 287; splmts, 288
Doctors, nutritional, 117, 163, 249, 310–13, splmt for, 204
Dogs, 297–98, 300, 303, 317; vitamins, 28, 51, 61, 296–97
Dong Quai, 159, 235
Dopamine, 239, 240
Drinking Man's Diet, 261
Drugs, 254, 289, 318; alternatives, 252–53; caffeine in, 246–47; depression/stress/anxiety causing, 241–42; nutrients

depleted, 255–57; skin problems and, 285; *See also* Alcohol; Aspirin; Caffeine; Cocaine, Marijuana/Hashish

Ear, 63, 168, 316
Eating disorders, 42, 316–17, 318
Echinacea, 149
Eczema, 41, 42, 54, 57, 65, 179. *See also* Skin
Eggs, 41, 42, 124, 183, 302
Endorphins, 107–09
Endurance, 51, 89, 114, 120
Energy, 2, 36, 37, 61, 75, 77, 81, 85, 109, 111, 118, 138, 143, 146, 290–91
Enzymes, 4, 8, 10, 12, 79, 93, 119, 132–33, 221
EPA, 126, 128, 129
Epileptics, 56, 317, 318
Esophagus, 7; cancer of, 13
Estrogen, 13, 31, 32, 34, 36, 42, 47, 48, 53, 56, 58, 60, 61, 65, 82, 217, 222, 295
Evening primrose oil, 125, 152
Exercise, 82, 111, 117, 146, 208–09, 218, 269, 277, 278, 290, 293–94, 304
Executives, drink/splmt, 199
Exhaustion, 42
Eyes, 27, 31, 49, 110, 168, 231, 187–88, 318

Fast food, 186–87
Fat, body, 57, 77, 84, 110, 111, 118
Fat, dietary, 42, 54, 57, 71, 85, 122, 125, 127, 129, 177, 179, 303, 308; fake, 129–30
Fatigue, 2, 39, 46, 52, 79, 83, 109, 113, 117, 120, 138,

150, 169, 244; splmts, 169, 292, 293–94; high-pep reg., 290–91
Fatty acids. *See* Vitamin F
Feet, cold, 212–13
Fenugreek seed, 125
Fever, 96, 149, 150, 223
Fiber, 84, 126, 140–42, 145; for seniors, 200
Flatulence, 137, 139, 142, 150, 153, 216
Flaxseed, 157
Fluorine, 13, 76–77
Folic acid, 11, 12, 37, 55–56, 64, 65, 115, 170, 172, 177, 238, 239, 302–03, 305
Food additives, 12, 126, 308–09
Food processing, 30, 34, 42, 47, 48, 52, 56, 58, 59, 65, 78, 89, 94
Free radicals, 67, 114, 118, 288
Fructose, 263, 272
Fructose Diet, 263
Fruits, cancer-fighting, 307; dieting, 265; storage, 185, 186; tart, craving, 184
Fungus infections, 137, 141; herbal remedies, 149

Gallbladder, 10, 47, 151, 153, 169–70, 184
Gallstones, 81, 122, 128
Gamblers, splmt for, 203
Garlic, 12, 126, 139, 157, 227
Gastrointestinal problems, 115, 169–70; splmt for, 170
Gatorade, 278
Gelatin, 110, 282
Germanium, 159
Ginger, 126, 217
Ginseng, 45, 138, 222, 247, 294; Brazilian, 159
Glossitis, 34

Glucose, 115, 131, 139, 272, 278

Glutamic acid/Glutamine, 101, 113, 117, 120; caution, 113

Glycine, 101, 112, 115, 118

Glycogen, 9, 115, 120, 131

Goiter, 78

Golfers, splmt for, 205

Gout, 62, 143, 304

Grapefruit, 269–70

GRAS, 20, 24, 194

Growing pains, 71

Growth, 29, 31, 36, 46, 54, 73, 77, 79, 85, 94, 110, 268

Growth hormone releasers, 111–12, 117, 118–19

Growth, retarded, 177

Gum (chewing), 264, 278

Gums, 63, 64, 86, 212, 289

Hair, 31, 41, 42, 53, 55, 57, 64, 65, 72, 75, 78, 91, 111, 115, 120, 150, 163, 170–72, 211, 281–82

Handicapped, splmt, 205

Hands, healthy, 282

Hay fever, splmt, 214

Headaches, 60, 104, 108, 129, 151, 152; splmt, 214

Healing, 110, 111, 120, 121, 145, 149–53, 180, 219; vit./min., 43, 46, 52, 85, 94, 180, 213

Heart, 172, 231, 303

Heartburn, 136, 215, 221

Heart disease, 39, 85, 87, 107, 108, 118, 122, 127, 129, 139, 245, 274, 302, 318; attack prevention, 231–32, 289

Heart disease-fighting: foods, 13, 14, 68; HDL, 124; herbal

remedies, 149, 151; vit./ min. 51, 52, 54, 66, 69, 92

Heat exhaustion, 90

Hemorrhoids, 141, 150, 215

Herbal: remedies, 148–60, 286, 318; tea, 247

Herpes simplex, 109, 110, 111, 120, 213, 229, 237, 268

Herpes zoster, 29, 235

High-pep regimen/splmt, 290–91

Histidine, 100, 101, 120

Hormones, 60, 83, 123, 159

Hydrochloric acid, 8, 33, 133, 221

Hypoglycemia, 46, 71, 87, 115, 118, 120, 138, 232, 244, 273, 274, 317

Ice craving, 187

Ice cream, craving, 183

Immune system, 12, 110, 118–19, 120, 129, 144, 145, 149, 150, 289, 293; vit./ min., 27, 39, 43, 46, 56, 63, 79, 91, 229

Impetigo, 232–33

Impotence, 95, 113

Indigestion, 81, 135, 138

Infants, splmt for, 197

Infection, susceptibility to, 115, 173

Infertility, 94, 109, 110, 120

Inosine, 293–94

Inositol, 11, 57–58, 61, 122, 166, 172, 179, 252, 280, 304

Insect repellant, 211–12

Insomnia, 70, 76, 138, 152, 173–74, 215

Intestine, 8, 9, 137

Insulin, 10, 35, 73, 93, 112, 115, 120, 263

Iodine, 11, 77–78; deficiency, 78, 169, 171, 179, 304

Iron, 11, 14, 15, 43, 52, 53, 70, 71, 75, 79–80, 84, 86, 169, 187, 303

Itching, 215, 216, 218, 245

Jet lag, splmt for, 216

Joggers, splmt for, 199

Jojoba oil, 285–86

Jumping rope, 290

Juniper berries, 151

Kelp, 59, 72, 78, 90, 142

Kelp, Lecithin, Vinegar, and B6 Diet, 142, 263

Ketosis, 132, 259

Kidney, 82, 85, 86, 118, 120, 129, 280

Labels, 189–94, 274, 276; abbrev., 191; "sugarless," 264, 273

Lactose, 137, 138

Laetrile, 11, 40–41

Laxatives, 43, 138, 139, 149–53, 157, 214, 253, 256, 276

Lead, 70, 86, 97, 304

Lecithin, 48, 49, 57, 58, 122, 124, 193, 265, 280

Leg pain, 216–17

Lemon grass oil, 126

Leucine, 101, 115, 119

L-glutathione (GSH), 118

Licorice, 151, 234, 309

Lignin, 141

Lipotropics, 122–23, 128

Liquid Protein Diet, 261–62, 270–71

Liver, 9–10, 37, 39, 48, 49, 72, 91, 118, 122, 151, 158, 184

Locust bean, 193

Lunch, 266–67, splmt with, 291

Lupus erythematosus, 129

Lysine, 101, 104, 109–10, 120

Magnesium, 11, 12, 14, 15, 33, 35, 45, 69, 70, 71, 81–83, 86, 88, 94, 97, 104, 105, 112, 176, 180–81, 240, 303

Manganese, 14, 15, 79, 83–84, 95, 167, 168, 240, 303

MAO inhibitors, 117, 304, 305

Margarine, 13, 27, 129, 308

Marijuana/hashish, 250

Mayonnaise, 308; craving, 184

Measles, splmt for, 233

Meat, 84, 276, 308; cured, 276

Memory, 106, 174–75; vit./ min., 36, 47, 48, 49, 83, 84, 175

Men, 12, 110, 88–89, 95, 291–93; splmt for, 196–97

Menopause, 53, 64, 89, 159–60, 217, 222

Menstruation, 37, 58, 71, 76, 149–52, 175, 217

Mental disorders, 94, 238–43

Metabolism, 4, 77, 90, 268; vitamins to aid, 31, 36, 41

Methionine, 101, 104, 115, 120–21, 122

Microwaving food, 188

Milk, 12, 50, 132, 185–86, 216, 288, 304; craving, 184

Milk thistle, 158

Mind, 106, 109, 110, 113, 120, 121; vit./min. for, 36, 47, 57, 60, 77, 87, 91, 93, 94

Mindell Vitamin Program (MVP), 164, 195

Minerals, 11–12, 14–15, 19, 238–39, 280

Mint leaves, 87
Molybdenum, 84–85
Mononucleosis, splmt for, 233
Mood, 107, 116, 120, 121
Motion sickness, 12, 29, 217
Mouth, 7, 31, 175
MSG, 12, 113, 184, 276, 309
Multiple sclerosis, 37, 119, 152
Mumps, splmt for, 234
Muscle, 52, 79, 81, 83, 87, 88,
    90, 93; amino acids and,
    111, 112, 115, 121; pain,
    41; spasms, 33, 108, 175–
    76; splmt, 176; toning, 110–
    11, 112, 120

Nails, 120, 152, 181, 286; vit./
    min. and, 31, 78, 91, 94,
    181, 282
Nausea, 33, 110, 253
Nervousness, 176–77
Nervous system, 114; disorders,
    36, 39, 238–39; drugs and,
    241–42; herbal remedies,
    149–52; irritability, 83,
    116; vit./min. and, 36, 48,
    49, 60, 70, 81, 83, 85, 87,
    90, 239–40
Neuralgia, 90, 108
Neuritis, 33, 143
Niacin, 10, 41, 42, 60–62, 85,
    103, 104, 105, 116, 126,
    165, 167, 176, 179, 238,
    240, 303
Niacinamide, 10, 11, 60–62,
    104, 106, 112
Night blindness, 27
Night workers, splmt, 202
Norepinephrine, 116, 117, 239,
    240
Nosebleeds, 59, 177
Numbness (hands/feet), 33, 47
Nurses, splmt for, 204

Nursing mothers, 96, 157–58,
    198, 314; vitamin/mineral
    needs, 26, 30, 31, 32, 33,
    36, 43, 53, 55, 60, 77, 79,
    85, 89, 93
Nutrients, 6–7
Nurtri/System, 270
Nuts, craving for, 183

Obesity, 142, 309
Octacosanol, 292–93, 294
Ohsawa, George, 262
Oil, dietary, 52, 53, 54, 126,
    127–29, 193, 198, 308
Olive, craving, 183
Omega 3, 126, 128, 129, 157,
    214; Omega 6, 129
Onions, 183, 265, 288, 307
Oral contraceptives, 75, 117,
    126, 218, 240–41, 257,
    285; vit./min. and, 12, 28,
    30, 32, 34, 45, 53, 82
Orange juice, 99, 116, 188
Ornithine, 101, 110, 112–13,
    119, 121, 268
Osteoarthritis, 108, 144
Osteoporosis, 15, 70, 71, 83;
    senile, 50
Oxidation, 63, 67, 88

PABA, 11, 46, 55, 64–65, 169,
    170, 171, 176, 303, 304
Pain, 107; reducing, 55, 64,
    104, 107–09, 121, 149–53
Papain, 119, 135, 221
Papaya, 135, 305, 306
Parkinson's disease, 121; B6
    warning, 35, 301
Parsley, 71, 152
Pau D'Arco, 160
Peanut butter craving, 182
Pectin, 126, 137, 141, 193
Pellagra, 61, 238

Penicillin, 66, 257
Pennyroyal, 152
Peppermint, 152–53
Pepsin, 8, 132
Personality changes, 60
Phenobarbital, 56
Phenylalanine, 101, 106–07, 110, 116, 121, 240, 273, 304
Phenylpropanolamine, 117–18
Phosphorus, 11, 14, 15, 28, 49, 51, 71, 81, 82, 83, 84, 85–86, 95, 139, 164
Pickles, craving for, 183
Pituitary gland, 111, 115, 119, 268
PKU (phenylketonuria), 106, 108
P.M.S., 234, 235
Poison ivy, remedy, 218
Poke weed, 149
Pollutants, 49, 50, 59, 66–67, 75, 98, 126; vitamins for, 12, 37, 40, 45, 51, 66–67
Polyps, splmt for, 218
Polysorbate 60, 193
Potassium, 14, 15, 72, 81, 87–88, 90, 112, 139, 168, 173, 235, 275, 303, 168, 173
Potatoes, 44, 68, 87, 295, 306
Pregnancy: cautions, 21, 108, 150, 152, 157–58, 208, 245, 250, 301; cravings, 183, 184; morning sickness, 33, 217; splmt for, 198; vit./min. req., 26, 30, 31, 32, 33, 35, 42, 43, 53, 55, 77, 79, 81, 85, 89
Prickly heat, 219
Propolis, 293, 294
Prostate gland, 89, 93, 94, 95, 308; splmt for, 219
Protein, 12, 13, 14, 39, 55, 73, 92, 93, 102–20, 122, 164, 169, 177, 193; high-/heavy diet, 12, 33, 34, 37, 122, 260–62; high drink, 290; how much, 101–02; liquid diet caution, 261–62; splmts, 103
Psoriasis, 120, 219–20
Pycnogenol, 67, 288–89

Quercetin, 13
Questran (cholestyramine), 29

Racketball, splmt for, 205–06
Radiation, 45, 59, 114, 118, 145
RDA/U.S. RDA, 192–93
Relaxant, natural, 105–06
Renin, 8, 132
Reproductive: disorders, 52, 83, 94; organs, 93
Retin-A, 28
Rice, tips on, 185
Rickets, 50, 70, 86
RNA-DNA, 2, 55, 287–88, 304
Rosemary, 153
Runners, 278; splmt for, 198

Saccharin, 273
Salespeople, splmt for, 203–04
Salt, 13, 72, 78, 90, 91, 183, 275–77; foods high in, 91, 276–77
Saw-Palmetto (berries), 149
Scarsdale Diet, 260–61
Schizophrenia, 93, 111, 113, 115, 121, 268
Selenium, 11, 14, 15, 51, 66, 67, 68, 89–90, 119, 171, 300
Seniors, splmt for, 200
Serotonin, 104, 215, 240, 243, 249

Sex: aphrodisiacs, 292, 294–95; enhancement, 144; food/splmts for, 292; interest in, 106, 120, 121; STD hotline, 318; vits. and, 291–92

Shark cartilage, 144

Silica, 286; silicic acid, 135

Silymarin, 158

Singers, splmt for, 204

Skin: cancer, 106; discolor., 56; vits., 17, 27, 33, 41, 46

Skin care/health, 120, 137, 279, 288, 318; cosmetics, 283–85; herbal remedies, 149–53; drugs that harm, 285; problems, 178–80, 214; protein drink, 279–80; scarring, 52; sunlight, 62, 64; splmts for, 280–81; vit./min. for, 31, 41, 53, 55, 60, 75, 78, 79, 91, 92, 178–80, 214

Sleep, 104, 105, 111–12, 121, 215–16, 317

Sleeping pills, 36, 47, 61; alternatives, 252, 255

Smell, loss of, 174

Smoking, 12, 13, 30, 43, 45, 64, 68, 75, 114, 118, 126, 220, 257, 308; nicotine gum, 222; splmt, 206; stop, 220

SOD, 2, 288

Sodium, 13, 14, 15, 72, 81, 87, 90–91, 164, 176, 275, 303

Soft drinks, 71, 106, 274, 276, 277. See also Cola

Sorbitol, 264, 273, 278

Soybeans, 103

Spanish Fly, 294

Spirulina, 144

Stillman Diet, 260

Stomach, 7–8, 9, 139, 149–53

Stress, 104, 120, 121, 126, 133, 138; drugs and, 241–42; vit./min. for, 2, 30, 31, 32, 47, 56, 81, 87, 223, 239–40

Students, splmt for, 199

Sudden Infant Death Syndrome (SIDS), 43; hotline, 318

Sugar, 5, 73, 88, 126; dangers, 273–74; depression and, 243; foods with high, 273–74; hidden, 274; kinds, 272; in med., 275; vit. for users, 30

Sulfa drugs, 30, 32, 42, 47, 48, 56, 58, 61, 65, 66, 257

Sulfur, 41, 91–92, 282–83

Suma, 159

Sunburn/sunscreening, 64, 66, 150, 220

Sunstroke, 90

Surgery, second opinion, 318

Sweating, 93, 277, 303

Sweeteners, artificial, 264, 273

Taste, sense of, 94

Taurine, 116–17

T-cells, 119, 149, 229

Tea, 76, 81, 234, 246, 247

Tea tree oil, 211

Teachers, splmt for, 206

Teeth: decay, 50, 76, 274, 277; health, 78, 81, 86; loss, 72; softening, 180; splmt, 180

Teeth grinding, 220

Tennis players, splmt, 205

Threonine, 101, 121

Thyme, 153

Thymus gland, 119, 293

Thyroid gland, 77, 83, 286, 304

Tissue salts, 133–35

Tonsillitis, 236

Tranquilizers, 48, 57, 81, 214, 240, 243, 252, 253
Travelers, splmt for, 207
Trauma, 111
Tremors, 180–81
Triglycerides, 61, 125, 129
Trihalomethanes, 98
Truck drivers, splmt for, 202
Tryptophan, 33, 60, 101, 104, 105–06, 112, 121, 215, 216, 240, 241, 243, 249
Tumors, 115, 118, 144
Turkey, 71, 104, 127, 216, 266
TV watchers, splmt for, 207
Tyrosine, 75, 112, 116, 121, 240, 252, 304

Ulcers, 32, 46, 66, 113, 120, 133, 139, 169–70, 202, 236, 305
Urinary tract infections, 43, 71, 149, 151
Urine tests, 45, 163, 304
Uterine cancer, 222

Vaginal itching, 181
Valium, 107, 109
Vanadium, 92–93
Varicose veins, 141, 221
Vasectomy, splmt for, 221
Vegetables, 132, 185–86, 306–07; dieting and, 265; eating, 76, 86, 88, 96, 185
Vegetarians/ism, 25, 35, 37, 75, 129, 263, 318
Venereal disease, 236–37
Vitamin A, 5, 9, 10, 14, 16, 17, 22, 26–28, 41, 42, 49, 51, 71, 83, 95, 119, 139, 164, 168, 169, 171, 173, 174, 178, 179, 194, 301, 305
Vitamin B1, 1, 5, 10, 12, 29–31, 35, 60, 83, 105, 114, 116, 164, 169, 175, 187, 245, 239, 301
Vitamin B2, 10, 31–32, 35, 41, 42, 60, 83, 105, 116, 167, 168, 170, 177, 179, 181, 301–02
Vitamin B6, 10, 12, 32, 33–35, 41, 42, 60, 83, 95, 103, 104, 105, 112, 139, 163, 171, 175, 176, 178, 181, 239, 301
Vitamin B10/B11, 11
Vitamin B12, 8, 11, 12, 33, 35–37, 74, 103, 129, 165, 171, 172, 175, 176
Vitamin B13, 11, 37–38
Vitamin B15, 11, 38–40
Vitamin Bt, 11
Vitamin C, 1, 5, 11, 12, 14–15, 16, 17, 18, 22, 23, 28, 32, 35, 41, 43–45, 51, 56, 62–64, 66, 67, 68, 71, 75, 79, 81, 83, 94, 107, 112, 114, 116, 119, 126, 137, 138, 164, 166, 169, 170, 172, 177, 180, 214, 216, 219, 238, 239, 303
Vitamin D, 9, 11, 12, 15, 17, 22, 28, 49–51, 64, 85, 86, 123, 139, 169, 176, 180, 303
Vitamin E, 11, 12, 15, 17, 18, 22, 23, 28, 51–53, 54, 58, 66, 67, 68, 72, 80, 88, 89, 119, 126, 128, 139, 239, 280, 291–92, 303
Vitamin F, 11, 12, 109, 167, 171
Vitamin K, 17, 18, 22, 58–59, 139, 167, 177, 303
Vitamin L, 11
Vitamin P4, 11
Vitamin T, 11, 66

Vitamin U, 11, 66, 139

Vitamins, 3–4, 10–11; getting the most from food, 184–86; metabolism, 4; min. and, 11–12, 14–15; oil soluble, 17

Vitamin supplements, 5–6, 16, 17–24, 34, 45, 55, 65, 173, 207; allergies, 189, 194; anti-aging, 288, 289–90; dieting and, 259–63, 267–68; forms/recommend, 16–17, 23, 24–25; high-pep, 291; for illness, 223–37; labels, 189–94; multis, 189; MVP (Mindell Vitamin Program), 164, 195; RDA/U.S. RDA, 192–93; regimens, individual, 196–207; sex/fertility, 291–92; special situation, 210–22; what to look for, 193; when/how to take, 22–23

Warts, 221

Water, 13, 53, 72, 76, 77, 82, 87, 95–99, 276, 285, 288

"Water Diet, The," 260

Water retention, 88, 181

Weight reduction, 54, 111, 112, 144, 145, 259–71, 289

Weight training, 112, 117, 119–20, 146, 201–02, 218

Weight Watchers, 261

Weights and measures, 190–91

Whiplash, 108

Wilson's disease, 114, 304

Women, 12, 13, 53, 69, 71, 79, 80–81, 97–98, 124, 295, 317; splmt for, 196

X-rays, 54, 59, 114, 118

Yeast, 142–44

Yeast infections, 145, 160, 227–28

Yogurt, 59, 72, 126, 227, 264

Yucca, 140

Zen Macrobiotic Diet, 262–63

Zinc, 11, 14, 15, 28, 73, 76, 93–95, 112, 119, 164, 165, 169, 174, 177, 181, 240, 292, 304